T0256157

DANGEROUS MEDICINE

DANGEROUS MEDICINE

The Story behind Human Experiments with Hepatitis

SYDNEY A. HALPERN

Yale

UNIVERSITY PRESS

New Haven and London

Published with assistance from the Louis Stern Memorial Fund, and
from the foundation established in memory of William Chauncey
Williams of the Class of 1822, Yale Medical School, and of William
Cook Williams of the Class of 1850, Yale Medical School.

Copyright © 2021 by Sydney A. Halpern.
All rights reserved.
This book may not be reproduced, in whole or in part, including
illustrations, in any form (beyond that copying permitted by Sections
107 and 108 of the U.S. Copyright Law and except by reviewers for
the public press), without written permission from the publishers.

Yale University Press books may be purchased in quantity for
educational, business, or promotional use. For information, please
e-mail sales.press@yale.edu (U.S. office) or sales@yaleup.co.uk
(U.K. office).

Set in Janson Text type by IDS Infotech Ltd., Chandigarh, India.
Printed in the United States of America.

Library of Congress Control Number: 2021937560
ISBN 978-0-300-25962-9 (hardcover : alk. paper)

A catalogue record for this book is available from the British Library.

This paper meets the requirements of ANSI/NISO Z39.48-1992
(Permanence of Paper).

10 9 8 7 6 5 4 3 2 1

Contents

Preface

MY FIRST ENCOUNTER with documents from human infection experiments was at the library of the American Philosophical Society, a redbrick building that sits across a cobblestone street from the Liberty Bell in Philadelphia's Independence Park. I was perusing the archived papers of Joseph Stokes Jr., who was chair of pediatrics at the University of Pennsylvania between 1939 and 1963 and a tireless infectious disease researcher throughout his career. He oversaw human tests of numerous experimental immunizing agents, preparations designed to prevent measles, mumps, influenza, and polio. I was collecting material for a book—completed before this one—on how mid-twentieth-century researchers managed risks when conducting vaccine trials. Investigators began human studies of new immunizing agents with high hopes that their preparations would protect against serious disease; but experimental vaccines sometimes had harmful, even fatal, results. Stokes's papers were rich with information on how scientists assessed and responded to vaccine hazards.

I was standing before a mahogany table illuminated by diffuse light from the reading room's tall windows, sifting through hundreds of folders; a cart of archive boxes was to one side. From an open container with materials on immunization against measles, I pulled a folder with a label that included the word *volunteers*. I thought it would hold lists of vaccine recipients, and perhaps information on a preparation's effectiveness. I half opened the file, expecting to take a quick look before moving on.

What I saw stopped me short. The top page was labeled "WAIVER AND RELEASE" and read in part: "*For the purpose of experiments on hepatitis, I hereby consent to be infected and reinfected in an attempt to discover the cause, transmission, and prevention of hepatitis.*"

My initial surprise gave way to the gravity of what I was reading. I sat down and surveyed the folder contents in full. It contained a stack of consent statements, their legally worded text in black typescript. All were for human experiments with hepatitis. The signatures of research subjects were scrawled on the documents in blue fountain-pen ink. The distinctive script of each signature made a striking contrast to the formal text. Each typescript page had spaces for additional entries: the date, the subject's name and age, the signature of a witness. The documents were dated 1944 and 1945 and showed that the subjects were conscientious objectors to the military draft, young men in their late teens and early twenties. Some of the forms—for subjects not yet twenty-one—had a section displaying the signatures of parents.

I had seen waiver and release forms for many vaccine trials, but the studies described here were different. In midcentury vaccine experiments, researchers inoculated subjects with pathogens they had weakened or killed in hopes of conferring immunity without symptoms. If a vaccine caused illness, investigators stopped the human trial and returned to the laboratory.

In the hepatitis studies referred to here, the pathogens were unmodified and fully virulent. The predictable outcome of these experiments would be to *cause* a serious illness, not prevent it. Even knowing about dangerous experiments in the country's past, I was stunned and perplexed: stunned that researchers had exposed subjects to risks so much greater than what was acceptable in routine vaccine trials, and perplexed that healthy people had agreed to participate in studies that promised them harm without benefit.

In the months after discovering the waiver forms, I began hunting for additional materials on the hepatitis infection experiments. I soon realized that Stokes's work with hepatitis was part of a large-scale U.S. government-sponsored program of virus transmission studies that spanned World War II and the early Cold War. As I located more records, unraveling questions about the invasive hepatitis studies became a mission. How did the research program begin? What allowed it to continue for decades? How did scientists justify the studies' hazards and how did they manage to gain access to subjects? Who were the enrollees and what happened to them? And what, finally, brought the experiments to a close?

Pursuing answers, I sought out informants for in-person interviews and pored over oral histories, newspaper articles, scientific reports, and documents from dozens of libraries and archival repositories. The search took me from Illinois to Pennsylvania, New York, New Jersey, Connecticut, Michigan, Virginia, Texas, and California. My most frequent destination was the Washington, DC, area, where I made repeated trips to collections at the National Academy of Sciences and the National Library of Medicine. I lost count of my visits to the National Archives in College Park, Maryland, where I spent months combing through the records of federal agencies.

What I unearthed reveals the inner workings of federally sponsored human experimentation in midcentury America and the political and cultural developments that shaped its conduct. Among the findings are that, with funding and approvals from government agencies, elite scientists pursued disease-inducing studies with members of multiple institutionalized and disadvantaged groups, raising troubling questions about inequities in the conduct of biomedical research. I also discovered a trail of unanticipated and unaddressed injuries.

Hepatitis investigators insisted that knowledge from their studies was critical for advancing disease prevention. They recognized the immediate danger of fatalities their interventions posed, yet declared that subjects were either benefiting from participation or were freely choosing to make sacrifices for the common good. While the experiments were ongoing, researchers were aware that some people infected with blood-borne hepatitis retained the viruses, but investigators did not realize that many who failed to clear these pathogens would experience serious delayed harm. What scientists unwittingly did was create a pool of hepatitis carriers at risk for slowly simmering, life-threatening liver diseases.

The titanic global health emergency unleashed by COVID-19 has galvanized new calls for extremely hazardous human research. In spring of 2020, within weeks of the pandemic's arrival in the United States, well-placed commentators were advocating human infection studies with the novel coronavirus. In March and April of 2021, two groups of British researchers, working separately, announced the launch of human transmission procedures with SARS-CoV-2. Proponents have argued that such experiments will hasten understanding of how the disease spreads and speed or otherwise facilitate the testing of vaccines. Their claims echo those made by hepatitis investigators many decades ago: that knowledge gained from high-risk interventions will save lives and serve the greater good.

Like hepatitis at midcentury, the maladies SARS-CoV-2 cause are both menacing and obscure. The long-term consequences of infection are unknown and are not likely to be fully understood for years. Amid the zeal for research aimed at controlling COVID-19, it is vitally important to understand human experiments with dangerous viruses conducted during a previous national and international emergency: how these studies came about, what they did and did not accomplish, and what the consequences were for human subjects.

Acknowledgments

WRITING AND PUBLISHING *Dangerous Medicine* was a very long journey. Regrettably, I am unable to name all of the great many people who helped me along the sometimes tortuous route. I have gone here for brevity instead.

A Grant for Scholarly Works in Biomedicine and Health from the National Library of Medicine (NLM), National Institutes of Health, was invaluable in allowing me to gather the wide array of archival materials I draw upon in the book. My thanks to Robert Cook-Deegan, Jonathan Moreno, and Susan Reverby, who wrote letters in support of my application to NLM.

I met or otherwise communicated with half a dozen senior hepatitis or vaccine researchers in the course of my work. I am tremendously grateful to Donald M. Jensen, professor of medicine and liver disease specialist at the University of Chicago and then Rush University, who served as consultant on my NLM grant and, in addition to providing sources, sat patiently while I peppered him with questions about the complex hepatitis viruses. Special thanks also to Anna Suk-Fong Lok, distinguished university professor in hepatology and internal medicine at the University of Michigan, who read a draft of *Dangerous Medicine* and offered thoughtful observations. Any mistakes in the book and all opinions are mine alone.

Others commented on parts of the evolving manuscript, including Wendy Foster, Joel Howell, Howard Kushner, Sarah Rodriguez, Anthony Somkin, Carol Somkin, Sandra Sufian, and Carol Tsang. Two outstanding anonymous reviewers for Yale University Press provided detailed suggestions that I greatly appreciated. I also benefited from informal input on sources, research presentations, and publishing matters from a range of fellow scholars. From the history and history of medicine communities: John Eyler, Lara Freidenfelds, Laura Hein, Susan Lederer, Paul Lombardo, David J. Rothman, John Swann, and Arleen Tuchman. From the disability studies community: Steven J. Taylor. And from the bioethics community: Alice Dreger and Katie Watson. My thanks to other colleagues and also students in the Program in Medical Humanities and Bioethics at Northwestern University's Feinberg School of Medicine for stimulating feedback on talks that drew on material from the book.

I owe debts of gratitude to my superlative freelance editor, Anna Fenton-Hathaway, for providing an unflagging combination of incisiveness and cheer, and to Michael Gold who, in addition to handling a more than full-time day job, provided bountiful assistance with images, file transfers, software, and Web matters. My thanks to Jean Thomson Black, my editor at Yale, and to the press production staff who shepherded *Dangerous Medicine* through review and publication processes amid hurdles created by the ongoing COVID-19 epidemic.

It was a privilege to hear about the experiences of the four interviewees who appear in the book as well as those of people whose narratives are preserved in archives and oral histories. I am grateful to informants and family members who allowed me to report personal stories and related images. Meeting and learning about people whose lives intersected with America's hepatitis program has been one of the great pleasures of writing this book.

I could not have gathered materials for *Dangerous Medicine* without the assistance of a multitude of archivists and librarians. These range from seasoned professionals at major repositories who assisted me in navigating complex record groups to workers at small-scale public libraries who forwarded me obituaries from regional newspapers or clippings from local history collections. I feel remiss in failing to name all of those who helped with documents, but I fear if I start doing so, the list would not be complete, nor would my expressions of gratitude be adequate. It is to all of these keepers of the historical record that I dedicate this book.

Abbreviations

ACP:	American College of Physicians
AEB:	Army Epidemiology Board
AFEB:	Armed Forces Epidemiology Board
AFMPC:	Armed Forces Medical Policy Council
AFSC:	American Friends Service Committee
AMA:	American Medical Association
APHA:	American Public Health Association
CDC:	Centers for Disease Control and Prevention
CPS:	Civilian Public Service
DHEW:	U.S. Department of Health, Education and Welfare
IHD:	International Health Division of the Rockefeller Foundation
JAMA:	*Journal of the American Medical Association*
JCDH:	Jewish Chronic Disease Hospital
MCHR:	Medical Committee on Human Rights
NAS:	National Academy of Sciences
NIH:	National Institutes of Health
NRC:	National Research Council
NYU:	New York University
OSRD:	Office of Scientific Research and Development
OTSG:	Office of the Surgeon General–Army
Penn:	University of Pennsylvania
PHS:	U.S. Public Health Service
R & D Command:	Research and Development Command–Army
WMA:	World Medical Association

DANGEROUS MEDICINE

Introduction

A Sobering Story

FOR THIRTY YEARS, 1942 through 1972, American biomedical researchers deliberately infected people with hepatitis. Their aims were to discover basic features of the disease and the viruses causing it and then to develop immunizing agents. Ordinarily scientists conduct research of this type with laboratory animals. But attempts to transmit hepatitis to animals repeatedly failed, and investigators resorted to experimenting on people. Ten federally funded research teams undertook hepatitis infection studies; the number of physician-investigators involved in the program exceeded sixty. These scientists were from the mainstream of U.S. biomedicine, prominent infectious disease specialists holding appointments at major universities and government laboratories. In hundreds of studies conducted during the program's three decades, researchers enrolled more than thirty-seven hundred people in hepatitis-inducing experiments. All of the subjects lived in institutional settings on U.S. soil. The great bulk of them were men, although some were women. Most were white, although a portion, perhaps 20 to 25 percent, were African American. The majority were adults, although more than eight hundred were children.

Hepatitis is characterized by inflammation of the liver; its symptoms include abdominal pain, loss of appetite, nausea and vomiting, diarrhea, muscle and joint aches, fever, and exhaustion. A widely recognized sign of the disorder is jaundice—yellowing of the skin and eyes—although hepatitis can occur without jaundice. Three strains of the virus—hepatitis A,

B, and C—are the most common cause of liver inflammation. People contract hepatitis A from contaminated food or water; blood or other bodily fluids carrying the viruses are the usual sources of hepatitis B and C. Midcentury researchers infected their subjects with specimens from patients with known or suspected cases. Under medical supervision, some enrollees ingested materials containing hepatitis A; others received inoculations with blood-borne hepatitis B and even—unbeknown to investigators at the time—hepatitis C.

The short-term result was that many participants contracted cases of hepatitis, a nasty illness that when severe can drag on for six to eight weeks. A number of subjects receiving hepatitis B developed fulminant hepatic failure, an overwhelming, often fatal condition in which the patient's immune system, in an effort to eliminate the virus, attacks and destroys massive numbers of liver cells. Over the course of the research program, four prison inmates died of fulminant hepatitis B after receiving experimental inoculations; a fifth lay in a coma for more than a week before slowly recovering.

The damage did not stop there. Some patients sickened with blood-borne hepatitis continue to harbor the viruses; these carriers can be infective to others and are at risk for developing cirrhosis and liver cancer two or more decades after initial exposure. Among adults infected with hepatitis B, a small portion becomes carriers. Among those with hepatitis C, the vast majority retain the virus indefinitely. Scientists did not suspect that C existed until the 1970s; at that time they discovered a third strain—then called non-A, non-B—lurking in blood specimens that earlier investigators had transferred to subjects. The full implication of the carrier status was not clear until years after hepatitis infection studies had ended. Yet even when the dangers facing carriers did become evident, no researcher or agency tracked, acknowledged, or addressed slowly developing liver diseases and resulting deaths among past hepatitis subjects.

Records from the hepatitis program that I first stumbled across—the waiver and release forms among Joseph Stokes Jr.'s papers at the American Philosophical Society (APS)—exemplified the stance researchers with federal contracts adopted toward research injuries. The documents included wording intended to exempt investigators and their sponsors from liability for harm to subjects—this was the meaning of *waiver and release*. While researchers occasionally used waiver provisions before the Second World War, it was during the 1940s that these clauses became standard issue; they remained so through the early 1970s. When experiments were hazardous, federal sponsors had agency lawyers reviewed the wording of waiver statements and required researchers to have subjects sign approved documents. The prevalence of waiver provisions was consistent with a more general pattern: scientists and their government patrons distanced themselves from all but immediate research-related maladies. Throughout the hepatitis program, investigators provided medical care for enrollees' illnesses while the studies were ongoing, but participants were on their own if their symptoms did not completely resolve or if they developed lasting disabilities.

America's hepatitis infection experiments were one feature of a much broader program of federally sponsored biomedical research. With the country's entry into the Second World War, the U.S. government unleashed a flood of resources for defense-related science. The influx of funds and accompanying administrative support transformed medical research from an assortment of small-scale efforts into a systematically organized program. A new group of investigators coalesced, a military-biomedical elite that included university researchers with federal contracts, physicians in the U.S. Public Health Service (PHS), and medical officers in the armed forces. These diversely situated actors came together at the meetings of scientific committees, councils, and boards that government agencies convened and sustained. Their ties to defense agencies allowed national security priorities to shape the conduct of medical research. When evaluating the risks and benefits of human experiments, they placed unprecedented value on expected gains for science in the interest of the country at large.

Experiments that exposed human subjects to virulent pathogens, while not new, became increasingly common during and after the Second World War. Two units managed the bulk of federal contracts with civilian scientists for wartime biomedical studies: President Roosevelt's Office for Scientific Research and Development (OSRD), through its Committee on Medical Research, and the Army Epidemiology Board (AEB), overseen by the Office of the Surgeon General–Army (OTSG) within the Department of War. Both agencies supported human infection studies with scientists pursuing a variety of goals.

Among the uses of interventions exposing subjects to unmodified pathogens was to evaluate new immunizing agents. These measures were widely known as "challenge" inoculations. Early vaccine researchers administered challenge procedures to individuals who had already received an experimental immunizing agent; the person's ability to withstand exposure to disease microbes without succumbing to illness demonstrated the vaccine's effectiveness. By the 1940s, scientists sought systematic evidence of vaccine efficacy and began administering virulent pathogens to both immunized and unimmunized subjects—termed, respectively, experimental and control groups. During the war, AEB investigators employed challenge interventions with both vaccinated and unvaccinated subjects to test new preparations against influenza and measles, while OSRD scientists carried out controlled challenge trials of vaccines against dysentery. Researchers conducting these studies fully expected that a great many participants would become ill.

Wartime human infection procedures served other purposes as well. AEB-funded investigators sickened subjects with sand-fly fever and dengue to clarify mechanisms of disease transmission. OSRD investigators exposed enrollees to atypical pneumonia in an attempt to identify and isolate the pathogen. The agency also began malaria infection studies to evaluate the efficacy of new pharmaceuticals; the army assumed responsibility for this program after the war and continued the experiments through the early 1970s. Meanwhile, the AEB or its postwar successor, the Armed Forces Epidemiology Board (AFEB), sustained hepatitis infection research with investigators addressing multiple scientific issues.

The notorious Tuskegee Syphilis Study was not among the government's disease transmission studies. In that project, ongoing between 1932 and 1972, PHS physicians enrolled more than four hundred African American men in rural Alabama with late-stage syphilitic disease and an additional two hundred subjects as controls. The men with latent disease agreed to participate with the understanding that they would receive medical care for their condition; instead, investigators were examining the course of untreated syphilis. The researchers deceived subjects about the nature of the study and denied them available medical therapies. Inducing syphilis, however, was not among the project's violations against subjects. In another set of experiments, PHS physicians did infect human subjects with sexually transmitted diseases. These took place between 1946 and 1948 in Guatemala, where the researchers induced STDs, including gonorrhea and syphilis, in enrollees. Their objectives were to better understand serological tests for the diseases and to clarify the efficacy of penicillin for treatment and prevention.

Most human infection experiments were small in scale, limited in duration, and involved one or two categories of subjects—prisoners typically among them. The U.S. malaria infection program was unusual in continuing for more than thirty years but unexceptional in drawing all but a handful of its subjects from prison populations. America's hepatitis program was distinctive in its size and longevity and also in the variety of its human participants. I know of no series of problematic infectious disease studies that involved a wider array of devalued and stigmatized groups. The subjects included scores of draft objectors routinely derided as "yellowbellies"; thousands of prison inmates, a substantial portion of them African American; several hundred mental patients; and well over a thousand adults or minors with intellectual impairments. In one of the last of the hepatitis projects, a seventeen-year series of studies at Willowbrook State School on Staten Island, researchers transmitted hepatitis to hundreds of developmentally disabled children.

Issues of social justice are at the heart of the story of America's hepatitis transmission program. The use of such a broad range of marginalized groups is astounding, and the fact that the program proceeded for years with apparent public acquiescence demands explanation. Researchers were well aware that enrolling these populations in disease-inducing experiments could provoke what the investigators' military sponsors referred to as "public relations problems." Scientists were uneasy about public reactions to experiments, even those conducted with nonstigmatized adults, when study interventions were potentially controversial, but the use of children and members of marginalized groups generated particular concern.

Hepatitis investigators devoted substantial effort to both arranging access to diverse subject pools and to normalizing experiments with these groups. They did so by appealing to currents in the culture at large while also customizing their messages to the ideals of particular institutional communities. They encouraged conscientious objectors and their Peace Church sponsors to consider involvement in medical experiments as a form of altruistic service, and told prisoners and correctional officers that participation was a route to rehabilitation. With the physician directors of mental hospitals and training schools, they promised assistance with outbreaks of infectious diseases. Throughout, scientists emphasized the urgent need to quell hepatitis outbreaks that undermined military operations and national security. They insisted that knowledge from the research was crucial for advancing disease prevention and promoting the greater good.

When addressing outside audiences, researchers showcased studies using conscientious objectors and prisoners, declaring that these recruits freely chose to make patriotic contributions to the country's war efforts. Where possible, investigators concealed experiments with children and the disabled, anticipating that these studies might generate disquieting questions. When pressed, they argued that underage and impaired persons benefited from planned exposure to hepatitis under medical supervision. Scientists' authority and skills at persuasion allowed them to secure buy-in from managers of multiple custodial facilities and sympathetic coverage from the press, which portrayed the experiments as consistent with American values. Two features of the historical context facilitated researchers' efforts at normalization: at midcentury, U.S. medicine was at the height of its legitimacy; and invocations of patriotism held great sway during the war and early Cold War years.

Dangerous experiments with the disempowered did not go uncontested. After the Nuremberg Medical Trial, physicians in Europe opposed enrolling captive and vulnerable groups in nontherapeutic experiments. And from the outset, some in the United States who were close to the experiments raised questions about the level and acceptability of risk and about the use of subjects whose capacity for consent was in question. For years, scientific leaders were able to keep this dissension at bay or behind closed doors. But their unified edifice collapsed with the cultural shifts of the 1960s. Rights activists inside and outside medicine opposed using vulnerable people in experiments unrelated to their medical care, and they objected to prioritizing scientific ends over the health of subjects. Progressive-minded physicians challenged the old guard of biomedicine and took their critiques into public arenas. Reports of research abuses gained dominance in the mainstream media. It was when elite scientists lost control of the public conversation that hepatitis transmission studies finally came to an end.

My analysis illuminates the rise and fall of a moral framework that enabled dangerous experiments with marginalized people as it valorized sacrifices for the good of the nation. It elaborates the motivations of powerful actors who promoted this moral narrative, the cultural imagery deployed to sustain the scaffolding, and the social transformations that led to the ascendance of an alternative ethic, one grounded in notions about individual and group rights.

Normalizing narratives, underlying injustices, and emerging realizations about research injuries are central themes in the story of America's hepatitis infection program. Also integral to my account are the perspectives and experiences of people whose lives intersected with the experiments: the scientists who conducted or oversaw the studies, institutional managers who opened their doors to researchers and, as much as available sources allow, the individuals who received experimental interventions. The circumstances of the program's human subjects diverged sharply. Some were swayed by investigators' calls for patriotic service and chose to enroll in the research. Some acquiesced reluctantly or were coerced. The institutionalized children and adults with intellectual impairments likely did not grasp that they were part of a medical experiment. What I learned about the situations of most of the subjects came solely from written materials. A handful of participants I had the good fortune to speak with in person. My conversations with four interviewees display a wide range of sensibilities about the experiments—I relay the experiences of three of them in this introduction.

In the cache of waiver and release forms among Stokes's papers was one bearing the signature of Warren Sawyer. When he enrolled in Stokes's study, Sawyer was a twenty-three-year-old conscientious objector working as a ward attendant at a state mental hospital in the Byberry neighborhood of north Philadelphia. I tracked him down and reached him by phone in the spring of 2014. A name on a worn archival document came alive.

I asked Sawyer if he would sit down with me for an interview and he cheerfully replied, "Oh, sure, but you'd better come soon—I'm ninety-four." I took his advice and made a hasty trip to the retirement community where he lived on the outskirts of Philadelphia.

Sawyer was tall, white-haired, affably talkative, and by his own account flattered to be interviewed. He told me that, as a child, he had lived in Greenwich Village in New York City and attended Catholic Mass at St. Patrick's Old Cathedral, where he and his two brothers were altar boys. His parents separated when he was in primary school. As a teenager he was unhappy at home and moved to upstate New York to stay with an aunt. There he attended Quaker meetings and, as he put it, "I got acquainted with their beliefs and it suited me fine."

His brothers both served in the military during World War II, one of them in the U.S. Marines. But when his draft notice arrived in 1941, Sawyer applied for conscientious objector status and entered Civilian Public Service (CPS), a system of camps in which draft objectors performed alternative service. Sawyer was interested in pursuing a career in social work and requested the mental hospital unit as his second camp posting.

Nine young men in the Byberry conscientious objector camp enrolled in Stokes's first round of hepatitis experiments. They lived and
worked at the hospital, and on days when they were scheduled for experimental procedures, they traveled by bus to the University of Pennsylvania, where Stokes's project was based. During Sawyer's tenure as a
subject, he had a mild bout of hepatitis B; he hardly remembered being
sick. What he recalled most vividly were the needles and accompanying
equipment investigators used when drawing blood for laboratory tests.
The research staff had trouble locating his veins, and he developed a
loathing of needles as a result. "In those days," he recalled, "they didn't
have valves that they get several samples of blood with one injection—
the valve that turns off to get another bottle in there for a sample. So you
got injected two or three times each time you were there. I got so nee-
dle-shy that I gave up after a year."

I asked Sawyer how he became a hepatitis research subject. He told
me that John Neefe, an army doctor assigned to Stokes's project, visited
Byberry to talk with the draft objectors there about participating. Neefe
had enrolled in the Army Medical Corps to fulfill wartime military duty;
he had only recently completed medical training and was barely older
than the CPS men. Sawyer continued: "He told us what we'd be doing—
needle work, taking blood samples, and getting injected with this and
that." Neefe "mentioned that it could be a risky thing," Sawyer said. "Bad
things could happen . . . a person could die." Some of Sawyer's friends
"had the idea of trying to prove that we were not afraid to die, like the
service people in the army."

I prompted him to confirm that Neefe had told the men there was a
chance the experiments could prove fatal. Sawyer responded, "Well, yes,
okay, but doctors were right there to try to prevent that. . . . The idea
that I might die was just a passing thought so far as I was concerned." He
continued: "The thing that moved me was that it would be helping mankind get rid of a bad thing, a bad disease. That was my major reason. . . .
My motivation was just to be of service to mankind."

For Sawyer and other conscientious objectors, participating in hepatitis studies was an expression of personal moral convictions, a way of em-
bodying a valued identity. They were also deferring to medical authority,
accepting on faith investigators' claims about how important the experiments were for science and the common good. When seeking institutional access and recruiting subjects, researchers appealed to the core
beliefs of their audience. With Quakers like Sawyer, they emphasized that

participants would be assisting the war effort in a manner consistent with their pacifism and contributing to a humanitarian cause of the utmost importance. In these accounts, researchers were forging critical advances in medicine, and their subjects were making heroic sacrifices for science and country.

Sawyer and his CPS comrades were young and healthy; few of them would suffer lasting harm from their part in the research. They had other options for alternative service and willingly chose to enroll in hepatitis experiments. But the circumstances of others whose lives were touched by the hepatitis experiments were more fraught. I spoke with the mother of a child who participated in hepatitis infection studies at Willowbrook State School during the early 1970s. At that time, researchers from New York University (NYU) were testing preparations for generating immunity to hepatitis B and using challenge procedures with the unmodified virus to test the preparations' effectiveness. The investigators insisted that parents had consented, but Diana McCourt felt she had given her permission under duress.

I met with McCourt at the apartment she shares with her husband in an unassuming prewar building in Manhattan's Upper West Side. Eighty-two years old, with short graying hair and wide-set eyes, she told me she had grown up in a town in Westchester County, New York, graduated from Smith College, and then moved to New York City, where she worked on a literary magazine. After her experiences with Willowbrook School, she turned her attention to grassroots community development programs.

McCourt spoke in a subdued voice about her daughter from her first marriage. Nina was born autistic with severe cognitive impairments and never developed language. She was prone to self-harming behavior when frustrated and needed constant supervision. At the time, public schools made no accommodations for children with special needs, so when her daughter was five, McCourt began arranging for a series of group programs. When Nina reached ten, available private placements became unworkable. By then, McCourt had two small children from her second marriage, a teenage stepson, and a husband who worked nights. She was overwhelmed. "I thought I was having a breakdown," she told me. "I just couldn't do it. . . . I was drowning."

She recalled meeting with a social worker at Willowbrook School who told her the facility was overcrowded, and that the only way to get in was to enter the hepatitis research unit. "He said it would be safe there . . . safer than anywhere else at Willowbrook." The staff showed her pictures of a model classroom where Nina might eventually go; it "looked deceptively clean and colorful," McCourt remarked. She told herself it would only be a few months before her daughter was moved to a regular child's unit. "I guess they held the children's unit up in front of my eyes, and I thought it would all be over with soon," McCourt said. "It's horrifying for me to think about, but I felt that I had to participate. . . . I was desperate and I had no choice."

McCourt and Nina's stepfather visited their daughter on Sundays and were distressed by her condition while on the research unit. "She was in a daze," McCourt said. "She had obviously been heavily drugged." The researchers kept her isolated in a closed room.

As McCourt learned more about appalling deficiencies in care on other Willowbrook units, she became involved with an activist group composed of professionals and parents determined to effect change. The dissidents initiated a lawsuit and won a consent decree that shut down the institution and required New York State to provide services in community settings for former residents.

When I spoke to McCourt, Nina was fifty-six years old, residing in an apartment with one other person, and receiving care tailored to her needs. To McCourt's great relief, Nina left Willowbrook without contracting hepatitis B.

Other child subjects at Willowbrook were likely not spared. Experiments NYU researchers conducted between the mid-1960s and early 1970s involved transmitting hepatitis B to susceptible children. Investigators believed that hepatitis B was a milder illness in children than in adults. But they would learn later that children exposed to this virus strain are far more likely than adults to become permanent carriers. When Willowbrook was closing, a good number of youngsters left the facility as hepatitis B carriers, asymptomatic but highly infective to others. Researchers never addressed whether the children had become carriers as the result of experimental interventions or from contact with other Willowbrook residents. Nor did scientists seek information on long-term health outcomes for the carrier children.

NYU scientists were not the first to transmit hepatitis to impaired children. Stokes enrolled the full range of subject populations in his hepatitis infection studies, including adult mental patients and developmentally disabled minors. For a decade, he held leadership positions in the AEB and ran the largest of the agency's hepatitis programs, by his own account enrolling fourteen hundred participants. Some of his subjects— the CPS men—were inoculated with hepatitis viruses as many as four times and then underwent surgical liver biopsies. Stokes was an outspoken advocate for the transmission experiments, arguing that the studies involved minimal risk. He stated proudly that no deaths had occurred in the many hepatitis experiments under his watch.

To better understand the mindset of a major hepatitis investigator, I arranged to speak with Stokes's daughter, Eleanor Stokes Szanton, at her retirement home, a train ride from Washington, DC. On the day of our appointment, Szanton and her husband welcomed me into their living room, where I sat across from a sensibly dressed woman of eighty, whose handsome face reminded me of pictures I had seen of her father.

The Stokeses were a prominent Quaker family from Moorestown, New Jersey, which traced its roots to settlers in the province of William Penn. Szanton, the youngest among her siblings, told me they were brought up to believe the world could be made a better place. She and her two brothers pursued service-oriented careers. Her chosen area was early childhood development; she completed a doctorate in the field, wrote books on the subject and, for many years, directed a child advocacy group. She had devoted her entire professional life to promoting the well-being of infants and toddlers.

She described her father as a person of tremendous optimism who spoke with unselfconscious enthusiasm about his research. He belonged to the fifth generation of Stokes physicians, all of whom placed great value on medical innovation. One of his accomplishments was an outgrowth of wartime hepatitis research, although not from the virus transmission experiments: Stokes was the first to show that administering the blood product gamma globulin during an outbreak of hepatitis A created sufficient temporary immunity to slow the appearance of new cases. Szanton recalled that her father and a co-investigator were thrilled with this finding.

One piece of Stokes's history that Szanton shared illuminated her father's deep-seated commitment to human experimentation. According to family lore, the first Stokes doctor carried out his own experimental challenge demonstration of Edward Jenner's method of vaccinating against smallpox using cowpox specimens as the immunizing agent. To help overcome local resistance to the procedure, the Stokes progenitor vaccinated his own young daughter and then put her to bed with one of his patients with active smallpox—without ill effect.

Szanton said her father referred to that story as inspiration for his work. He embraced the belief, foundational to experimental medicine, that progress in disease control is possible through empirical observation, reason, and human experimentation. If he was convinced that an unorthodox intervention would produce benefit with what he judged to be minimal risk, he would proceed with its use, even on members of his family. In fact, Szanton told me, when she was two years old, Stokes inoculated her with an experimental measles vaccine. At fifteen, she contracted a case of measles her father found so concerning that he took her to the hospital for evaluation. "It was a failed experiment," she reported.

I asked her how old she was when she learned about the experimental inoculation. "I was six, and I was very proud to be a guinea pig." When we spoke, Szanton was still proud of her father's accomplishments and dedication but also disturbed by practices that might have placed defenseless or unknowing people in jeopardy. And she was keenly ambivalent about having been a child subject herself. Her divided sentiments were emblematic of broader struggles over appropriate experimental practices, particularly when the subjects are children or otherwise in need of protection.

After my conversation with Szanton, I found written versions of the family's smallpox vaccination story in histories of New Jersey's Burlington County. These accounts identified the girl as Hannah Stokes and the physician as John Hinchman Stokes, who practiced medicine in Moorestown between 1786 and 1816. Jenner described his method of smallpox vaccinations and his success with the procedure—including his own soon-famous challenge interventions, the first conducted on the eight-year-old son of his gardener—in a pamphlet distributed in his native Britain in 1798; it made its way across the Atlantic the following year.

John Hinchman Stokes lived contemporaneously with the Enlightenment-inspired authors of the U.S. Constitution. His use of clinical demonstration was entirely consistent with the Founders' embrace of empirical methods. Many signers of the Declaration of Independence and the Constitution were members of the APS, the country's first scientific society, an association devoted to empirical inquiry and the advancement of useful knowledge. Thomas Jefferson was a gentleman scientist and an APS member. In 1801, just after his inauguration as president, he became a very early adopter of Jenner's method. He arranged to have his slaves at Monticello vaccinated with cowpox specimens and for one of the recipients to be challenged with human smallpox. When this individual remained disease-free, Jefferson promoted broad application of Jenner's procedure. I found in these accounts of early vaccine demonstrations a reminder that risky experimental interventions for the purpose of advancing public health and nation building—often conducted on persons without power and in no position to consent—are as old as America itself.

During the hepatitis program's three decades, its researchers voiced enormous confidence that human experiments would yield tools for controlling the disease and repeatedly claimed that preventive measures were imminent. They greatly underestimated the difficulties they would face. They had initial successes in distinguishing the A and B strains and their routes of transmission. But when investigators moved to work on immunizing agents, their efforts continually fell short. Techniques used in developing vaccines for other viruses did not work with hepatitis. The first hepatitis vaccine, a preparation against the B strain formulated through a highly unconventional method, was not licensed until the early 1980s, four decades after scientists started human and laboratory studies with the pathogen. Since then, researchers have introduced new vaccines for hepatitis A and B as well as a cure for hepatitis C carriers. But as of 2021, three-quarters of a century after research efforts began, there was still no cure for carriers of hepatitis B and no vaccine for hepatitis C.

Misjudgments about long-term injuries are as glaring. At the time they were infecting subjects with blood-borne hepatitis, scientists were unaware that they were creating a pool of virus carriers at risk for cirrhosis and liver cancer. Delayed harms from America's hepatitis program might be considered a metaphor for limitations in assessments of experimental hazards when researchers are working at the boundaries of medical knowledge. But the problem was not only that medical science had yet to evolve; it was also that by research harms, scientists meant immediate fatalities or serious injuries. Delayed illnesses and disabilities were not part of their calculus.

The program's defense sponsors instructed hepatitis researchers to be done with their subjects when experiments were over; military officials did not consider compensation or care for subsequent research-related illnesses to be their responsibility. And even when researchers realized that some hepatitis patients developed chronic symptoms, few investigators showed interest in contemplating the long-term health consequences for human subjects. At the program's outset, scientists and their federal patrons had more pressing concerns. America was facing an immediate crisis: hepatitis was ravaging its soldiers and the country was at war.

1942–1946

We are now in this war. We are in it—all the way. Every single man, woman and child is a partner in the most tremendous undertaking of our American history. We must share together the bad news and the good news, the defeats and the victories— the changing fortunes of war.

—FRANKLIN D. ROOSEVELT, Fireside Chat, December 9, 1941

CHAPTER ONE

In the National Interest

AMERICA HAD BARELY ENTERED World War II when the U.S. military confronted a massive outbreak of hepatitis B, the largest ever single-source outbreak of the disease. Yale researcher John Rodman Paul called it the "the great epidemic of serum hepatitis of 1942," remarking that it "fell upon the troops like another unsuspected bombshell within four months of Pearl Harbor." The Office of the Surgeon General–Army in Washington, DC, began receiving reports of illnesses at military bases early in March and new cases quickly multiplied, reaching a peak in June. The press caught wind of the spreading affliction, forcing Secretary of War Henry Stimson to acknowledge the seriousness of the outbreak. In July he reported that 28,500 servicemen had contracted hepatitis and 62 had died. By year's end, the army and air force had hospitalized more than 50,000 personnel with jaundice, while subsequent estimates placed the total number of infected personnel at well over 300,000. After Stimson's July disclosures, the War Department withheld information about hepatitis-related fatalities on grounds of national security.

The expanding epidemic during the spring of 1942 sent waves of alarm through the top brass of the military. Stanhope Bayne-Jones, second in authority at the OTSG's Preventive Medicine Division, recalled later that military leaders were unnerved by the outbreak's rapid progression. "It was more shocking to the commander of the Army, I think, than any bombardment . . . because so many people were sick, and there were so many critical things in the offing." One of the military's earliest war-time engagements was the Battle of Midway, fought in June 1942 against Japan for control of the Pacific. American forces did prevail. In retrospect, Bayne-Jones observed that the battle "was won by air pilots some of whom were suffering from hepatitis."

It would turn out that the epidemic was a crisis of the War Department's own making. The source of infection was a hepatitis-contaminated yellow fever vaccine that the military was administering to all service personnel. Decisions about that vaccine's adoption involved a spiral of miscalculations. Assumptions made by the lead scientist responsible for the vaccine's formulation proved to be both faulty and avoidable. And the War Department hastily ordered universal use of the immunizing agent because officials were persuaded that Japan might deploy yellow fever as a biological weapon—an event that never transpired. Missteps in the preparation and rushed adoption of an immunizing agent were the prelude to the nation's first hepatitis infection experiments.

The context was America's mobilization for war. As the U.S. government prepared for armed conflict, it greatly enhanced its support for defense-related biomedical research and empowered a new constituency of scientists to make decisions about the conduct of human research. Key members of this military-biomedical elite determined that human transmission studies were crucial for verifying the source of the hepatitis outbreak. In their assessment, advancing knowledge of a disease among soldiers was more important than the well-being of institutionalized persons who would serve as research subjects.

In 1940, it appeared ever more likely that the United States would become a combatant against Axis forces. During the spring, Hitler's troops overran Belgium, Luxembourg, and Holland; in early June, they occupied the streets of Paris; in September, the German air force began bombing London. That month, the U.S. Congress enacted a peacetime draft so that, well before Japan's attack on Pearl Harbor, the army's ranks swelled from 200,000 to 1.5 million. By 1941, the federal government more broadly was fully absorbed in gearing up for war.

The Roosevelt administration saw American scientific expertise as a critical resource for the war effort, and engaging civilian scientists in defense-related research was part of the ongoing mobilization. In June 1941, the president created an Office for Scientific Research and Development, best known now for projects that resulted in radar systems for air defense and the world's first atom bomb. The agency also dispensed $25 million—more than $437 million in 2020 dollars—to university scientists for a wide range of medical studies through its Committee on Medical Research. The OSRD's medical subcommittees worked closely with the medical department of the National Research Council (NRC), a division of the National Academy of Sciences (NAS) that provided expert advice to federal agencies.

The War Department set up its own structures for supporting the war-related research of civilian scientists. This included the Army Epidemiology Board, formally constituted in January 1941 and composed of a central oversight panel and multiple disease-focused working groups called commissions. The purpose of its projects was improving control of infectious diseases affecting military personnel. In previous wars, more soldiers had died from combat conditions and communicable diseases than from battle injuries. The scourge of World War I was influenza; the 1918 pandemic sickened between 20 and 40 percent of American military personnel, and tens of thousands of them died from either the flu or the pneumonia that followed. The AEB's original name was the Board for the Investigation and Control of Influenza and Other Epidemic Diseases in the Army.

University researchers affiliated with these agencies, together with physicians in the armed forces and the U.S. Public Health Service, formed a military-biomedical elite. Its members convened at OSRD, NRC, and AEB advisory panels where they set agendas for advancing biomedical science in the national interest. These committees made decisions about research funding and determined which human experiments would be conducted and with what groups of subjects. The new agencies sponsored a large volume of risk-laden human studies. OSRD projects included studies of conditions that soldiers might encounter—hypothermia, starvation, ingestion of seawater, and exposure to high altitude—as well as malaria infection studies aimed at evaluating drug therapies. The AEB pursued research on human transmission of pathogens causing poorly understood diseases. The agency—or its postwar successor, the AFEB (Armed Forces Epidemiology Board)—had a hand in virtually all of America's hepatitis infection experiments. It also sponsored a large number of trials testing the efficacy of experimental vaccines.

Immunization was the military's primary strategy for controlling infectious diseases among soldiers. Before the war started, recruits routinely received vaccinations against smallpox, typhoid, and paratyphoid.

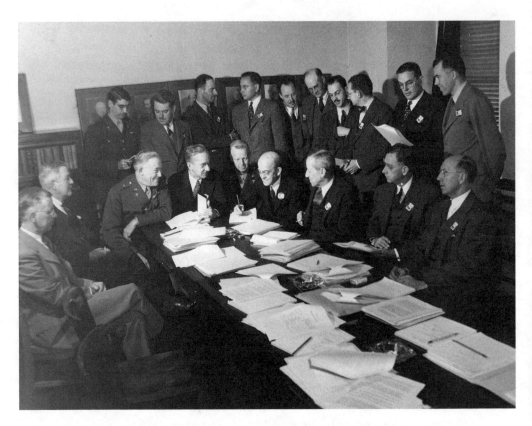

Members of the Army Epidemiology Board in May 1943, including several who were central figures in the hepatitis research program: James Stevens Simmons (*seated, third from left*), Stanhope Bayne-Jones (*seated, fifth from left*), Thomas Francis Jr. (*standing, fifth from left*), and Joseph Stokes Jr. (*standing, second from right*). (Courtesy of the Tennessee State Library and Archives. Image is available on the National Library of Medicine's website, Profiles in Science, Oswald T. Avery Collection.)

By war's end, the armed services had added immunizations for influenza, tetanus, B encephalitis, and yellow fever. The yellow fever vaccine was by far the most problematic and its initial, ill-advised adoption would have the most far-reaching consequences.

The architect of the War Department's yellow fever vaccine initiative was James Stevens Simmons, head of the OTSG's Preventive Medicine Division and Bayne-Jones's immediate superior. Simmons was a career medical officer with training in public health and experience in tropical diseases from postings in Panama and the Philippines. In February 1940, the OTSG transferred him to its Washington office, where he applied his abundant energies to reorganizing and expanding the department's preventive medicine services. Among his early activities at the OTSG was navigating approvals for creation of the AEB. One commentator described Simmons as high-strung, a person of burning enthusiasms, and a big-picture man impatient with detail. Bayne-Jones—soon to be Simmons's second-in-command—would call him "a preventive medicine evangelist."

Simmons was especially evangelical when it came to prevention of yellow fever, a mosquito-borne viral disease common in South America and central regions of Africa. Yellow fever had not been seen in the continental United States since 1905, and it was unclear whether American troops would be deployed in tropical regions where they would be exposed to mosquito carriers. Nonetheless, Simmons was tireless in promoting yellow fever immunization and began lobbying the War Department for mandatory vaccination even before Congress enacted the peacetime draft. His stated logic was that some soldiers might pass through or be posted in areas where yellow fever was endemic and, if an outbreak occurred, returning personnel could bring the disease back to the United States.

At Simmons's urging, the War Department referred the matter to the NRC's Subcommittee on Tropical Diseases. Its chair was Wilbur Sawyer, head of the Rockefeller Foundation's International Health Division (IHD). Sawyer and the IHD had years of experience with yellow fever abatement. In the early 1920s, the organization had launched campaigns in South America to eradicate the disease by exterminating the mosquito carrier. When these efforts failed to stop recurring epidemics, the IHD turned to vaccine development. It set up a Virus Laboratory on the Manhattan campus of the foundation's sister organization, the Rockefeller Institute for Medical Research, and began work on an immunizing agent.

With Sawyer at the helm, IHD scientists followed then-routine procedures for formulating an immunizing agent: cultivating the pathogen in a growth medium; killing or weakening it (with a virus, the latter was often achieved by passing it serially through an animal host or a laboratory culture); and administering the resulting preparation to a susceptible animal. If that animal remained free of symptoms, investigators then exposed it to unmodified pathogens—a challenge procedure—to see whether it was able to resist infection. Researchers had an available animal model for yellow fever—monkeys. But viruses do not multiply in laboratory media used for bacteria, and developing a culture that would sustain yellow fever microbes took years. After extensive trial and error, an IHD investigator succeeded in growing the virus in a culture of fetal monkey tissue and found that, after more than a hundred passages, the pathogens were attenuated.

In 1937, the Rockefeller Virus Lab had a preparation it felt was ready for human use: vaccine 17D. Along with the weakened microbes, it contained serum that researchers thought was necessary for stabilizing the virus. The IHD conducted field tests of the vaccine in Brazil, where yellow fever epidemics were ongoing. It then continued using the preparation in areas of Brazil and Colombia where the disease was prevalent and distributed stocks of the immunizing agent more widely, including to researchers in Britain.

In June 1940, the NRC Tropical Diseases Subcommittee recommended that the War Department vaccinate personnel traveling into regions where yellow fever was expected to exist. The IHD would manufacture the vaccine at its Virus Lab and supply it to the government free of charge in support of the war effort. The military's initial request was for one hundred thousand doses.

Then in February 1942, two months after Pearl Harbor, Secretary Stimson abruptly ordered yellow fever immunizations for *all* military personnel, vastly expanding the scope of the War Department's yellow fever vaccine mandate. The IHD geared up production and manufactured more than 4 million doses of the 17D vaccine, supplying a good portion of them to the government in 141 numbered lots. The *New York Times* declared that the new vaccine directive would mean that soldiers could be dispatched anywhere without risk of infection. But ease in posting soldiers was not the principal reason behind the revised vaccine policy. Rather, the War Department was responding to the perceived threat of germ warfare.

Some military men, Simmons among them, believed that Japan or Germany would attempt to use microbes, yellow fever in particular, as biological weapons. A pair of episodes at the IHD helped stoke their fears. On two occasions in 1939, Japanese scientists had asked Virus Lab researchers for specimens of the yellow fever strain being used in vaccine development. With America's entrance into the war, Simmons became increasingly outspoken about the possibility that Japan might find a way to deploy yellow fever as a tool of combat.

In August 1941, the NRC appointed a new committee, the War Bureau of Consultants, to evaluate the threat. (Officials gave this and later biological-warfare committees opaque names to mask their focus.) Simmons was among the liaison personnel on the committee and he attended its meetings. The bureau issued a report in February 1942—the same month as Stimson's revised immunization order—recommending actions for reducing vulnerability to biological weapons. The report stated that yellow fever virus was "one of those most to be feared" as a possible vehicle for germ warfare, and that vaccination was "the method of choice" for protecting soldiers. It also recommended that the United States begin its own biological weapons program, advice the Roosevelt administration followed.

While Japan did have an active germ warfare research program during the war, neither it nor Germany weaponized yellow fever. Bayne-Jones later remarked that Simmons had seized on the IHD incidents and "used this scare to persuade the general staff and others to sanction vaccination of American soldiers against yellow fever." Bayne-Jones's biographer observed that the hepatitis epidemic of 1942 "could be traced to American leaders' belief in the possibilities of biological warfare." A profound irony underlies the 1942 hepatitis epidemic: in an effort to address a disease threat that never materialized, military leaders approved measures that caused an outbreak of yet another serious illness.

Bayne-Jones was a central figure in investigating the 1942 epidemic and in orchestrating the hepatitis transmission experiments that followed. He arrived at the OTSG in February 1942, just as the Army Medical Department began grappling with the outbreak. A seasoned medical researcher and administrator, he had earned his medical degree at Johns Hopkins, served in the Army Medical Corps during World War I, and then held professorships in bacteriology at the University of Rochester and Yale University. Before returning to the army, he completed a five-year stint as dean of Yale Medical School.

With his leadership position in academic medicine and ties within the War Department, Bayne-Jones was exemplary of America's military-biomedical elite. His central responsibility at the OTSG would be to serve as the AEB's first executive director. His skills and connections to university researchers made him well suited to the job. His biographer described him as able "to master the detail of day-to-day operation without . . . losing grasp of overall policy." Genial and witty, Bayne-Jones was also a shrewd and tough-minded scientist; on matters of biomedical research he was focused, meticulous, and insistent on exactness. Before he could fully engage in overseeing the AEB's research program, there was an immediate crisis to be resolved. During his first six months at the OTSG, Bayne-Jones was almost totally absorbed in identifying the cause of the hepatitis outbreak and bringing the epidemic to an end.

In March and early April 1942, the Army Medical Department was scrambling to identify what was causing the illnesses. Early cases of jaundice were concentrated in the West Coast military bases. The OTSG dispatched a small group of consultants to affected bases with instructions to investigate and report back. One of two lead figures on the team was Sawyer who, in addition to his other posts, was also director of the AEB Commission on Tropical Diseases. The other was Karl Meyer, professor of bacteriology at the University of California, San Francisco, and a recently appointed army consultant on Sawyer's AEB Commission. Bayne-Jones remained in Washington, but kept close track of the West Coast investigation.

Meyer knew about cases of hepatitis following use of vaccines containing serum and, when he arrived at affected bases, he immediately focused on the immunization histories of soldiers hospitalized with jaundice. All had been vaccinated against yellow fever two to three months before the appearance of symptoms; all had received particular lots of the vaccine. Meyer had no doubt that the vaccine was the source of the outbreak. But Sawyer resisted attributing the problem to the vaccine and instead looked for infection in civilian populations surrounding the bases that might have made its way to military personnel. As the investigation proceeded, Sawyer had to acknowledge that the IHD vaccine was likely generating the epidemic. But in the meantime, he was withholding information about problems with the 17D vaccine.

This was not the first time that the immunizing agent had caused hepatitis. Jaundice had followed use of IHD yellow fever vaccine in both South America and Britain. Journal articles appearing in the late 1930s described some of these episodes. Sawyer was well aware not only of these incidences but also of later cases of jaundice in Brazil, about which no reports had yet been published. The IHD laboratory in Brazil stopped using vaccine with serum in December 1940, and was conducting field trials with a serum-free preparation. But Sawyer considered the serum-free vaccine to be insufficiently tested for broader use. The protocol for preparing 17D vaccine for government use included an extra precaution; the serum was heated to 56 degrees centigrade for at least half an hour before being added to the immunizing agent. Sawyer was confident this measure would inactivate any jaundice-causing agent. But the new hepatitis outbreak was proving him wrong.

In early April, the OTSG gathered information from a variety of sources about hepatitis following use of 17D vaccine. Some of the information came from members of the IHD Board of Scientific Directors. By mid-April, OTSG arranged to suspend yellow fever vaccinations until the investigation of the outbreak was completed. But this did not mean abandoning yellow fever vaccination altogether.

After attending a meeting at the OTSG on April 10, Johannes Bauer, then head of the IHD Virus Laboratory, wrote to his boss, Sawyer, who was still in California. Bauer reported that Simmons held out against terminating the program: "Col. Simmons was particularly emphatic on this point and stated that if vaccination was once discontinued, it would be exceedingly difficult to start it again and he said that it took them a whole year to convince the general staff of the importance of this protective measure."

The investigation of the outbreak moved to a new phase in late April. Bayne-Jones never believed that heating serum to 56 degrees would neutralize hepatitis pathogens. Now he urged the IHD to closely examine blood components used in manufacturing the vaccine. The IHD had obtained serum from a laboratory at Johns Hopkins that had relied on blood donations from medical and other health science students. The Hopkins lab had pooled donated blood and processed it into serum before delivering it to the IHD. In May, Bauer and several other IHD scientists went to Baltimore to examine both blood donor records and procedures used in generating serum pools. When they compared these records with rates of hepatitis associated with disease-causing vaccine lots, they found a pattern. Only those lots of vaccine receiving serum from a handful of serum pools generated high rates of hepatitis. The implication was that some donors contributing to those pools were carrying hepatitis. Evidence that serum in the 17D vaccine was the source of hepatitis was now overwhelming.

Shock and dismay were among the initial reactions to news that the yellow fever vaccine had caused the epidemic. Both the IHD and the

Rockefeller Institute had stellar reputations. The Rockefeller Institute had played a major role in establishing the United States as an international leader in biomedical research during the interwar years. The IHD was widely known for yeoman's work on disease eradication throughout the developing world. Meyer later reported that when he telephoned Simmons early in the West Coast investigation to say that the vaccine was causing hepatitis, Simmons blurted out, "Can't be. . . . It's perfectly safe. The Rockefeller made it." The hepatitis epidemic would be, in the assessment of an IHD historian, "the most embarrassing episode in Health Division history."

That the IHD vaccine had caused the epidemic was also a tremendous personal blow to Sawyer. It had been his decision alone to provide the government with vaccine made with serum. He did so knowing that serum-containing preparations had previously caused outbreaks of hepatitis. He was so sure that heating the serum was an adequate protective measure that he assumed the vaccine was safe even when new illnesses began appearing.

Imputations of blame circulated through the biomedical community. Meyer felt it was unpardonable that Sawyer had concealed information about post-vaccination hepatitis. A number of virologists, including some among the IHD's scientific directors, faulted Sawyer for not providing the army with the serum-free immunizing agent already being used in Brazil. Virus Laboratory researchers criticized Sawyer less for making a decision that turned out to be calamitous than for making it unilaterally and without consultation. In their view, Sawyer had placed insufficient weight on the judgment of scientists at the IHD laboratory in Brazil; he had deflected advice from his colleagues at the New York laboratory; and he had failed to seek advice from his own Board of Scientific Directors. Sawyer had been insular in his decision-making and overconfident in his scientific judgments.

Criticism was not confined to scientific circles. The hepatitis outbreak created a public relations nightmare for the army. The War Department tried to suppress news of the epidemic, but by June, stories were proliferating in the mainstream press about the widespread illness and deaths at military bases. When Stimson released information about the scale of the outbreak in July, it was an attempt at damage control. He acknowledged the epidemic and its cause but emphasized that the vaccine was no longer in use, and that the situation was now under control.

But the press was not mollified. The *Chicago Tribune* responded with a scathing editorial headlined "A Grievous Error." The paper demanded to know, "How did it happen that wholesale inoculations were undertaken with a vaccine which quite obviously had not been thoroughly tested in advance?" The editors continued, "In the war thus far, some 1,400 American soldiers have been wounded. Twenty times as many have fallen victim to yellow fever vaccinations." The *Tribune* called for a congressional investigation, as did a member of the U.S. House of Representatives. The denouncement of military decision-making was short-lived, but for the war's duration, the OTSG would be on notice: it was not to create any further public relations problems for the War Department.

As this controversy was unfolding, critical decisions had yet to be made about the future of the yellow fever vaccine program. The IHD Board of Scientific Directors convened a meeting in Manhattan with Virus Laboratory scientists on June 13 to bring together available information on the source of the hepatitis outbreak. The directors then held a closed session during which they issued a request for a meeting in Washington with representatives of the army, navy, and PHS. The IHD would provide a full accounting of what it knew about the infective vaccine and the serum-free immunizing agent. The scientific directors were not comfortable with sending Sawyer to Washington alone and insisted on accompanying him.

Two meetings on the fate of yellow fever vaccination took place in the summer of 1942 at the NAS headquarters in Washington, DC. The first, on June 17, was the conference requested by the IHD board. The AEB president chaired this meeting. The fifteen attendees included members of the IHD Board of Scientific Directors and representatives from the army and navy, among them Simmons and Bayne-Jones. Top officials from the PHS were also there: the surgeon general, the director of the National Institutes of Health (NIH, the research branch of the PHS), and the chief of the NIH Division of Biologics Control, the governmental unit responsible for licensing immunizing agents and ensuring vaccine safety. The PHS was at the time facing its own problems with vaccine 17D; the agency had distributed the immunizing agent in the U.S. Virgin Islands, and in late May a hepatitis outbreak had occurred there.

The assembled scientists issued a statement saying that, until the problem of the outbreak was fully resolved, vaccination against yellow fever should be limited to persons traveling to or through areas where yellow fever was endemic. It was a stopgap measure. Still to be determined was whether the military would reinstate universal yellow fever vaccinations and, if so, with what immunizing agent. Scientists were considering use of the serum-free vaccine and looking into possible sources for its preparation.

Further decisions about policy on yellow fever vaccination would be made at an upcoming meeting of the NRC Tropical Diseases Subcommittee. It would take place on July 8 in the Lincoln Board Room of the NAS. At that meeting, leaders of America's military-biomedical elite would also launch plans to conduct human transmission experiments with hepatitis.

The NAS headquarters is a stately neoclassical structure on Constitution Avenue at the west end of the Washington Mall. It was dedicated in 1924, but plans for its construction date to the First World War and the creation of the NRC. Its location and bearing speak to the aspiration that science would be an essential contributor to a broad range of national policies. The building stands within view of the Lincoln Memorial, and its pale marble façade echoes the memorial's exterior. The site is a short walk from the White House and the Executive Office Building; just to the north on C Street is the State Department in a structure that, until the late 1940s, housed the Department of War.

The board room occupies the southeast corner of the building's elegant first floor. To arrive there from the Constitution Avenue entrance, a visitor passes through a bronze- and mahogany-flanked entry foyer into the towering Great Hall with its elaborately painted domed ceiling. The board room itself has warm-hued wood paneling and contains a huge oval conference table with rows of surrounding armchairs. Above the table hangs a large light fixture in the shape of a globe; on its surface is a map of the world. A large marble-framed fireplace adorns the room's west wall; above it is a mural of Abraham Lincoln and the academy's nineteenth-century founders.

On July 8, 1942, forty members of America's biomedical elite filled the Lincoln Board Room. Among those attending were members of the NRC's Tropical Disease Subcommittee and senior officials from its Division of Medical Sciences. All the agencies affected by or studying the hepatitis outbreak sent representatives: the IHD and the army, navy, and NIH. Simmons, Bayne-Jones, and Sawyer were there, as were the director of the NIH and the NIH chief of Biologics Control. The meeting minutes report the outcome of deliberations concerning the military's vaccine program: "The consensus ... is that yellow fever vaccine manufactured without human serum is effective and should be used instead of serum-containing vaccine used heretofore." The War Department would now be using vaccine that the PHS manufactured at its Rocky Mountain Laboratory.

Not all of what transpired appears in the minutes. In correspondence, NRC officials reminded Sawyer, who was responsible for producing the written record, that some of the matters discussed were of a secret nature. This very probably included information about the threat of biological warfare. But conversations about another sensitive matter were also taking place during the meeting. Under the mural of Lincoln in the academy's board room or in nearby hallways, scientific leaders were making arrangements for the PHS to serve as lead agency in experiments using lots of hepatitis-contaminated vaccine to deliberately infect research subjects. The human participants in these studies would be residents of a Virginia state institution for the intellectually impaired. The ostensible purpose was to verify that the IHD's original immunizing agent was the source of the hepatitis epidemic.

The problem of the hepatitis outbreak had, in fact, already been solved. Using the methods of epidemiology, researchers had determined that all the soldiers who became sick had been vaccinated; that only certain lots of vaccine generated symptoms; and that those lots contained serum from the same set of blood donors. From these patterns, scientists inferred that the blood of these donors contained a jaundice-causing agent. When they stopped using vaccine with serum and substituted a serum-free preparation, the number of new cases steadily declined and the serum-free vaccine generated no new illnesses. Yet it was precisely at this moment that human infection experiments began.

The reason for undertaking the experiments was that biomedical leaders saw a scientific opportunity too promising to forgo. They had long suspected that pathogens—probably viruses—caused hepatitis, but they lacked laboratory evidence of a jaundice-causing agent. They were schooled to place their confidence in experimental medicine; epidemiological findings only whetted their appetite for empirical evidence that hepatitis was caused by a transferable pathogen. Lots of infective yellow fever vaccine were now readily available to be used as specimens in experiments that would demonstrate the transmission of hepatitis from person to person. In short, the faulty vaccine and subsequent epidemic had created a compelling scientific opening, and the exigencies of war provided justification for pursuing experiments to advance medical knowledge, even at the cost of deliberately sickening human subjects.

In the normal course of events, scientists would conduct experiments of this type with laboratory animals. But several groups of investigators had already tried to do so without success. When investigators in Brazil and Britain realized that yellow fever vaccine triggered jaundice, they inoculated animals with both the vaccine and serum from symptomatic patients. The most recent attempts at animal transmission accompanied the investigation of jaundice at U.S. military bases. With Meyer's help, an IHD researcher working in California inoculated numerous animal species, among them horses, with infective materials. These attempts had also failed. Scientists would now bypass an animal model and conduct basic research on human participants.

While not routine science, inoculating human subjects with unmodified pathogens for basic research had historical precedents. In 1900, in the aftermath of the Spanish-American War, a U.S. Yellow Fever Commission led by army surgeon Walter Reed initiated studies in Cuba with the intention of showing that bites from yellow fever–infected mosquitoes caused the disease in humans. When the group's transmission demonstration had succeeded, affiliated investigators infected research subjects in an effort to generate immunity. The combined efforts triggered multiple cases of yellow fever and several deaths. Two decades later, just after World War I, a team of U.S. scientists tried to infect human participants with influenza with the goal of identifying the pathogen and its means of infection; their attempts to transmit influenza failed. With both the yellow fever and influenza studies, disease outbreaks accompanying war had emboldened scientists to place greater weight on hoped-for advances in knowledge of epidemic illnesses than on the prevention of injury to human subjects.

In May 1942, Bayne-Jones was actively lobbying for human infection studies with hepatitis. That month, Bauer sent Bayne-Jones a progress report on the IHD's investigation of the donated blood used in tainted lots of vaccine. Bauer stated, "One thing is quite definite: the agent [causing hepatitis] was present in normal human serum used in manufacturing the vaccine." Bayne-Jones responded by asking Bauer whether his statement was based on statistical correlations or experimentation. Bayne-Jones continued: "It would be a great achievement if the presence of a jaundice-producing agent in human serum could be demonstrated by designed and controlled experiments. I hope work along that line will go ahead as rapidly as possible, in spite of difficulties." By "difficulties," Bayne-Jones meant the lack of susceptible animals and impediments to obtaining human subjects for a study of this type.

The AEB had already signed on to the idea of human infection experiments. At its May 12–13 meeting, the AEB oversight committee took a clear position on the matter. Meeting minutes include the following statement: "After thorough discussion the Board, without formal vote, approved plans outlined for further etiological investigation, using suspected lots of yellow fever vaccine, blood serum of donors with histories of jaundice, and materials from patients. *If experiments on human volunteers can be arranged, such experiments are desirable.*"

Not all scientists were enthusiastic about the prospect of human infection experiments. Meyer—in California but aware that human studies were in the works—voiced trepidation in a July 1 letter that underscored the hazards such research would entail: "Experiments in human volunteers appear imperative but in light of recent deaths at several camps, one would hesitate to undertake such tests." However, other members of the biomedical elite had reached a consensus—and they were not hesitating.

Scientists took concrete steps to begin hepatitis transmission studies within days of the July 8 meeting in the Lincoln Board Room. The NIH was directly responsible for the experiments. On July 10, Bauer sent NIH director Rollo E. Dyer yellow fever vaccine from lot 331—one of two infective lots that investigators would use as inoculants. Several weeks later, Milton V. Veldee, head of Biologics Control at the NIH, wrote Bauer asking for additional vaccine from a lot that had generated large numbers of illnesses. Veldee urged that the vaccine be shipped via airmail express, "since our work is about to begin." The hepatitis transmission studies in fact started the following month.

Agency leaders assigned the task of conducting the experiments to PHS commissioned officer John W. Oliphant. In July, Oliphant and two other PHS physicians were on assignment in the Virgin Islands investigating the hepatitis outbreak there that followed use of vaccine 17D. As soon as the group returned, Oliphant attended a meeting at the OTSG with Bayne-Jones, Simmons, Dyer, and Veldee.

The following day, August 4, 1942, Oliphant submitted a three-page memo on NIH letterhead requesting formal approval for hepatitis infection experiments. The memo provided an overview of the initial experiments to be conducted. Researchers would give fifty patients yellow fever vaccine from either lot 331 or another lot with a record of high jaundice production. Once illnesses appeared among those inoculated, freshly drawn serum from jaundiced patients would be given to new subjects. A separate group of participants would receive a variety of other hepatitis-tainted specimens.

A good portion of Oliphant's memo is devoted to justifying the experiments. He wrote that yellow fever was a serious menace for both military and civilian populations: "A safe and reliable vaccine is of utmost national urgency." He continued: "A prompt solution to the problem of the etiology of jaundice following vaccination against yellow fever is a matter of extreme national urgency. Because of the national importance of the problem" and because no animal model was available for hepatitis research, "it is deemed by us to be justifiable and necessary to use human beings as experimental subjects."

Oliphant addressed the memo to Lucius F. Badger, chief of the NIH Division of Infectious Diseases. Text added to the memo shows that on August 12, Badger approved the proposal and forwarded it up the organizational ladder. A handwritten scrawl on the final page of the document is evidence of the NIH director's authorization: "Approved by R. E. Dyer."

If Oliphant's memo is taken alone, it would appear that he had initiated the human experiments with hepatitis. But when he submitted the document, the decision to proceed with human studies had already been made, and the machinery for accomplishing them was already in motion. With Bayne-Jones in the lead and the AEB and NIH senior scientists concurring, members of America's biomedical elite had decided that immediate military exigencies justified disease-inducing human experiments. Oliphant's memo was pro forma—official paperwork to be completed before embarking on the next assignment. Oliphant was a mid-level PHS commissioned officer. He had earned his medical degree from Indiana University, finished his training at PHS hospitals, and then joined the agency's medical corps. In early evaluations, his supervisors described him as thorough, industrious, and dependable, though unoriginal. He was an agency man, relocating frequently to carry out assignments officials above him deemed important. His stated preference was for clinical work and field investigations. In this case, Oliphant had the job—unappealing to most—of making frequent trips to a custodial institution and sickening its residents with virus-containing specimens.

What remains of the Central Virginia Training Center is located on the outskirts of Lynchburg, Virginia, 180 miles southwest of Washington, DC. The facility sat on a plain above the James River, near the foot of the Blue Ridge Mountains. Founded in 1910 for residential care of epileptics, it soon opened its doors to persons with intellectual impairments and was known as the Virginia State Colony for Epileptics and Feebleminded. In 1942, it housed a population approaching two thousand and went by the name Lynchburg State Colony. At that time, all of its residents were white; Virginia would not desegregate its state hospitals until the 1960s. Among disability rights scholars, the facility is best known for its history of eugenic sterilizations: between 1927 and 1972, in America's single largest sterilization program, institutional officials sterilized more than eight thousand inmates. The Lynchburg State Colony was also the location of the first U.S. experiments in which scientists deliberately transmitted hepatitis to human subjects.

Oliphant's publications state that PHS researchers conducted three rounds of hepatitis transmission experiments. The first started in August 1942 and involved 189 subjects, both males and females, between the ages of thirteen and fifty-seven; of them, 30 developed symptoms of hepatitis. The second and third rounds, begun during July 1943 and June 1944, raised the total number of subjects to 303 and the number contracting hepatitis to 44. According to Oliphant, most of the illnesses were mild. In his journal articles, he referred to his human subjects as *volunteers;* midcentury investigators routinely used this term for study participants, regardless of the circumstances surrounding recruitment. His publications did not disclose that Lynchburg Colony was the site of the studies or that the subjects were intellectually impaired.

Documentary records on the studies at Lynchburg are sparse. Brief entries in the colony's annual reports do confirm that PHS physicians began work related to the yellow fever vaccine at the facility in August 1942, and that they had left the institution by June 1945. Initially, a doctor and a technician were at the colony "the entire year working on yellow fever." One passage reads that the PHS "selected the institution to do some original research work trying to find the cause of . . . fatalities from yellow fever vaccine." The annual reports never state that the research involved infecting Lynchburg residents with hepatitis.

Records of the state hospital board, a body composed of a commissioner and the physician superintendents of state institutions, provide hints as to how the experiments came to be located in Virginia. In February 1944, an observer sent to Lynchburg reported that two PHS physicians were working and living at the colony two days a week without reimbursing the facility for their room and meals. At the next meeting, a board member who had been Lynchburg superintendent in 1942 stated that when arrangements were made for PHS research at the facility, he had invited the investigators to stay at the institution. The commissioner added, "Several of the hospitals have cooperated with the Public Health Service from time to time and ... they have done very valuable work at the institutions." He continued, "It was the expressed wish of the Board that the institutions continue to cooperate with the United States Public Health Service in such matters." In other words, Virginia state health officials had reciprocal relations with the PHS, and their willingness to have Lynchburg Colony serve as the site for hepatitis infection studies was part of an ongoing pattern of cooperation.

Prevailing attitudes toward persons with intellectual disabilities afforded these individuals minimal protection. Those classified as feebleminded were widely seen as incompetent, untrustworthy, and unfit for the privileges of citizenship. Advocates for eugenic sterilization depicted their targets as morally degenerate burdens on society. And while some of the professionals who staffed state facilities no doubt sought to equip their wards to reintegrate into society, the great bulk of these institutions became little more than repositories of social castoffs. For medical investigators seeking study sites, the isolation—both geographic and social—of state colonies was an advantage. With the assistance of institutional officials, scientists could shape what information about their experiments reached the outside world.

A great deal about the experiments at Lynchburg remains a mystery. This includes how subjects were selected and recruited; what they were told—and what they understood—about the experiments; whether enrollees had any choice about participating; and who, if anyone, provided consent. It is also unclear to what degree caregivers at Lynchburg were aware of the experiments and how they felt about resulting illnesses. Later hepatitis researchers would justify experiments with intellectually impaired persons by arguing the interventions were therapeutic in intent and aimed at controlling hepatitis at a facility. But hepatitis was not endemic at the Lynchburg Colony—at least not before the experiments were conducted—and Oliphant claimed no therapeutic purpose when it came to Lynchburg subjects.

While few answers can be found in the available records, sources do reveal that others pursued some of these questions. In 1995, an enterprising local journalist wrote a story about the experiments for the *Lynchburg News & Advance*. The reporter interviewed Bertha Corr, a nurse at the colony during the 1940s who had worked with Oliphant.

Corr, eighty-nine years old at the time of the interview, remarked that some Lynchburg residents would not have understood the word *volunteer*; and that the facility's nurses "did as we were told and did not ask any questions." On the matter of documents, Corr reported, "They took their records with them when they left." Those materials apparently never made their way to an archival repository.

From afar, Bayne-Jones was pleased with the course and outcome of the Lynchburg experiments. He had designed and promoted the initial human transmission studies and, when these were completed, he sent Oliphant specimens from sickened soldiers for use in further human inoculations. As the project proceeded, its focus expanded to include testing interventions that might inactivate the virus. Bayne-Jones followed the experiments with keen interest, corresponding with Oliphant and Dyer about the interventions and their outcomes. Oliphant sent Bayne-Jones progress reports, with both the NIH director and the chief of Infectious Diseases signing off on his communications. Meanwhile, the OTSG monitored what information about the studies would be disclosed in publications. Before allowing the team to forward its first paper to a medical journal, Dyer sent a copy to Bayne-Jones asking whether there was "anything in this article which should not be published."

Bayne-Jones was an appreciative audience. In July 1943, Oliphant sent Bayne-Jones a summary of findings from early experiments; the memo was stamped "*CONFIDENTIAL*." Oliphant reported that after sickening participants with infective lots of yellow fever vaccine, he had used specimens from these patients to induce hepatitis in another group of subjects. This work demonstrated the existence of a transmissible pathogen. Bayne-Jones responded effusively: "I am greatly obliged to you for your . . . condensed summary of results obtained in your investigations of jaundice. Yours is the best work I know of on the subject and it seems to me it settles some of the most important questions. I want to express appreciation to Dr. Dyer and to you for the directness of the attack on the problem."

The appearance of the project's first publication in August of that year generated more praise. Bayne-Jones wrote Oliphant: "I think this is the most important contribution which has been made to knowledge of the nature of the agent causing this type of jaundice. Please accept my high regard for this work." Oliphant's work at Lynchburg Colony greatly raised his professional standing. Agency officials no longer viewed him as an unremarkable commissioned public health officer; members of the biomedical community were now recognizing him as a fellow scientist. In April 1945, Oliphant received a meritorious promotion to senior PHS surgeon on the basis of his hepatitis infection research.

Writing in 1944, Bauer summarized the contributions of the Lynchburg experiments: "Jaundice following yellow fever vaccination can be passed serially from person to person by the injection of extremely small amounts of serum." The jaundice-causing "agent can be inactivated by ultraviolet irradiation, but . . . heating it to 56 C for one-half hour will not destroy activity." Researchers would discover later that Oliphant had been wrong about ultraviolet radiation; it did not inactivate hepatitis pathogens. The failure of this and all other methods for neutralizing the blood-borne virus would lead to another military and public health crisis, this one occurring in the early 1950s.

Leaders of the U.S. biomedical elite envisioned and approved America's first hepatitis infection experiments. Patterns of cooperation among major biomedical institutions made the studies possible; initial collaboration among the OTSG, IHD, and PHS was essential, as was subsequent cooperation between the PHS and Virginia state health officials. From the research community's perspective, the experiments at Lynchburg were very successful. Investigators achieved their scientific goals without visible criticism or complaints from the War Department about public relations. The isolation of their subjects combined with circumspection on the part of Virginia health officials helped researchers contain information about the experiments. Hepatitis infection studies at Lynchburg Colony would set a new precedent. Once experiments of this kind proceeded without incident, it would be easier to conduct them again.

CHAPTER TWO

Logistics on the Medical
Battlefront

OLLOWING THE VACCINE-INDUCED epidemic, hepatitis continued
to be a problem for the military, particularly in what the War
Department called the Mediterranean Theater of Operations.
During the fall of 1942, American troops joined the British
in North Africa, intent on pushing into Axis-occupied Europe from the
south. In subsequent months, the Allies expelled German and Italian
forces from Africa's northern coast, gained control of Sicily, and established a foothold in southern Italy. Meanwhile, soldiers were contracting
illnesses that military doctors had few tools to manage. In the spring of
1943, the Office of the Surgeon General–Army sent a group of medical
researchers to the region to investigate diseases among Allied personnel.
Yale scientist John Rodman Paul, who headed the team, encountered a
great deal of hepatitis there—it would prove to be largely hepatitis A.

As he toured field hospitals in Sicily after the Allied landing, Paul
saw facilities equipped to treat 750 patients that were handling twice that
number, with hundreds of cots overflowing into hallways and auxiliary
tents; it seemed to him that every other patient was jaundiced. Paul
reported that, in the Mediterranean arena, "hepatitis is the disease of
this war . . . and it dwarfs all other investigative problems as the disease
which is so prevalent and yet so obscure." He continued: "The nature of
its cause is unknown, its manner of spread is unknown, its manner of

prevention is unknown, and little is known about therapy." The Army Medical Department was especially concerned about hepatitis—with its liver inflammation and symptoms of fever, malaise, abdominal pain, nausea, vomiting, and diarrhea—because in severe cases the disease could remove soldiers from duty for weeks, even months. For the OTSG, epidemic jaundice on the battlefield was ample reason to press forward with basic research on hepatitis using human subjects.

One year after the PHS dispatched Oliphant to conduct preliminary transmission studies at Lynchburg Colony, the Army Epidemiology Board launched a hepatitis infection research program under the military's direct control. The army surgeon general approved the initiative in the summer of 1943, and human inoculations began in the fall. For the next two and a half years, the AEB supported three groups of researchers that conducted basic research on hepatitis using disease-inducing procedures. A civilian medical consultant for the army directed each of the teams: Joseph Stokes Jr. at the University of Pennsylvania, Paul at Yale, and Thomas Francis Jr. at the University of Michigan.

The three were experienced scientists and well-positioned members of the biomedical elite. Each headed one of the AEB's research commissions and led ongoing studies of viral diseases other than hepatitis. Stokes, chair of pediatrics at Penn, oversaw the AEB Commission on Measles and Mumps. He had earned his bachelor's degree from Haverford College, a Quaker institution, before studying medicine at Penn. Stokes was distinctive in his ardent advocacy for hepatitis transmission experiments. When later confronted with criticism for enrolling some categories of human subjects, he sent impassioned defenses of these procedures to his scientific peers. Colleagues at Penn would remember him for bringing wartime émigré scientists to Philadelphia's Children's Hospital, where he was medical director, and for setting the institution on a path to becoming a major pediatric research center.

Paul's AEB commission focused on neurotropic virus diseases; his particular interest was poliomyelitis. From an upper-crust family, Paul had graduated from Princeton and earned his MD from Yale before joining the Yale faculty in preventive medicine. He was contemplative, understated, and intellectually inclined. While on assignment in the Mediterranean region, Paul contracted hepatitis B from an experimental skin test administered by a member of his research team. In the wake of his illness, Paul said he would think twice about transmitting hepatitis to

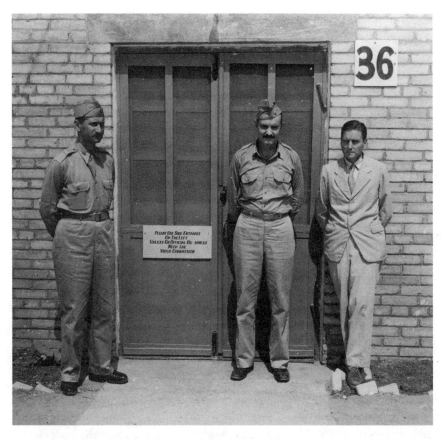

John Rodman Paul, head of an army scientific mission to the Mediterranean region in 1943, leans against a laboratory building at a military base in Cairo. With him are research team members Albert Sabin (*left*) and Cornelius Philip (*center*). (John Rodman Paul Papers [MS 1333]. Manuscripts and Archives, Yale University Library.)

subjects. He went ahead with such interventions nonetheless, although he did curtail transmission procedures at a major study site when the war was ending. Paul would be known for research on polio; work by his team at Yale on the epidemiology and transmission of poliovirus upended long-standing orthodoxies and contributed to vaccine development.

Francis, who signed letters as "Tommy," was the son of a Welsh immigrant. Colleagues found him both amiable and hard-driving. Having trained in medicine at Yale, he had distinguished himself as a young scientist at the Rockefeller Institute by developing the first influenza vaccine. His AEB commission was devoted to influenza; through it, he conducted large-scale studies of new immunizing agents. He would gain public visibility in the 1950s for evaluating the huge field trial of Jonas Salk's polio vaccine. Francis's involvement in hepatitis research was the briefest and entailed the fewest subjects, yet he was the only wartime researcher to confront the death of a subject from acute liver failure.

Overseeing them all was Stanhope Bayne-Jones, executive director of the AEB. He shaped the program's scientific aims, arranged for researchers to receive specimens from soldiers sickened with hepatitis, made determinations about what groups of subjects investigators could use, and helped negotiate access to potential recruits. To provide adequate staff for the projects, Bayne-Jones had the OTSG assign doctors attached to the Army Medical Corps to work as junior investigators. It was these physicians—in the army to satisfy their wartime military duty—who performed experimental interventions, cared for sick subjects, and produced a stream of reports on study procedures and outcomes. They also wrote scientific papers on which their names appeared as joint authors. For his part, Bayne-Jones commanded, guided, and cajoled, periodically issuing a well-placed rebuke to an investigator he felt had stepped out of line.

The program's senior scientists convened several times a year as a hepatitis study group, chaired by Stokes, and were in frequent contact with one another and with Bayne-Jones through an abundance of memos and correspondence. The experiments they conducted and their accompanying discussions addressed basic features of hepatitis and the pathogens causing it. Through human infection studies, they sought to discover how hepatitis spread, what bodily specimens were infective and for how long, how much time elapsed between exposure and the appearance of symptoms, and whether infection generated immunity to subsequent exposure. The clinical literature of the day identified two disease entities, then called "infectious (epidemic) hepatitis" (hepatitis A) and "serum hepatitis" (hepatitis B). Central among researchers' goals was to determine whether different strains of virus caused these illnesses. Meanwhile, they were also assessing what laboratory tests were best for identifying liver inflammation and its remission.

The methods at their disposal were rudimentary. The scientists proceeded by exposing subjects to specimens from infected patients; these specimens included serum, stool, urine, nasal washings, and a variety of biopsied tissues. Researchers tried multiple routes of transmission: ingestion, inhalation, and injection. The oral route generated some grimly humorous comments from subjects; here investigators instructed participants to swallow "milkshakes" made of hepatitis specimens—typically stool—mixed into chocolate milk.

After the inoculations, investigators followed subjects for three to six months, taking frequent blood draws for liver function tests and recording the details of resulting illnesses. In immunity and cross-immunity studies, researchers exposed subjects to specimens multiple times to see if the recipients were resistant to later exposures. The cross-immunity experiments—aimed at distinguishing two strains of the virus—were the most taxing for subjects; participants in these studies endured as many as four or five separate inoculations with hepatitis viruses, and their tenure as subjects could extend for well over a year.

While scientific matters were the preeminent concern of hepatitis investigators, the logistics of carrying out human experiments were a close second. Research logistics were multifaceted; they included persuading managers of custodial facilities to open their doors to scientists, convincing potential recruits to participate, and either concealing dangerous experiments with institutionalized persons or winning public support for such studies.

Bayne-Jones and his scientists pursued several strategies for handling the public interface of human infection research. At first, anticipating criticism, they suppressed information about the studies, particularly those with subjects whose capacity for consent was in question. But they soon came up with a more ingenious strategy. With Bayne-Jones taking the lead, they sought public favor by advancing accounts that portrayed research subjects as freely choosing to make vital contributions to the war effort. Their narrative logistics rested on the selective release of information and cooperative relations with a press already deferential to scientific expertise and sympathetic toward military priorities. But before they could begin these efforts, program scientists had to secure a resource indispensable for their work: human subjects.

Arranging for access to subjects was a perpetual headache. Researchers would begin promising discussions with institutional overseers only to encounter delays and obstacles. At one point, Paul felt stymied in his efforts to gain entrance to custodial facilities in Connecticut reasonably close to the Yale campus in New Haven. He wrote Bayne-Jones saying he wanted to enroll soldiers at a nearby military installation. Although soldiers would serve as subjects in wartime and postwar studies of chemical warfare agents and ionizing radiation, federal sponsors avoided recruitment of military personnel for disease-inducing interventions taking place on U.S. soil. Bayne-Jones immediately vetoed Paul's idea: "Use of soldiers for jaundice experiments is too risky." He insisted that the studies be conducted in "a *suitable* institution."

Stokes proposed housing hepatitis subjects on farms in western New Jersey, where he had long-standing contacts. Bayne-Jones quickly rejected this plan also, citing "the possibility of the spread of the disease in a community, the attendant publicity, and the possible bad effect of the experiment upon public relations of the War Department." "Suitable" institutions were ones in which the spread of both infection and information could be controlled.

Sometimes disqualifying complications arose after experiments at a site had begun. Francis drew most of his subjects from inmates at the Michigan State Prison in Jackson—also called Jackson State Prison—not far from the University of Michigan's Ann Arbor campus. During the summer of 1945, when Francis's team was still at the prison, the warden at Jackson, who ran a de facto patronage system, became embroiled in a battle with state officials. A crime syndicate with members both inside and outside the prison was implicated in the murder of a state legislator. The Michigan attorney general accused the warden and his senior staff of colluding with the syndicate, and the accompanying scandal attracted national attention; *Newsweek* carried a page-long story about corruption at the prison. Bayne-Jones reacted with alarm—soon after, Francis discontinued experiments at the facility.

Paul ran into a different type of problem when conducting experiments with inmates at the Federal Correctional Institution in Danbury, Connecticut. Paul's team enrolled eight prisoners in an early hepatitis transmission study; at least four of them were conscientious objectors, men who either rejected or failed to qualify for legally sanctioned alternative service. Militant draft resisters at the prison staged a series of political protests, including a hunger strike aimed at desegregating the dining hall. Their social activism disrupted institutional routines and made it difficult to proceed with medical experiments at the prison.

Ultimately, each of the AEB research teams drew on a combination of subject groups: Stokes used conscientious objectors and mental patients; Paul recruited conscientious objectors and prisoners; Francis enrolled prisoners and a small number of long-term-care patients at Eloise

Hospital in Michigan where he and Jonas Salk—then a young investigator with Francis's commission—were testing influenza vaccines. Together the AEB researchers enrolled approximately 320 subjects in hepatitis infection experiments: 6 hospital patients, 70 prisoners, 75 mental patients, and more than 170 conscientious objectors who were performing work deemed an acceptable alternative to the military draft in a system of Civilian Public Service camps.

The institutional context of these groups' participation varied, as did the character of their involvement in the research. Conscientious objectors were of critical importance both because of their relative numbers and because accounts of their enrollment would be of great assistance in winning public favor for hepatitis infection experiments during the war. But CPS was a complex entity, and arranging for these men to enroll as hepatitis subjects required investigators to navigate a formidable array of governmental and nongovernmental agencies.

President Roosevelt established CPS by executive order in February 1941. Legislation creating the peacetime draft in the fall of 1940 had stipulated that men with religious or moral objections to bearing arms would be allowed to perform work of national importance under civilian direction. The provision was an accommodation to lobbying by the historic peace churches—the Mennonites, Brethren, and Quakers. But the bill did not specify what form alternative service would take, and the task of presenting a design to the president fell to officials at the newly created Selective Service System: Director Clarence Dykstra and Associate Director General Lewis Hershey. Their plan was to create a network of work camps run jointly by the Selective Service and the peace church community. Draft objectors who wished to avoid jail could accept noncombatant roles in the military or apply to Selective Service for admission to CPS. Roosevelt reportedly felt the proposal was too easy on men who sought to evade military service, but the plan's architects pointed out that, during World War I, conscientious objectors had caused problems for the military disproportionate to their numbers; it was better to keep them busy in out-of-the-way locations.

CPS rested on an uneasy relationship between the Selective Service and the peace church leadership. Church organizations handled the day-to-day administration of the camps. One of the denominations sponsored each of the units and carried the cost of its operation; the churches financed CPS with combined expenditures exceeding $7 million. But the

Selective Service determined camp procedures and policies, and while the agency was formally a nonmilitary unit of government, Hershey, who became director in April 1941, was a retired general. When he set up a Camp Operations Division in the agency's Washington headquarters, Hershey installed a military colleague, Lewis Kosch, as its chief. Though the peace churches had hoped that they would have substantial input in decisions about running the camps, from the outset Kosch made it clear that he was in charge, and Selective Service rules would prevail: "The peace churches are only camp managers," and CPS men "are draftees just as soldiers are."

The first CPS camps opened in May 1941. Many of them were converted New Deal Civilian Conservation Corps sites, where men worked at tasks related to soil conservation, reforestation, fire prevention, and national park maintenance, with a variety of federal agencies providing technical assistance. After some months, Kosch approved a category of "detached service" units located at state mental hospitals and training schools where CPS men would serve as ward attendants. With the draft and wartime industries depleting the availability of patient aides, conscientious objectors filled in as an unpaid substitute labor force. Then, during the summer of 1942, Kosch's Camp Operations Division agreed to endorse another form of special service: participation in government-sponsored human experiments. CPS men called these the "guinea pig projects."

The church community itself initiated use of conscientious objectors as subjects in wartime medical research. An early proponent of the arrangement was Paul Comley French, a Quaker leader and director of the National Service Board for Religious Objectors—a coalition of peace church organizations. In June 1942, French wrote to the PHS surgeon general and Kosch at Camp Operations saying that conscientious objectors in Britain were participating in research directed by the Ministry of Health and suggesting that American draft objectors also serve as experimental subjects. He offered to help recruit CPS men for this purpose.

French's initiative was in part a response to complaints from some conscientious objectors that the camp system offered too few options for work of genuine social value. Church leaders had religious grounds for enabling men under their watch to participate in medical research. Their theology placed great value on the testimony of pacifist Christian beliefs through work. For young men so inclined, the experiments were a vehicle for enacting a commitment to life without war.

Scientists receiving funds from the president's Office of Scientific Research and Development began enrolling CPS men as research subjects in July 1942. Six months later, conscientious objectors were serving as participants in eight different OSRD medical studies. By the fall of 1943, AEB researchers were also recruiting from CPS camps. The numbers of both government-sponsored human studies and experiments using draft objectors grew rapidly. Over the course of the war, more than five hundred CPS men—the figure may have been closer to a thousand—enrolled in four-dozen wide-ranging research projects.

Bayne-Jones approached Kosch in June 1943 about access to CPS men for AEB hepatitis infection experiments. Stokes had already laid the groundwork for cooperation from peace church organizations through his connections within the American Friends Service Committee (AFSC). Stokes had long been active in the Quaker organization, and was now medical advisor to its CPS division. The Quaker branch of CPS, through the AFSC, sponsored four of five camps where hepatitis transmission studies took place during the war.

Even with the AFSC's cooperation, arranging for access to men in CPS camps was laborious. Each request for subjects required approvals from both Camp Operations and the National Service Board. Initially Stokes and Paul drew subjects for hepatitis experiments from CPS units at mental hospitals where men were working on the wards. Because these camps ran under the auspices of state agencies, researchers needed the assent of state officials before proceeding. But some of these officials had serious reservations.

When Paul was planning experiments with conscientious objectors stationed at state psychiatric hospitals in Middletown and Norwich, towns not far from New Haven, approvals from Hartford were not forthcoming. Connecticut officials wanted first to know who would cover the expense of treating conscientious objectors sickened with hepatitis. But their primary concern was the loss of workers. One official insisted that the state's hospitals were "in such a depleted condition . . . that any loss of the services of its personnel cannot be justified." He also feared that assigning conscientious objectors to a research project would jeopardize the state's future allocations of CPS men for institutional work.

Stokes ran into similar problems when seeking access to draft objectors working at Philadelphia State Hospital at Byberry. S. M. R. O'Hara, Pennsylvania's secretary of welfare, demanded that a number of matters be clarified before she gave researchers the go-ahead. She sought assurances that the state would not be paying for the care of sick research subjects and that its allotment of CPS men would increase to make up for the loss of workers due to the men's participation in medical studies. Most prophetically, O'Hara wanted an accounting of who would be responsible for any disabilities or continuing illnesses that might result from the research.

Bayne-Jones engaged in what he described as "long, drawn-out negotiation[s]" with state officials. The outcome was that the AEB agreed to carry the costs of medical care for conscientious objectors during the experiments, with funds coming from investigators' research accounts, and Camp Operations and the National Service Board would endeavor to supply the states with supplementary CPS workers as quickly as possible. But regarding responsibility for research-related disabilities, Bayne-Jones was adamant that remediation for injured subjects was out of the question. On this matter, he issued a blunt statement: "I have been informed that the Government does not provide compensation for religious objectors who may be disabled in the course of work on projects or in service of the type contemplated in these experiments on jaundice." This prohibition would extend to the purchase of life or disability insurance for research subjects. The government's solution was to have the AEB provide states with protection from liability by extending waiver and release provisions to cover state agencies.

After hard-won approvals were secured, hepatitis researchers moved on to the next challenge: persuading potential subjects to sign on. Investigators recruited conscientious objectors by distributing project announcements to CPS units. On several occasions, Stokes had his junior researcher John Neefe visit CPS camps to solicit applications. Initial efforts to generate applicants yielded meager results. The expectation that men undergoing experimental interventions would also serve as mental hospital aides impeded recruitment. Compounding the problem was that, by the time hepatitis investigators began seeking subjects, multiple OSRD and AEB projects were competing for CPS men willing to enroll as research participants.

Persistent recruitment efforts did eventually yield recruits. Stokes was able to start hepatitis experiments with CPS men at Byberry Hospital in September 1943. Paul began studies with draft objectors working at psychiatric facilities in Middletown and Norwich in the spring and

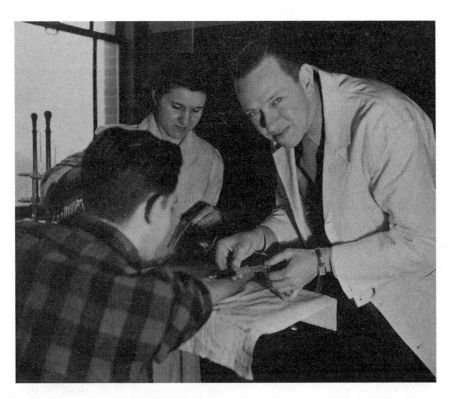

John Neefe, an army corps physician on Stokes's project, performs an experimental procedure in 1943 on a conscientious objector from the CPS camp at Byberry Hospital. (Courtesy of Swarthmore College Peace Collection.)

summer of 1944. But as the experiments proceeded, conflict flared within CPS over the dangers of hepatitis and the lack of provisions for compensating research injuries.

In November 1944, a vocal minority of CPS men raised objections to the presentation of risks in a circular that the AFSC was distributing for Stokes's upcoming hepatitis studies. The text stated that hepatitis was seldom fatal: the mortality rate was low, around one in a thousand. The flyer was silent on the matter of possible long-term disabilities. Two CPS men at the soil conservation camp at Big Flats, New York, considered this account of hepatitis risks inadequate. One, Sandy Clarke, believed that the announcement minimized the dangers of hepatitis. He had learned from doctors in New York City that inoculations with hepatitis, particularly in repeated doses, could cause permanent liver damage. He wanted to know whether men transferred to project sites would have the opportunity to withdraw from the study when the full facts were given to them. The camp director at Big Flats warned the AFSC central office that Clarke felt so strongly about the matter that "if he is not given some assurance that the men are getting all the facts … about the possible complications, and the chance to withdraw, he will … take it upon himself" to warn them of the risks.

Another draft objector at Big Flats, Al Kane, complained that the AFSC was not doing enough to protect CPS men and their families from the impact of possible disability. He felt hepatitis research subjects should be covered by insurance that would provide compensation in the event of death or debilitating injury. As Kane put it, "The Service Committee ought to have more regard for human life."

By this time, the AFSC had already repeatedly asked Selective Service about purchasing disability or life insurance for CPS men enrolled in hepatitis experiments, and had even found a company willing to issue policies at regular rates. But Camp Operations had flatly denied these requests. The complaints from the Big Flat men now triggered disquiet at the AFSC central office about its handling of medical research hazards. In an internal memo, the personnel director of the AFSC's CPS division reviewed measures for protecting research subjects from death or permanent impairment. These provisions included obtaining medical advice on the suitability and importance of the projects, ensuring high-quality medical care, and allowing adequate time for convalescence. In every case the AFSC tried to give the men as much information in advance as possible, inviting them to talk directly with the doctors where feasible. Most important, all participation in research projects was voluntary.

The AFSC referred the complaints of the Big Flats men to Alex Burgess, a young physician serving as medical director of its CPS division. Burgess was in frequent contact with Stokes, who was Burgess's senior in both age and position in the medical hierarchy; Stokes's assessment of hepatitis risks was sure to prevail. Burgess responded to the Big Flats protesters by saying that, in his view, the chance of long-term disability from the hepatitis experiments was low, and the judgment of researchers in charge of the experiments "outweighs that of any number of anonymous New York physicians who do not know the conditions of the experiment." AFSC leaders echoed Burgess in their rejoinder to the Big Flats men: "It is our judgment that the possibility of permanent or even protracted or severe impairment of liver function following participation in the jaundice experiment is very slight. This has been well stated by those who are in charge."

After Burgess's death, his brother, Samuel, also a physician, would say of Alex's involvement in the project: "If he knew then what he knew later, he would never have approved that hepatitis experiment. A number of people who were in the hepatitis experiment never were well again."

The intertwined issues of hepatitis injuries and compensation came to a head when Francis faced the cruel reality of a research death. Between February and May 1945, Francis's team enrolled thirty-one inmates at the Michigan State Prison at Jackson in hepatitis infection studies. In a round of experiments begun in April, the researchers inoculated eight inmates with specimens Bayne-Jones had provided from a soldier in Italy. Six weeks later, four of the subjects developed jaundice. One of the men became acutely ill and, on May 29, he died from fulminant hepatitis. The deceased was Herman Lee Ford, a twenty-four-year-old African American man from Detroit who was serving a sentence of three to five years for receipt of stolen property. Ford's death was not the first to occur in World War II medical research. In September 1942, a twenty-seven-year-old white inmate at Norfolk Prison in Massachusetts succumbed to serum sickness while participating in the OSRD study testing bovine albumin as a substitute for the human blood product. The fatality at Michigan State Prison was apparently the first in an AEB-sponsored experiment.

The prison warden signed Ford's death certificate, a document that listed Helen H. as the deceased man's common-law wife. The warden asked researchers at the prison whether they would be arranging a financial contribution to Ford's family. The warden—soon to be accused of collaborating with inmates—may have been in league with a crime syndicate, but he believed that when powerful actors cause serious harm, they owe the injured restitution.

Several weeks later, Francis received a letter from Helen H., a twenty-three-year-old African American woman. She wrote: "I understand my husband took tests for the Government.... I would like to know under what conditions ... he submitted." She continued, the prison warden "told me to write you for further information before I can take other steps." She asked for a copy of the agreement she was told Ford had signed, adding, "I do not believe my husband would foolishly place his life in jeopardy without making some provision for his family."

The letter unnerved Francis; he sent it and related documents to Bayne-Jones, who forwarded the material to War Department lawyers. Through Bayne-Jones, legal officers instructed Francis on how to respond. They noted that Helen H. might "try to make a claim against the Government" and advised that all communication with her should be coordinated with the army's Legal Division and the Claims Division of the Judge Advocate General. They provided Francis with carefully worded text to send to Helen H. The statement noted that she had a different surname than Ford and that he had told researchers he was unmarried. It instructed Helen H. to forward a copy of her marriage certificate—a document they knew she did not have.

Ford had in fact signed a waiver and release form; it stated that he voluntarily consented to be infected with hepatitis, and that he, his representatives, and heirs exempted the government from liability for "any ill effects" resulting from the experiment, including "permanent disability or death." Waiver statements of this type might not have held up if challenged in a court of law, but they appear to have been effective in discouraging injured parties—most of them with limited resources—from pursuing claims against the War Department.

The government's response to Helen H. did not even mention Ford's waiver form. What it did convey was that she had no legal standing. The last of available correspondence on the matter is Francis's letter to Helen H. relaying text from the Legal Division. With that, the paper trail goes cold. Helen H. apparently gave up her efforts to gain compensation from the War Department.

Francis's communications with the OTSG about hepatitis experiments at Jackson Prison continued through the fall, now focusing on press coverage of the studies. To Bayne-Jones's displeasure, both the *Detroit Free Press* and the *Ann Arbor News* had reported Ford's death, identifying him by name. Neither paper revealed that investigators at the prison were injecting subjects with an unmodified virus; their articles stated instead that Ford had received "a new serum for jaundice," suggesting that the study was therapeutic in intent. In the months following the fatality, however, local reporters and prison staff pressed Francis for more information about his hepatitis experiments. The prison's head physician warned that, without an officially sanctioned account, "wildcat type of publicity" might reoccur. On Bayne-Jones's instructions, Francis delayed his response; then finally, in October 1945, Bayne-Jones allowed Francis to release a preapproved statement to the press. It highlighted the subjects' contribution to understanding a disease afflicting soldiers and made no mention of Ford's death.

Stokes's use of mental patients as human subjects was yet another grim feature of America's program of hepatitis experiments. In the early spring of 1944, when he needed more recruits but the enrollment of CPS men had slowed, Stokes initiated arrangements for access to inpatients at New Jersey State Hospital in Trenton—also called Trenton State Hospital. During the war years, his research team enrolled seventy-five of the facility's patients in virus transmission studies; a good portion of these were persons classified as criminally insane.

Stokes wrote Bayne-Jones in March 1944 saying that he had met with New Jersey officials, including the commissioner of institutions and agencies and members of the hospital's board of directors and medical staff; Stokes reported, "They showed great interest in the work and agreed to assist." They would provide the Philadelphia research team with laboratory facilities and sixty patient-subjects, with a larger number to follow if things progressed satisfactorily. Bayne-Jones responded approvingly: "I hope these plans will work out as they have every promise of doing." The OTSG was fully aware of Stokes's experiments with psychiatric patients. The army surgeon general himself later wrote the Trenton State director to thank him for his continuing cooperation with the research.

In his March 1944 letter, Stokes had made a point of telling Bayne-Jones that hospital physicians had suggested "that they use the [hepatitis-causing] agents as a means of treatment" for the facility's patients. The claim that inducing hepatitis might be therapy for psychiatric conditions sounds entirely disingenuous. But sources on the history of treatments for severe mental disorders provide an eye-opening picture of appalling practices that were common before the introduction of psychotropic drugs in the early 1950s. During the preceding three and a half decades, hospital psychiatrists had experimented with a variety of radical methods for suppressing symptoms of psychoses.

One type of treatment was based on the theory of focal infections, which held that bacterial toxins from diseased bodily tissues triggered psychotic symptoms. Some physicians who subscribed to this notion conducted surgeries—removing teeth, resectioning colons, and performing hysterectomies—to eliminate the presumed source of mental illness. Other radical treatment methods included prefrontal lobotomy, fever therapy, and induction of shock by administering electrical current, a convulsive agent, or insulin. Fever therapy—generating high fevers by infecting patients with malaria—had its own distinctive history. The practice of inducing malaria for treatment of syphilitic infections of the brain began in the 1920s. An Austrian researcher received the Nobel Prize in medicine in 1927 for introducing the method. When the procedure worked with a portion of cases of neurosyphilis, some mental institutions extended its use to patients with a range of other psychiatric disorders.

Trenton State Hospital had a long history of draconian interventions with its patients. Henry Cotton, the hospital's director between 1907 and 1930, believed in the theory of focal infection and, beginning in 1918, oversaw invasive surgeries on several thousands of the institution's residents. After his retirement, the hospital pursued an aggressive program of fever therapy on patients *without* signs of syphilis.

Given the facility's ongoing interventions, it was not a great stretch to use infection with hepatitis as an experimental treatment. Stokes had assured state officials that "the risk of serious or fatal illness" from hepatitis was "very small." The hospital director welcomed the prospect of a new therapeutic technique, suggesting to his Board of Managers that jaundice might be even more effective than their current fever-therapy procedures using malaria and the injection of foreign proteins.

The arrangement was to have Stokes's team handle matters related to disease transmission, with hospital physicians evaluating the effects of hepatitis on patients' psychiatric condition. In the hospital director's view, "it was to our advantage to enter into the study." The experiments were to begin in April 1944 and staff had already selected a group of adult males younger than thirty-five who were among 250 patients at the hospital classified as criminally insane. Available records do not identify the race of hepatitis subjects at Trenton State Hospital.

Not all members of America's biomedical elite were comfortable with conducting experiments with the mentally impaired. Some scientific advisory panels rejected enrolling persons with either mental or cognitive impairments. In 1943, the OSRD's Committee on Medical Research was planning a study of a chemical treatment for gonorrhea that would require infecting subjects with the disease. The NRC's Subcommittee on Venereal Disease devoted considerable attention to the choice of a subject pool, eventually deciding to use prisoners. Joseph E. Moore, the subcommittee's chair, excluded from consideration "the insane" and "the feeble-minded" because these were "persons incapable of providing voluntary consent." But Moore's judgment about appropriate subject pools was not a widely shared standard—indeed, at the war's end, he reversed his position on the matter and endorsed STD infection experiments with mental patients in Guatemala. During the 1940s, federal agencies sponsoring medical experiments had no standard policy governing the selection of subject populations. Decisions on the matter were highly decentralized, and the AEB imposed no set restrictions.

Stokes's research group apparently had its own reservations about enrolling psychiatric patients. In memos and unpublished reports, the investigators consistently referred to the conscientious objectors participating in hepatitis studies as *volunteers*, but they called the mental patients *"volunteers"* (with added quotation marks). Through this singular feature of their written communications, team members were acknowledging that they did not consider Trenton State patients to be willing subjects.

Anticipating that the use of mental patients in hepatitis research would be controversial, Stokes and his OTSG sponsors advised New Jersey officials to treat experiments at Trenton State as a war secret. When the State Board of Control approved the experiment in March 1944, the commissioner informed board members that the details of the program were to be kept confidential. And from the outset, the Trenton director told his own hospital board, "At the request of the War Department we are refraining from giving any information and making any comments" about the presence of army medical staff at the hospital.

Stokes himself took elaborate measures to prevent the spread of information about hepatitis infection experiments with mental patients, carefully hiding the use of this subject pool even in journal articles. Stokes and other AEB researchers routinely included notes in their publications acknowledging institutions that provided access to subjects. In one early article, Stokes's team even thanked conscientious objector subjects from Byberry Hospital by name, adding, "It is a pleasure to express our appreciation of the whole-hearted collaboration of these men." While some of the group's publications report that Trenton State Hospital cooperated with the research by providing laboratory facilities, none make any mention of mental patients' participation in hepatitis experiments.

Stokes was following Bayne-Jones's lead in concealing the use of mental patients as hepatitis infection subjects. It was part of a more general policy of controlling the presentation of information about hepatitis

infection research. Bayne-Jones's administrative purview included review
of articles prepared for medical journals. OTSG protocol required that
AEB scientists submit scientific papers to him prior to journal submission.
Failure to do so triggered a testy reminder. In November 1944, Bayne-
Jones dispatched a scolding letter to Walter P. Havens Jr., the highest-
ranking medical corps physician on Paul's team, who had neglected to
seek approval for a manuscript submitted to a scientific journal. Bayne-
Jones wrote, "You are required by Army regulation to submit every article
bearing your name to the Office of the Surgeon General for approval and
release by the Bureau of Public Relations of the War Department." Havens and Paul quickly sent Bayne-Jones separate letters of apology. In
practice, the Bureau of Public Relations was Bayne-Jones himself.

On another occasion, Bayne-Jones insisted that Neefe, one of the
army corps physicians assigned to Stokes's project, make alterations to a
journal submission about chlorination of water for hepatitis prevention.
Bayne-Jones instructed Neefe to change the paper's title and remove ref-
erence to the army in relation to the chlorination method, "as this appeared to invite unwarranted criticism" of the War Department. In his
efforts to influence presentations of AEB research in scientific journals,
Bayne-Jones was following an already established pattern. During the interwar years, the editor of a major medical publication had advised authors to avoid language that might prompt objections in the event details
of human experiments were to become public.

Bayne-Jones's foremost concern was disclosures to newspapers and
popular magazines, and his initial stance was to reject all press coverage.
In June 1943, when Stokes began negotiating with the AFSC to recruit
CPS men for hepatitis studies, the *Baltimore Sun* and *Washington Evening
Star* announced that a draft objector in Maryland had "volunteered to be
a guinea pig in a jaundice experiment" that Penn researchers were conducting with support from the AEB. One of the articles quoted Stokes as
saying that hepatitis was such a serious problem that "all blood banks are
in continuous danger of being contaminated." Bayne-Jones sent a dispatch to AEB president Francis Blake, with a copy to Stokes, complaining that Stokes's statements to the press overstated the threat of hepatitis
and had "already caused trouble and undue anxiety." The OTSG had
once before precipitated a public relations debacle involving hepatitis,
and it was determined to avert another.

Stokes responded by insisting he had never spoken to a reporter; the
quoted text was from a narrative he had sent to the AFSC for use in re-

cruiting men from CPS camps. A conscientious objector had released portions of it to newspapers "in direct defiance of camp orders," and the man was being disciplined. Meanwhile, the AFSC sent telegrams to a dozen CPS units warning, "CURRENT NEWSPAPER PUBLICITY ENDANGERS CONTINUATION OF JAUNDICE EXPERIMENT. URGE UTMOST CARE."

At the OTSG, Bayne-Jones forwarded Stokes's letter to his boss, James Simmons, with a handwritten message: "In the future Dr. Stokes will send me advance copies of any statement he plans to issue—at least he said he would." Simmons responded with a combination of bravado and—presumably—levity; he returned Stokes's letter to Bayne-Jones with his own handwritten note attached: "Col Bayne-Jones, Damn the objectional torpedoers! Full steam ahead!" Now that misbehaving parties had been reined in, Stokes's experiments would proceed.

Both the AEB and the OSRD's Committee on Medical Research sought to prevent disclosures about human experiments that the public might consider ethically suspect. While Stokes was effective at concealing hepatitis studies with mental patients, Bayne-Jones and his investigators were never entirely successful at suppressing news about studies with prisoners or conscientious objectors; nor were OSRD scientists. Managers of the facilities providing access to these subjects could not always be restrained, and some reporters were willing to circumvent War Department restrictions. Newspapers began publishing stories about some OSRD experiments with prisoners and draft resisters soon after the studies were under way. This coverage included accounts of the death in 1942 of the Norfolk Prison inmate who participated in a bovine-albumin experiment and a 1943 article in *Cosmopolitan* magazine describing OSRD-sponsored studies exposing conscientious objectors to seawater ingestion, hypothermia, and pesticides for control of lice. By February 1944, multiple press reports were circulating about prisoners participating in malaria infection experiments. In another OSRD project that attracted considerable media attention, conscientious objectors were enrolled in a study conducted at the University of Minnesota to assess the physiological impact of semi-starvation. *Life* magazine showcased the experiment in a piece appearing in 1945.

Bayne-Jones had hoped to forestall newspaper reports about hepatitis infection studies until the investigators' journal publications were in hand, when questions about the risks of transmitting the viruses could be countered by pointing to knowledge gained from the research. But the public was intensely interested in the wartime activities of draft objectors and prisoners. The *Hartford Courant* carried numerous stories about the work of conscientious objectors in state institutions and, in May 1944, just as Paul was arranging for hepatitis studies with CPS men, the *Courant* reported that draft objectors at Middletown Hospital would be study subjects. The paper's source was apparently the hospital superintendent. Efforts to suppress coverage were no longer working.

In the winter of 1944–45, Bayne-Jones changed his approach to media coverage and implemented a strategy for shaping accounts published in newspapers and magazines. It helped that scientific papers from the hepatitis program had begun to appear. Bayne-Jones now issued press releases about the experiments and also allowed researchers to disclose information so long as reporters and their editors agreed to submit articles to his Public Relations Bureau for approval before publication. He then sought to mold the content and tone of submitted pieces. He detested the term *guinea pig*. He wanted reporters to use dignified language and emphasize the scientific contributions achieved by the research. On a number of occasions, he wrote the science editors of major newspapers correcting inaccurate statements about the experiments. His letters often generated deferential responses. The mainstream press was willing to frame the experiments as efforts to advance national defense. With media cooperation, Bayne-Jones implemented narrative logistics aimed at affecting social perceptions and public sentiments about disease-inducing experiments.

Reverential depictions of human experiments were not new to the 1940s. Stories about heroes and martyrs of medical science had long been embedded in both professional lore and popular culture. In earlier decades, the characters spotlighted were typically researchers, some of them casualties of self-experimentation. But wartime narratives gave study participants top billing; now it was media descriptions of subjects' altruism that captured public attention.

In February 1945, the *Philadelphia Evening Bulletin* ran an article approved by Bayne-Jones titled "Fighting the War on Disease"; the subheadline added, "50 Conscientious Objectors Voluntarily Submit to Jaundice in Army Experiments Here to Combat Widespread Malady." The author, Don Fairbairn, the paper's feature editor, noted that hepatitis was a serious problem for the military, and that as a result of human experiments, scientists had learned a great deal about the disease and how it spread. The story focused on the men enrolled in research at Penn, depicting them as bravely volunteering for humanitarian service that in-

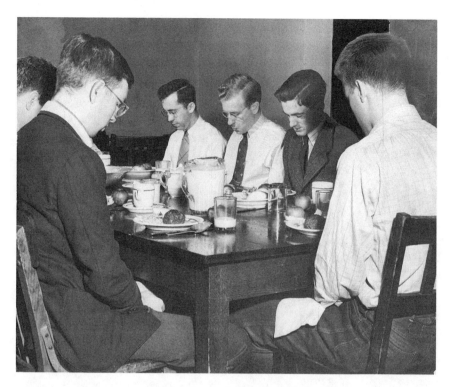

CPS men saying grace. This image accompanied a Philadelphia newspaper story praising the altruism of conscientious objectors who were subjects in Stokes's hepatitis studies. (George D. McDowell Philadelphia Evening Bulletin Collection. Courtesy Special Collections Research Center, Temple University Libraries, Philadelphia, PA.)

volved substantial risk. Fairbairn quoted one research participant as saying, "I feel that war is wrong. I could not kill a man or help others to take a human life. . . . But I would do anything possible to preserve life, to help combat disease, for instance. That is how we all feel here." The article included photographs showing men saying grace at a meal before their experimental inoculations began and a man sickened and bedridden in the course of the research.

Through such stories and imagery, the U.S. public came to accept both risk-laden human experiments and the use of draft objectors as research subjects. Given that American men were being involuntarily conscripted into military service, it seemed appropriate that conscientious objectors, excused from the draft, would take other risks in support of the

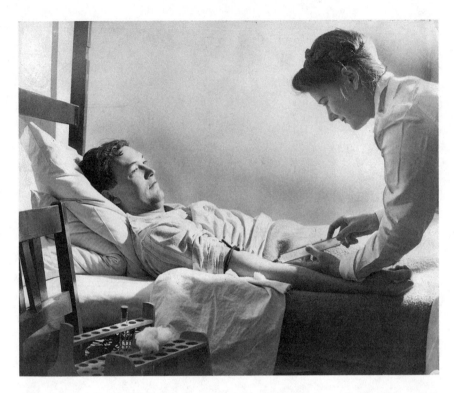

Appearing with the Philadelphia newspaper article about Stokes's hepatitis experiments, this photo shows a bedridden CPS man who, the story suggests, sacrificed his health for the good of others. (George D. McDowell Philadelphia Evening Bulletin Collection. Courtesy Special Collections Research Center, Temple University Libraries, Philadelphia, PA.)

armed forces. Accounts in the popular media portrayed both scientists and subjects as engaged in a quest to conquer disease and advance the war effort. The peace church community was pleased to have publicity that countered the prevailing construction of pacifists as no more than cowards. The scientific community was gratified by the highly visible presentation of study participants willingly submitting to hazardous research procedures. The well-orchestrated press coverage legitimized and normalized dangerous human infection studies.

CHAPTER THREE

Guinea Pig Camp

TIMOTHY HAWORTH ALIGHTED FROM a train in New Haven early in the overcast, blustery afternoon of February 5, 1945. The twenty-four-year-old conscientious objector was there to begin work as assistant director of a new Civilian Public Service unit at Yale University. The camp's sole purpose was to provide human subjects for army-sponsored hepatitis transmission experiments. George Mohlenhoff from the American Friends Service Committee office in Philadelphia accompanied Haworth to New Haven. The AFSC was the camp's peace church sponsor, and Mohlenhoff, thirty years old and himself a conscientious objector, was director of Special Service Projects for the organization's CPS division. From the train station, he and Haworth proceeded to the Yale Medical School to meet with Walter P. Havens Jr., a major in the Army Medical Corps and a full-time investigator on the Yale hepatitis project.

Later that afternoon, Haworth and Mohlenhoff made their way to the Beta Theta Pi house, a three-story brick building two blocks from Yale's Old Campus that was the designated headquarters for the CPS unit. Among Haworth's initial tasks was to get accommodations ready for the first batch of research subjects, twenty-six conscientious objectors who would be converging on the fraternity house during the following week.

On the day Haworth arrived in New Haven, Roosevelt, Churchill, and Stalin were meeting in Yalta. British and American air forces were poised

59

to bomb Dresden, and Allied ground troops were closing in on Berlin from several directions. The leaders were confident that they would soon subdue Hitler, and Germany in fact surrendered three months later. At Yalta, the Allied leaders were planning both the postwar disposition of Germany and Eastern Europe, and a swift end to hostilities in the Pacific.

Even as World War II drew to an end, army-sponsored hepatitis research was gaining momentum. The AEB's wartime hepatitis transmission experiments would continue well into 1946, more than six months after Japan's surrender in August 1945. Program scientists were on track to make full use of conscientious objectors as research subjects for as long as the system of alternative service camps remained open.

By December 1944, the Selective Service had approved the creation of two special CPS camps devoted to hepatitis transmission research: the one at Yale, headed by John Rodman Paul, and another directed by Joseph Stokes Jr. at the University of Pennsylvania. Stanhope Bayne-Jones, executive director of the Army Epidemiology Board, had lobbied for the new units for months. He and his hepatitis researchers had encountered continual problems getting approvals from state oversight agencies to enroll subjects from among CPS men stationed as attendants at mental hospitals. The new units gave Paul and Stokes greater control over recruitment and ready access to the men who agreed to be subjects.

The accompanying arrangements were truly novel: for a year at Yale, and fifteen months at Penn, the Ivy League schools were home to conscientious objectors receiving experimental inoculations of unmodified viruses. And at both campuses, the draft objectors lived and convalesced in an otherwise unused, university-owned fraternity house.

Fortunately for project scientists, a CPS assistant director handled a preponderance of administrative tasks associated with each of the camp's operations. Alternative service units ran under rules of the Selective Service—an agency that had, in the words of one commentator, "a bureaucratic passion for paper." Its Camp Operations Division required documents for every conceivable purpose: transfers in, transfers out, furloughs, discharges, and reports of assignee work activities—to name but a few. At Yale, Haworth would be keeping track of information for reporting requirements and spending a good deal of time at his typewriter, dispatching a steady stream of forms as well as memos and letters to the AFSC office in Philadelphia. He would also oversee the New Haven house and work with researchers on matters of concern to assignees.

Haworth was well suited to the job of assistant director. Sociable and garrulous, he excelled at organizational work. He also enjoyed playing the cutup. When applying for one alternative service project, he submitted, instead of a standard biography, a series of short written clips he titled "Myself in Briefs." Haworth had become a committed Quaker in his youth, after several years at a Friends boarding school. He graduated from Haverford College in the spring of 1942, and after receiving his draft notice that summer, he applied for conscientious objector status within CPS. One of his early postings was to a camp in Florida, where unit members elected him to a CPS executive committee, and from there he came to the attention of the AFSC central office.

His first administrative challenge at Yale was that the men transferring in had not been instructed to keep travel receipts, so his initial communications with the AFSC central office concerned payments for undocumented expenses. Haworth was happy to report that church coffers would be spared; he had persuaded project scientists to reimburse the newly arrived men without requiring the usual paperwork. He had even "palmed off"—his words—several of his own meals, for which he "could produce no evidence beyond a flabby midriff and a deflated purse." From the outset, his letters were cheery and buoyant.

The young recruits joining Haworth at the Yale camp in February 1945—with or without their travel receipts—had grown up in cities and towns across the country. All were white. Their draft boards were located in fourteen different states. One-third were Quakers; another third Methodists or Presbyterians; the others listed a variety of Christian denominations, with one Jewish draft objector from Brooklyn completing the roster. Whether their views arose from church doctrine or personal conscience, the men shared a commitment to both pacifism and altruistic service. Each had applied to be posted at a unit known among CPS men as one of the "guinea pig camps."

Archived documents relating to the Yale and Penn CPS units are abundant and offer insights into the assignees' concerns and motivations, their thoughts about the experiments, and their relations with project scientists. What emerges from these records is a more fully rendered picture of life for draft objector subjects than is possible to unearth for any of the other groups that participated in hepatitis infection research.

Conscientious objectors had multiple options for alternative service within CPS. After an initial assignment at a base camp, they could request transfers to other units they had learned about from peers or informational flyers. Most of the men who enrolled in the hepatitis transmission studies were responding to recruitment materials that circulated through the camp system. Paul and Stokes, who each conducted multiple rounds of hepatitis experiments, produced a succession of recruitment flyers. The Friends Committee distributed these appeals for research subjects and encouraged conscientious objectors to sign up.

While the wording of the flyers varied considerably, a typical recruitment announcement began with a statement about the urgency of the problem of hepatitis for the army, the purpose of the upcoming studies, and the opportunity that participation provided for humanitarian service. It identified the lead researcher, his institutional affiliation, and the federal agency sponsoring the study; described work that research participants would be doing when not undergoing experimental procedures; and noted any special conditions or rules that would apply to camp members.

The announcements also addressed research hazards. A circular for Stokes's first hepatitis experiments with CPS men, distributed midway through 1943, included a section titled "Chances for Survival": "There is a definite, though extremely small risk of mortality in the course of the experiment. . . . Fatal cases of the disease are very rarely seen and the vast majority of cases are extremely mild in nature, with only slight disability, frequently not requiring bed rest." Later announcements provided a mortality rate for hepatitis and a fuller description of what subjects might experience during a bout with the illness.

The circular for the first round of experiments at the Yale camp began, "FLASH: NEW OPPORTUNITY! The Connecticut guinea pig experiment has been reorganized into an attractive four-month project." An earlier appeal, which failed to attract applicants, stated that camp members were to spend nonresearch time as attendants at a nearby psychiatric facility. In the revised edition, potential recruits were offered laboratory positions or other jobs at New Haven General Hospital. As for research hazards, the New Haven flyer reported a death rate of one per one thousand for hepatitis and continued, "The period of illness usually is three to four weeks. The doctors are particularly careful to provide a thorough convalescent period. Recurrences of the disease are uncommon."

The flyer noted conditions that might discourage men from enrolling. Camp quarantine rules would prohibit alcohol, sex, and travel outside the New Haven area, even during furloughs. CPS men considered restrictions on furlough travel a significant hardship. But researchers also provided incentives, including relatively generous allowances and a promise of educational opportunities. Camp members would receive $15 per month, a larger allowance than provided in nonresearch CPS units and, in their spare time, they could participate in individual and group study. Perhaps most important, enrollees would know they were helping develop measures to control a disease that scientists described as a worldwide menace.

In statements they made at the time of the experiments or in later oral histories, CPS hepatitis subjects gave a variety of reasons for signing up. Some had hoped to work in noncombatant roles in war zones. William Rhodes, who became assistant director at the Philadelphia camp, envisioned driving an ambulance in combat areas, as some conscientious objectors had during World War I. He said that his aim was to "serve in areas of acute human suffering, preferably in zones similar to those the armed forces participate in," and that he wanted to go beyond what was required of soldiers. But in 1943, the government prohibited CPS projects outside the United States, so Rhodes and some like-minded draft objectors chose the dangers of medical research instead.

In a similar vein, a number of men reported a desire to show they were not cowards. They hoped to challenge the widespread depiction of conscientious objectors as yellowbellies. Several went so far as to say that, while they were not willing to kill for the country, they wanted to demonstrate that they were willing to die for it. Haworth himself made such a statement in his application for conscientious objector status.

For others, a desire for new experiences or the influence of peers was paramount. Paul Zimmerman grew up on a farm in the Midwest and was studying agriculture at the University of Illinois when his draft notice arrived. He was accepted into CPS and spent a year and a half at a camp in North Dakota doing land-reclamation work before requesting a posting at the Penn hepatitis unit in Philadelphia. He explained his decision to transfer: "One of my friends who was more sophisticated and educated thought I was dying spiritually and intellectually. He thought I should go someplace where there was more stimulation. . . . I had never lived in a city and I thought it was worthwhile work. I wasn't much afraid of the jaundice. I had researched it a bit. I just went there and it was very interesting."

Virtually all of the men serving as hepatitis subjects spoke of a desire to engage in meaningful and consequential humanitarian service. They believed their participation in the research mattered; they were confident that the experiments would generate knowledge valuable for preventing the disease among soldiers and civilians. For Rhodes, being a subject was a way to help alleviate suffering in postwar Europe. In a June 1945 letter to the Friends Committee main office, he lamented that his unit had vacancies that remained unfilled, urging that more be done to attract additional research subjects. "Thousands of cases of jaundice will occur in Northern Italy, Southern France, and Germany. . . . The number of cases prevented in war-ravaged countries is in direct ratio to the speed we complete our work here." Rhodes both believed in his narrative and wanted CPS to take more initiative in promoting enrollment in the studies so that further spread of the disease would be averted.

His expectations were unrealistic. Scientists could not translate experimental findings into preventive measures so quickly. But researchers did not discourage these ideas, which served to motivate men who wanted to do good. Fostering an oversized notion of medical progress was perhaps the greatest inducement researchers could offer young men of conscience.

The draft objectors assembled at Yale quickly formed a community. At initial camp meetings, they elected a personnel secretary to help coordinate work assignments and an education secretary to arrange outside speakers and facilitate group and individual study. Quaker-run alternative service camps attracted educationally accomplished men, and members of the New Haven unit exemplified this pattern. Of the twenty-seven in the first Yale contingent, fourteen held bachelor's degrees; of these, five had postgraduate degrees or experience—three men had master's degrees in history, one was a law student, and one a PhD candidate in mathematics. Among the other men, six had completed some college before draft notices triggered their entrance into CPS. Camp recruitment materials had promised educational opportunities, and more than half of the new arrivals wanted to audit classes at Yale even if course credit was not in the offing.

Bayne-Jones had warned researchers that if hepatitis spread to the general population from an experimental case it would create a public relations debacle for the army, and Paul did not want potentially infective hepatitis subjects mingling with Yale students. But he persuaded the Yale provost to allow CPS men to arrange tutorials with university professors willing to direct individual studies.

Haworth served as liaison with project scientists, presenting the assignees' requests for study opportunities, and arranged for additions to the camp's facilities: a pool table, a Ping-Pong table, and a piano for the house. The incoming recruits delighted him; in one dispatch he wrote,

"There is a truly terrific bunch of men here, in my opinion, and I have the highest hopes for a successful and rich experience."

By mid-February, Haworth was sending frequent communications to the AFSC office in Philadelphia. Along with the office memos were long letters describing events at the camp and detailing the men's interactions with Yale scientists. Mohlenhoff responded appreciatively to Haworth's news-filled and entertaining correspondence: "Your most recent letter is going the rounds of the office at the moment . . . and it is nice to hear the chuckles rising from room to room as the letter progresses."

Haworth provided a running account of early days at the New Haven unit. The men's induction as research subjects began within days of their arrival, and he described their initial encounters with Yale scientists as auspicious: "Both Major Havens and Dr. Paul have met with the men and seem favorably impressed, and vice versa. Dr. Paul spoke Friday evening giving the general background of the experiments to be done and the broad lines of the circumstances under which we will live and work. Today, Major Havens spent considerably longer and went into the details of the disease and discoveries concerning it, and answered questions until the guys couldn't think of any more. I mean he *answered* questions."

The men underwent initial physical exams and baseline laboratory tests the following week. But before the hepatitis inoculations began, the camp held a housewarming party, inviting women from the Yale School of Nursing. On the subject of female guests, Haworth quipped, "Ah me, the college life!"

The evening before the research team was scheduled to begin infecting men with hepatitis, the New Haven camp held a second event at the fraternity house. Haworth called it "a Pre-Inoculation Dance" and described the setting vividly: "The large room was cleverly decorated by our two artists . . . with a series of gaudy cartoon murals on the general subject of pigs, test-tubes, Dracula-like Doctors sucking blood from squirming patients, inoculations with pneumatic drills, while absolutely the most luscious blood hussy dressed in a nurse's uniform [also an artist's depiction] was coyly looking on. . . . Both Major Havens and Dr. Paul came to this party, and seemed to enjoy themselves a good deal."

The jocularity of this and other parts of Haworth's account may be jarring, but it is also consistent with observations of other settings in which subjects have confronted hazards and uncertain outcomes. A now-classic study of a hospital research unit describes patient-subjects responding to serious illness and possible death with comic horseplay and gallows humor.

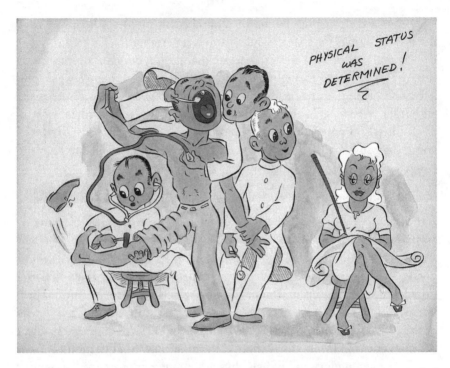

A New Haven camp cartoonist depicts the medical exams that preceded study interventions. (Drawing by David Hileman Miller. Courtesy of David H. Miller family.)

For their part, the twenty-seven young men thrown together in the Yale CPS camp produced their own distinctive antics and grim jokes.

The research team performed the first round of inoculations during the final week of February. Most of the men were part of an experiment aimed at determining the infectivity of specimens taken from a single case of hepatitis A during different phases of an infection—incubation, acute illness, and convalescence. When investigators completed the virus transmission procedures, strict quarantine went into effect. The rules required the men to eat all meals in the house, proscribed guests at meals, and prohibited the use of public gymnasiums, showers, or swimming pools. The usual incubation period for hepatitis A was three to six weeks; illnesses would not appear until well into March.

The New Haven camp settled into work and spare-time routines. Six men chose to be temporary laborers with the Connecticut Forest Ser-

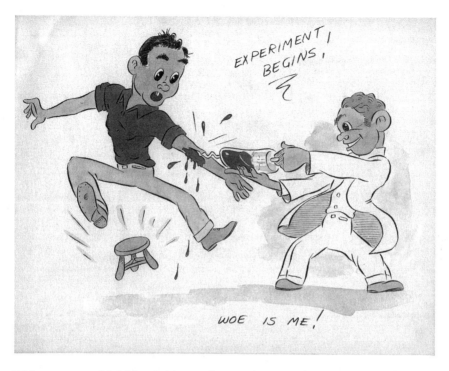

This cartoon of initial experimental procedures at the New Haven camp is in keeping with the assignees' gallows humor. (Drawing by David Hileman Miller. Courtesy of David H. Miller family.)

vice. Several others were on kitchen duty and exempt from experimental inoculations. Most camp members took positions as laboratory technicians or clerical workers at New Haven Hospital. Individual and group study began; assignees had access to Yale's library facilities, and seven of them set up individual tutorials with university professors on subjects ranging from elementary economics and Bible studies to personality development and eighteenth-century English history. Six camp members arranged for summer study on topics that included accounting, the history of biology, and Oriental history. The unit's educational secretary brought in outside speakers—the Yale chaplain, divinity professors, a spokesperson from the New Haven YMCA—and organized a lecture series on topics that included China studies. He referred to the camp's educational program as "Jaundice College."

In March, the camp produced the *Guinea Gazette*, a twelve-page mimeographed newsletter containing short articles about the camp

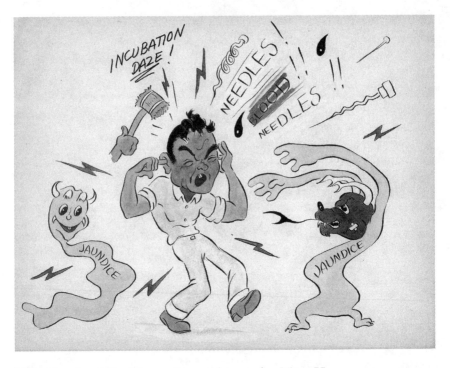

What lay beneath the apparent calm at the New Haven camp as men awaited the outcome of their inoculations with hepatitis viruses. (Drawing by David Hileman Miller. Courtesy of David H. Miller family.)

members' experiences. One piece discussed the ongoing experiment. Another chronicled camp events and outside speakers. Three others described the hospital units where CPS men worked: the clinical microscopy laboratory, the hospital X-ray department, and a "monkey room" housing animals for polio research. The *Gazette* reproduced imagery created by the unit's cartoonists that had appeared earlier on the walls of the fraternity house's great room: a squirming patient chased by a humongous needle, a desolate-looking man enclosed in a giant test tube. The grimness of the imagery was in sharp contrast to the men's good-natured bantering. A cartoon on the *Gazette*'s cover pointed to the disquiet just beneath the surface of the camp members' affability. The drawing showed a young man fleeing from an amorphous ghost that clutched at his coattails; the specter's name was Jaundice.

When the *Gazette* appeared, the project's laboratory regime was in full effect. Researchers collected blood and other specimens from

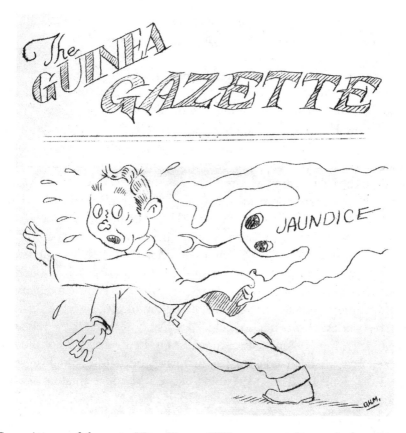

Cover image of the 1945 New Haven CPS camp newsletter, *Guinea Gazette*, depicting the specter of jaundice. (Drawing by David Hileman Miller. Courtesy of Swarthmore College Peace Collection.)

inoculated men several times a week. If a camp member failed to appear at the appointed time, Haworth delivered a reprimand, which sometimes came in the form of a comedic diatribe: "*YOU DID NOT SHOW UP FOR YOUR BLOOD COUNT THIS MORNING AT 9:30!!!!* What do you want, a special invitation? Well, you won't get one. Listen bub . . . get it into your mind and engrave it in your heart in words of fire. . . . 'Every Monday, Wednesday and Friday morning I must toddle up to Major Havens' lab and have my finger stuck. I must be on time. I must not forget. . . . I am a hero, and doing this for humanity and for Science and for Yale. . . . IWILLBETHERE. You can count on me. I am dependable!'"

By mid-April, results from the first round of interventions were in. Five of the infected men had contracted hepatitis; the illnesses were relatively mild. Most of the specimens used as inoculants had failed to produce clinical or laboratory evidence of infection.

In the spring, Yale researchers began preparations for a second round of experiments to start in July. Nine men were to leave the unit, and Paul requested replacements, plus a number of additional men. Haworth mobilized New Haven camp members to help with recruitment. As he apprised Mohlenhoff: "We now have a rather informal letter writing campaign underway. Men at present in this unit are writing the various friends in their base camp whom they think might be interested."

It was Haworth who drafted a new project circular that the Friends Committee distributed to CPS camps. His flyer provided considerably more information than previous versions; it included sections on the experiments, work assignments, living conditions, educational opportunities, recreation, and provisions for spiritual life. In a page-long section titled "Quotes from Veteran Pigs," two men who had contracted hepatitis described their illnesses, the medical care they received, and the pace of their recoveries. Haworth also included a testimonial about the researchers and their interactions with assignees. "Dr. Paul's direction of the unit has at all times been considerate and just," he wrote, and fostered a "spirit of cooperation" that prevailed between the investigators and the CPS men.

The AFSC completed transfers in and out of camp during the middle of July. The new census was thirty-two, with most of the men from the first round remaining in the unit. Except for men on administrative or household duty, all unit members held work assignments in Yale laboratories or hospital departments. The researchers proceeded with a new set of inoculations, this time using specimens from men at camp who had recently contracted hepatitis. The goal was, again, to determine the infectivity of specimens taken during different stages of an illness.

Haworth reported that camp morale was high, attributing this to a close relationship between the researchers and their subjects: "A better job was done in explaining to the men exactly what was being done, and the Major is now closer to the men than ever before. During the last experiment no one knew exactly the agent with which he had been inoculated, whereas this time each man knows exactly what has been done to him and the general purpose behind it. We seem to be more taken in to the confidence of the Doctors and more truly sharing in the experiment. There were five men working in the offices and labs on our experiment, doing all of the typing of reports, clinical data etc. which meant that we know everything that was going on."

The second round of procedures generated more serious cases of hepatitis and sent a number of the men to New Haven Hospital. Haworth made hospital visits and contacted the parents of one sickened subject to inform them of the severity of their son's condition. One feature of Haworth's account of these illnesses is especially striking. When the second group began contracting hepatitis, Haworth wrote: "The Chosen are dropping off like flies. . . . It appears that more men will actually become ill this time, which seems to add to the morale of the unit." In the ethos of the New Haven camp, an active case of hepatitis was a successful experimental outcome, and a personal badge of honor for the man afflicted.

The Philadelphia camp was larger, less cohesive, and more chaotic than the New Haven unit. Stokes opened his dedicated hepatitis unit several months earlier than Paul and handled nearly twice the number of subjects. The Philadelphia headquarters at the Delta Kappa Epsilon house had insufficient space to house all the assignees, so a number of the men lived off-site. CPS leadership at the camp was also more fluid. At Yale, Haworth was assistant director throughout the unit's existence; in contrast, the Philadelphia camp had a succession of three assistant directors during its operation.

The two units had commonalities as well. Recruitment materials for Philadelphia emphasized educational opportunities at the camp. One of the Philadelphia circulars announced, "Men interested in studying social work or premedical work in their spare time are especially invited to make application for the unit." As at Yale, men in the Penn unit held jobs as technicians or clerical workers at university hospitals. A number of them performed tasks related to the hepatitis project, compiling data and preparing charts and tables for the researchers' publications. Also like men at Yale, Penn assignees gave voice to gallows humor and the notion, conveyed with irony, that a case of hepatitis was an auspicious event. Rhodes, during his stint as assistant director, wrote the AFSC office to rescind a transfer-out request for a man who, after a long delay, had become ill: "Hold everything! While this man is on the list I gave you . . . he may not be transferred out right away. He is now a decidedly successful guinea pig—he's sick—isn't it wonderful! Anyway we need a replacement—some other poor duck."

At the Philadelphia unit, conscientious objectors extended their humanitarianism toward another class of research subjects. Six months into the Penn camp's operation, a group there set in motion a remarkable episode of research ethics activism. Their concern was scientists' use of mental patients as participants in virus transmission experiments.

In the spring of 1944, Stokes's team had begun hepatitis infection procedures with criminally insane inmates at Trenton State Hospital. In January 1945, Stokes expanded the scale of hepatitis studies with the hospital's patients, and arranged for a crew of men from the Philadelphia camp to work at the Trenton facility as laboratory technicians and ward attendants for sickened mental patients. The assignments precipitated debate and resistance, with draft objectors questioning the morality of enrolling mental patients in disease-inducing studies.

Conscientious objectors more generally were at the forefront of efforts to promote the welfare of the mentally impaired. By the war's end, more than a third of the alternative service units were located at mental hospitals or training schools, where the CPS men held positions as ward attendants. Conditions at the facilities shocked and appalled the draft objectors. Staffing levels, never generous, had plummeted to a new low during the war. Warren Sawyer, stationed at a CPS unit at Philadelphia State Hospital in the city's Byberry neighborhood, wrote letters home to his aunt describing the institution and his work there. A Building, the "incontinent ward," was a large open room with no chairs and a filthy concrete floor where several hundred men, many of them naked, wandered aimlessly or huddled against the bare walls. The accompanying odor was overwhelming.

Nearby B Building was the "violent ward," and there the staff routinely strapped and shackled patients to bed frames. "A few attendants have had their jaws smashed," Sawyer wrote, "but they're usually the ones who approached troublesome patients with broom handles." At Byberry, he and his comrades put into practice their commitment to nonviolence over brute force: "If you can convey to patients that you're not afraid of them and respect them as individuals—even though you're shaking in your boots—they return your respect."

As the war drew to a close, the Byberry attendants launched a campaign to bring public awareness to the deplorable care of the mentally ill. Their efforts, and those of conscientious objectors at other inpatient facilities, contributed to an eventual exposé in *Life* magazine, "Bedlam 1946: Most U.S. Mental Hospitals Are a Shame and a Disgrace," and to the creation of an advocacy organization, the National Mental Health Foundation.

Men from Stokes's Philadelphia camp were not working with the general patient population at Trenton State Hospital, and their complaints focused less on institutional conditions than on the use of disabled persons in medical experiments. Paul Zimmerman, who was among the draft objectors on work duty at the Trenton facility, recalled that the use of mental patients as subjects offended the men: "They were not getting permission from anybody to inculcate [sic] these people with hepatitis. . . . We thought we were volunteering for something good [by serving as subjects] and these guys [the mental patients] were just tricked into it." The conscientious objectors were deeply disturbed by the absence of genuine consent.

Dissatisfaction with the situation simmered for several months, finally coming to a head in July 1945. A Philadelphia camp announcement sheet that month carried this entry: "The constantly recurring question of the ethics involved in our carrying out work at Trenton will be taken up with Dr. Stokes within the next two weeks."

The resulting meeting was not with Stokes but rather with Sydney Gellis, the Army Medical Corps physician assigned to oversee research at the Trenton hospital. Rhodes reported that the work crew talked with Gellis, and that the question of ethics seemed to "revolve around the actual value of hepatitis as therapy."

At this time, malaria fever therapy was an accepted treatment for patients with syphilitic infections of the brain. But Trenton hospital physicians were inducing fevers as experimental treatment for an array of other psychiatric conditions. Their reason for collaborating with Stokes's virus transmission studies was to test hepatitis as an alternative to malaria as therapy for nonsyphilitic patients. The CPS men were unimpressed with this rationale; what they saw was the coercion of research subjects.

After talking with Gellis, the men went to see J. B. Spradley, the Trenton medical director and a psychiatrist who embraced the testing of experimental interventions. Spradley's reaction to the meeting is recorded in his monthly report to the hospital's Board of Managers. He became irate and demanded that Stokes replace the draft objectors with paid employees. These men, he complained, were "interesting themselves in hospital routines in which they should have no concern. Requests were made by them to be allowed to publicize their impressions of the hospital, which was denied."

Some weeks later, Rhodes reported that no men at the Philadelphia camp were willing to replace members of the outgoing Trenton work crew. The reasons given included "Experimentation on mental patients is out-of-bounds." The resistance of the Philadelphia study participants did not stop the experiments at Trenton State Hospital—hepatitis transmission studies continued at the institution for another eight years—but the CPS men's dissent was prescient. Postwar critics would argue that persons with mental disorders should not be included in medical experiments because their capacity for voluntary consent might be compromised.

By the fall of 1945, Japan had unconditionally surrendered, and U.S. armed forces were demobilizing. The hepatitis research camps were scheduled to close on March 1, 1946. Men not yet eligible for discharge from alternative service would relocate to other CPS units, some of which remained open through the end of 1946.

With the war over, the New Haven and Philadelphia projects took divergent paths. Paul had planned to conduct a third round of experiments with thirty subjects, and paperwork for the incoming men had already been submitted. But in late September 1945, Haworth cancelled the requests for new recruits. Paul had decided to scale back the project in New Haven, and for its remaining months, the Yale camp was limited to thirteen men already in residence.

In contrast, Stokes pressed on with another full round of studies. Philadelphia researchers were examining whether chlorination would inactivate water-borne hepatitis A, and Bayne-Jones was eager to have an additional chlorination trial. In late October 1945, Stokes's team member Neefe wrote to Bayne-Jones: "It appears . . . we have just sufficient time to carry out one more experiment using CPS men as volunteers."

A tragic event at the New Haven camp may have contributed to Paul's decision to curtail experiments there. Warren Dugan, a twenty-seven-year-old conscientious objector, died at New Haven Hospital in late August. He had not participated in the hepatitis experiments; rather, Yale scientists had brought him to New Haven from a CPS camp at Norwich State Hospital to work as a laboratory technician. Dugan had a master's degree in engineering, and researchers found him exceptionally capable at performing specialized laboratory procedures. He had worked in the Yale polio lab for nine months when he contracted paralytic polio and, within two days, succumbed to the disease. Exactly how he was exposed to poliovirus was unclear, but scientists classified it as a laboratory accident. Haworth reported that Paul and other physicians were with Dugan most of the night before he died, but were helpless to stop the progression of his illness.

In the morning Paul let it be known that Dugan would not recover. Haworth memorialized his deceased comrade in a letter to mutual friends. Dugan "laid down his life that others might live. . . . I know of no better example of the pacifist answer to the militarist than the story of Warren's life and work and sacrifice."

Dugan had married a year before his death, and Haworth described Paul as "truly wonderful" with the bereaved young widow. The loss of Dugan, Haworth observed, "hit Dr. Paul pretty hard." Three months earlier, one of Francis's hepatitis subjects at Jackson State Prison had died of fulminant hepatitis B. For investigators at Yale, the recent casualties and the severity of illnesses from their second round of hepatitis inoculations were an alarming reminder that inducing a serious infectious disease could have fatal results.

Haworth recounted what he understood to be the Yale scientists' reasons for changing course: "The time is no longer ripe for human experiments involving the possibility of a death. The end of the war and the increasing demobilization plans make such a risk far more serious than during the height of the war." He added, "I believe it is probable that the death of Warren Dugan has had some influence, although [nothing] has been said on this point." In the months that followed, others would question whether, with the war's conclusion, potentially life-threatening human experiments should still be considered morally acceptable.

As for the Philadelphia team, the researchers' determination to eke out all possible scientific gain extended beyond another round of hepatitis transmission procedures. During the last months of the camp's operation, physicians at Penn performed surgical liver biopsies on six men who had contracted hepatitis in earlier experiments. Initially, Stokes had sought permission for serial biopsies on hepatitis subjects, but Bayne-Jones rejected that proposal. Then, in September, Stokes requested approval of biopsies on two men to clarify the meaning of continued symptoms and abnormal test results, and to assist "in the further medical management" of the cases. The men had contracted hepatitis from experimental inoculations, recovered, and then relapsed. "We can see," Stokes wrote, "no valid objection to the use of biopsy as a diagnostic (not experimental) procedure." This time Bayne-Jones gave his approval, so long as the men signed a special waiver and release document developed

by the War Department's Legal Division. Stokes arranged for the biopsies to be conducted in October.

A month later, Stokes received approval for five additional liver
biopsies—four were performed—again with the provision that the subjects sign a special waiver agreement. The four subjects had participated
in cross-immunity experiments. Each had received four experimental inoculations, and had contracted both hepatitis A and hepatitis B. Each had
recovered and had no current symptoms. The rationale for these biopsies, conducted between December 1945 and early February 1946, was to
see whether microscopic findings suggested evidence of permanent liver
damage.

While needle biopsy was then an available technique, all six procedures on CPS men were open-abdomen surgeries performed with a scal-
pel, each extracting an inch-size wedge of liver. These were invasive
surgical interventions, at least four of them undertaken for purely experimental purposes, and entirely without benefit for the research subjects.
One of the biopsied men later told me that his surgery was conducted
with local, not general, anesthesia and that the incision was acutely pain-
ful. He said also that his recovery was prolonged by complications.

Jonathan Rhoads, head of surgery at the University of Pennsylvania,
oversaw the team of surgical residents that performed the procedures. At
Bayne-Jones's direction, Stokes had biopsy specimens sent to the Army
Institute of Pathology for analysis. According to the institute's assessment,
specimens from the two conscientious objectors with continuing symptoms
showed "subsiding inflammatory processes." Tissue from the four cross-
immunity subjects had "increased cellularity" in some areas, but Neefe later
commented that the meaning of this finding was "obscure." Researchers had
exposed six men to the hazards and pain of surgery, only to find that results
for the question of long-lasting liver injury were inconclusive.

Disturbing events at the Penn unit did not end with liver biopsies. As
the March 1, 1946, closure of the hepatitis units approached, researchers
at the Philadelphia camp faced a problem. Three of their hepatitis subjects were not fully recovered, but these men were not yet eligible for
discharge from CPS.

In the normal course of events, Selective Service would require that
the draft objectors complete their required time at another CPS unit.
But Stokes wrote to Bayne-Jones in early January saying the men were
experiencing continued symptoms of active hepatitis and that biopsy re-

sults on two of them showed residual inflammation—one of the men with persistent illness was not biopsied. Concerned that full-time duties at another CPS camp would aggravate their conditions, Stokes requested that the two be given medical discharges from CPS. He felt "the need for consideration of any man who may suffer sequelae of hepatitis. Despite the signing of waivers, there would appear to be some obligation in connection with these individuals."

Bayne-Jones was not encouraging. The Selective Service made decisions about medical discharges, and his staff had already spoken to officials there about the matter. Their response was that the medical discharge rules for army personnel also applied to CPS subjects. Bayne-Jones instructed Stokes to send medical reports on the two men in question to officials at the Camp Operations division of Selective Service, along with copies to him at the Office of the Surgeon General–Army. But he made it clear that the Epidemiology Board would not provide additional funds for medical oversight of hepatitis subjects with continuing symptoms. He added: "I will call your attention to the waivers signed by these men. It seems to me that the second paragraph would provide for your taking care of them under the medical research contract for your Commission until you feel that they are well enough to be removed from your medical care."

Selective Service denied the request for medical discharges. Stokes then worked with the AFSC medical director to develop plans for maintaining the Philadelphia camp beyond March 1, and secured private funds for expenses not covered by government agencies. Stokes's team was prepared to continue medical supervision for men needing it through June 30. Those remaining would also include conscientious objectors still convalescing from hepatitis or from liver biopsies, and four men who were assisting with analysis of project data.

However, the results of multiple liver function tests on the two subjects denied discharges were contradictory, and Bayne-Jones believed the men were malingering. In mid-March, he intervened, ordering that Philadelphia researchers immediately transfer those two unrecovered subjects to other units. In a terse message to Neefe, he wrote: "As we agreed this morning, you are to present these assignees to Colonel Kosch, Selective Service System, as now ready for return to another CPS unit."

Leaders of the peace churches that supported CPS—the Quakers, Brethren, and Mennonites—were clear-eyed in their later appraisal of the camp system's shortcomings. Church elders saw themselves as stewards of the young draft objectors, and deeply regretted their inability to obtain medical discharges for those CPS men in need of them. But the problem was larger than the failure to protect relapsing hepatitis subjects. In his post hoc assessment, one Quaker leader noted, "Directors of camps reported great trouble in securing medical discharges for men who were mentally or physically unfit for participation in camp life, and the camps did not have facilities or flexibility for taking care of such men." The source of this discontent was even broader: Selective Service exerted greater control over CPS than the church organizations ever envisioned when they embarked on their partnership with the agency. As a result, church leaders lacked leverage to successfully advocate for CPS assignees, and were often put in the position of being—as the Quaker elder put it—"instruments for carrying out Selective Service policies."

With alternative service camps disbanding, conscientious objectors returned to civilian life. Timothy Haworth gained release from CPS in March 1946, and immediately joined an AFSC medical project in China. After returning to the United States, he worked for many years as a management consultant for a firm in Philadelphia. George Mohlenhoff received his discharge in April 1946, and remained in Philadelphia, where he continued on at the main office of the AFSC. William Rhodes left CPS late in 1945. He went on to earn degrees in divinity at Yale and became a Methodist minister and a university chaplain in Denver. After Paul Zimmerman departed CPS, he earned a second undergraduate degree at Swarthmore College and returned to the Midwest, where he became an ordained minister and combined work with social activism, even participating in the Mississippi Freedom Summer. On leaving CPS, Warren Sawyer discovered that social work, his original career choice, was not his calling; after the war, he worked in sales, and eventually became a real estate agent in communities outside Philadelphia.

The Army Medical Corps physicians on the Yale and Penn projects also transitioned to civilian jobs. Havens secured a faculty position at Jefferson Medical School in Philadelphia; he remained active in hepatitis research but turned away from virus transmission procedures. Neefe stayed at the University of Pennsylvania and secured independent funding for further hepatitis infection studies. At a Liver Injury Conference in September 1946, he reported that three unrecovered subjects in the Philadelphia CPS camp had both symptoms and abnormal results from two lab tests that persisted for ten to twelve months. He classified the men as having chronic hepatitis. This was a diagnosis that a group of army physicians had introduced in the fall of 1945 for patients who failed to recover from an active infection after four months. Neefe estimated that 15 percent of hepatitis cases became chronic, and he made this condition a focus of his postwar research.

When recruiting subjects, investigators had depicted hepatitis as an often mild, self-limiting condition with a low death rate. By the war's end, they were realizing that some hepatitis patients were debilitated for extended periods of time, often without jaundice, or had symptoms return after an apparent recovery. Scientists were now confronted with evidence that the still poorly understood pathogens could be highly durable and generate long-lasting disabilities. It was an open question whether these findings would have any effect on the willingness of investigators and their government sponsors to continue human infection studies with the viruses. The answer would rest on developments unfolding far beyond the community of American hepatitis researchers.

1946–1954

The cold war is in fact a real war in which the survival of the free world is at stake.

—U.S. NATIONAL SECURITY COUNCIL, Report 68, April 7, 1950

CHAPTER FOUR

Nuremberg Notwithstanding

T HE CLOSE OF WORLD War II was a turning point that might
have ended the U.S. program of hepatitis infection experiments. Some with knowledge of the program felt that en-
dangering the health and lives of subjects for the sake of
scientific advancement was no longer justified now that armed conflict
was over. Revelations about Nazi concentration camp experiments and
the 1947 Nuremberg Code might have further discouraged dangerous
medical studies, particularly within institutional settings; during the
1950s, European scientists turned against using members of what critics
called "captive groups" in research unrelated to their medical treatment.
But many American investigators saw the Nuremberg Code as applicable
only to Nazi war crimes—not to their own scientific work. Meanwhile,
new defense imperatives spurred the reanimation of dangerous government-sponsored experiments using a wide range of human subjects. The
Cold War had arrived.

During the Second World War, American investigators had enlisted
more than six hundred subjects in hepatitis infection studies. Between 1946
and 1954, they recruited more than triple that number, all of them residents of closed institutions. With the disbanding of Civilian Public Service
camps, postwar investigators turned to correctional facilities as a major
source of research participants. Joseph Stokes Jr. continued his experiments
with mental patients and now, just as evidence of Nazi medical experiments
was emerging, added a new category of subjects: developmentally disabled

children. Expansion of the hepatitis program was emblematic of a broader pattern of emboldened nontherapeutic medical experimentation in the United States during these years. Researchers and their federal patrons were even more confident than they had been during the war that gains for science and national security justified grave risks to human subjects.

Germany surrendered in May 1945; Japan capitulated in August and signed a treaty early in September. Well before the hostilities were officially over, the Allies were planning war crimes trials against Nazi officials. The proceedings took place at the Palace of Justice in Nuremberg, a city located within the American-occupied sector of recently divided Germany. Between November 1945 and October 1946, an International Military Tribunal pursued cases against surviving senior officers of the Third Reich, men who had overseen Adolf Hitler's war machine and its methodical execution of Jews and others deemed racially impure.

After the International Tribunal had completed its work, the U.S. military authority conducted twelve additional judicial proceedings. The first of these was the Nuremberg Medical Trial, ongoing between December 1946 and August 1947. The United States, with assistance from Britain, prosecuted twenty-three German researchers—twenty-two men and one woman—for crimes against humanity in the name of medical science. The charges included murder, torture, and other atrocities.

Documents seized by invading Allied forces revealed that, with the support of the Third Reich, trial defendants had implemented a well-organized program of medical experiments with concentration camp inmates. Nazi scientists had exposed prisoners to freezing temperatures, conditions of extreme altitude, seawater ingestion, poisons, mustard gas, and phosphorous burns. They had created infected wounds and performed experimental surgeries involving sterilization, muscle and nerve grafts, and bone transplantation. They had conducted human infection experiments with unmodified pathogens including typhus, malaria, and hepatitis. The subjects were nonconsenting victims and, in many instances, researchers proceeded with the expectation that the prisoners would die.

The lead defendant in the trial was Karl Brandt, a senior medical officer for the Reich and Hitler's personal doctor. A panel of three American judges officiated and was empowered to determine trial outcomes. U.S. brigadier general Telford Taylor served as chief council for the prosecution. Taylor's team included two medical advisors who helped as-

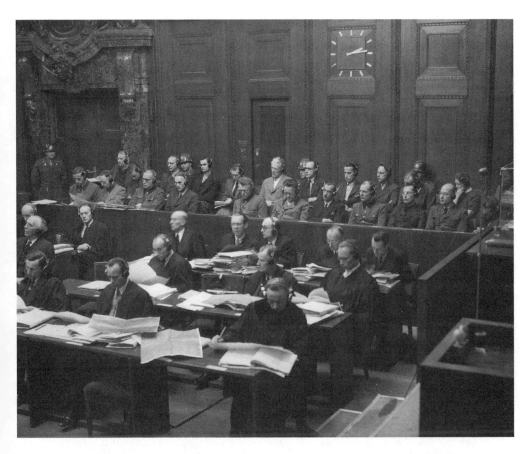

A view of the courtroom at the Nuremberg Medical Trial, 1947, showing defendants in the two rear rows and their lawyers in the foreground. (University of Washington Libraries, Special Collections, SOC9937.)

semble cases against those indicted. They were Leo Alexander, a neurologist and Austrian Jewish immigrant to the United States with an insider's knowledge of the German medical community, and Andrew C. Ivy, a physiologist well informed about scientific fields that Nazi researchers had investigated. During the war, Ivy had received funds from the Office of Scientific Research and Development to conduct studies exposing human subjects to ingestion of seawater and conditions of high altitude. He had recently assumed an administrative position at the University of Illinois Medical School and was known as a committed advocate for animal and human experimentation. U.S. authorities appointed

Ivy at the recommendation of the American Medical Association (AMA), and he reported back to the organization's leadership while the proceedings unfolded.

When trial preparations were under way, scientific leaders familiar with the evidence realized that revelations at the trial might turn the public against *all* human experiments. If this happened, restrictions on medical research more broadly might follow. The trial consultants understood that they faced a worrisome problem: how to demarcate a strong moral stance against Nazi research with concentration camp prisoners without discrediting human experimentation in general.

The strategy of defense lawyers put the consultants' concern into sharp focus. Attorneys for the Nazi doctors argued that the accused men were being condemned for practices used by medical researchers worldwide. The defense submitted abstracts of scientific papers and excerpts from popular magazines showing that American and British scientists had pursued some of the same types of research German investigators had conducted, and had done so using prisoners of the state. Documents they entered into evidence included reports from mass-distribution magazines describing U.S. government-supported starvation experiments with conscientious objectors and malaria infection studies with prison inmates. The evidentiary materials also included summaries of scientific papers from Stokes's team reporting on its hepatitis infection experiments with draft objectors.

Defense attorneys kept evidence bearing on Stokes's hepatitis experiments on hand for possible use as the trial unfolded. But it was malaria infection experiments in U.S. prisons that were in contention during the proceedings. In an arresting presentation, Brandt's lawyer, Robert Servatius, read from a *Life* magazine article describing experiments in which American researchers transmitted malaria to inmates at several correctional facilities, including Stateville Penitentiary in Illinois. The prosecution's position was that the prisoners had participated voluntarily and without coercion. Servatius challenged this claim, arguing that the inmates cooperated with the expectation of reduced prison time and thus their voluntariness was purchased. In Servatius's construction, medical studies with American prisoners were equivalent to experiments with concentration camp inmates.

Trial judges rejected the defense's claims of equivalence; they ultimately found sixteen of the defendants guilty and sentenced seven to death. At the urging of medical advisors, the judges issued along with their final rulings a ten-point statement on requirements for acceptable human experiments. Its purpose was to firmly differentiate Nazi experiments from ethically conducted human research. Both Alexander and Ivy composed draft provisions for the statement, at times in consultation with an international scientific commission, and submitted versions to prosecution lawyers and trial judges. The final statement of ethical principles issued at the trial's conclusion became known as the Nuremberg Code.

One of the code's provisions prohibits experiments "where there is an a priori reason to believe that death or disabling injury will occur." Another mandates the termination of ongoing experiments if their continuation will cause injury to a research subject. The document stipulates that experiments be conducted by scientifically competent investigators and be based on prior animal experiments. It requires that investigators avoid causing undue suffering and that risks not exceed the humanitarian importance of the research.

The code's cornerstone is the requirement of voluntary consent: subjects must participate by choice and do so without coercion. Its first provision reads in part: "The voluntary consent of the human subject is absolutely essential. This means that the person involved should have legal capacity to give consent; should be so situated as to be able to exercise free power of choice, without the intervention of any element of force, fraud, deceit, duress, overreaching, or ulterior form of constraint or coercion; and should have sufficient knowledge and comprehension of the elements of the subject matter involved as to enable him to make an understanding and enlightened decision." It would become a matter of debate whether this provision disqualified experiments with prisoners, children, and the intellectually impaired.

Ivy's efforts to distance the practices of Allied scientists from Nazi research in concentration camps went beyond his role in drafting the Nuremberg Code. While trial preparations were under way, he urged the AMA to issue principles for research conduct. The organization's leadership responded by arranging for its House of Delegates to release a brief statement on requirements for ethical human research; the first was voluntary consent. The date of adoption was December 1946, the same month the Medical Trial proceedings began. Ivy took additional measures after it was clear the trial defense would pursue an argument comparing American scientists' malaria experiments at Stateville Penitentiary with those Nazi researchers had conducted in concentration camps. During a brief visit to the United States after the proceedings had commenced, Ivy persuaded the governor of Illinois to appoint an advisory panel, the Green Committee—named for the governor, Dwight Green, and headed by Ivy himself—designed to exonerate the malaria infection studies with inmates at the state's prison.

Ivy testified at the trial as a witness for the prosecution, stating that the AMA principles for human research—freshly created at the start of the trial in response to the impending proceedings—were universally recognized standards that Nazi researchers had violated. When questioned about the timing of the document's issuance, he claimed that the ideas predated the statement's official formulation—that they were a matter of common practice. Servatius cross-examined Ivy about the participation of Stateville prisoners in malaria experiments. Invoking a draft of the yet-to-be-released Green Committee report, Ivy insisted that the inmates were motivated by humanitarianism and that they served as subjects voluntarily and without duress.

On his return to the United States, he attended to preparing the Green Committee's report. The final document, published in February 1948, praised the Stateville studies "as an example of human experiments which were ideal" in their conformity to the AMA's principles of research conduct. It conceded that some inmates might participate in experiments with the hope of gaining early release; excessive reductions in sentences, Ivy acknowledged, "can amount to undue influence." But he emphasized the rehabilitative potential of medical experiments in prisons. For an inmate to serve as a research subject, Ivy declared, was "an act of good conduct demonstrating social conscience of a high order."

Six months after the Green Committee report appeared, Ivy commented on the ethics of experimentation with persons having mental or cognitive incapacities. In a paper published in *Science* he wrote: "The ethical principles involved in the use of the mentally incompetent are the same as for mentally competent persons. The only difference involves the matter of consent. Since mental cases are likened to children in an ethical and legal sense, the consent of the guardian is required." According to Ivy, experiments with children and the developmentally disabled were morally acceptable so long as the researcher obtained the express consent of their legal guardians. With the Nuremberg Code interpreted in this manner, practices employed by American biomedical researchers were entirely compatible with that document's principles.

The Medical Trial and Nuremberg Code raised questions about experiments with members of what are now called vulnerable groups. Is an incarcerated or otherwise institutionalized person in a position to freely

choose to participate in a medical study? Is voluntary consent a meaningful concept for children or persons with mental or cognitive impairments,
and is the consent of a parent or guardian an acceptable alternative? In
the years that followed, medical experiments with prisoners, children, and
the cognitively impaired would be a source of contention among dispa-
rately situated medical professionals.

The Second World War left Europe shattered; it would be years before it recovered to the point of making substantial investments in medical research not directly related to patient care. The United States,
however, emerged from the war economically strengthened and with its
scientific capabilities fully intact. American investigators were eager to
proceed with human experiments, and the Nuremberg Code engendered
no immediate constraint on how they used human subjects. Their reactions to the Nuremberg principles were mixed. Some began addressing
ethical issues the document raised; evidence of these concerns appeared
in a 1953 issue of *Science* that included papers presented at a symposium
on the problems of human experimentation. But many others took little
notice of the code, or viewed it, in the words of one commentator, as a
"code for barbarians," unnecessary "for ordinary physician-scientists."
   European medical communities could not so easily divorce themselves from moral implications of the Medical Trial. German scientists
had been respected contributors to numerous investigatory fields. It had
been Germany, through its Ministry of the Interior, that in 1931 had issued the first written research ethics standards—provisions formulated by
the Reich Health Council before Hitler's ascendance. Many European
researchers were deeply troubled by the ethical violations and their
human consequences on display at Nuremberg. That the Nazi scientists
had disregarded a prior code of research conduct made the abuses even
more disturbing. In 1946, a number of European scientists convened
what would become the World Medical Association (WMA), largely in
response to the Medical Trial. Attendees expressed shock at the enormity
of the Nazi doctors' wrongdoing as well as their lack of remorse.
   In the early to mid-1950s, medical associations across Europe were
formulating country-specific guidelines for ethical medical research.
Two features of these various standards were consistent: one distinguished experiments providing innovative therapies from those conducted to advance science; the other imposed greater restrictions on the
latter category of research. The distinction between innovative therapies

and scientific experiments was not new. It had been embedded in medical traditions that predated written ethics codes and had also been a core feature of the German Health Council research regulations of 1931. The boundary between these categories would never be clear-cut—especially in vaccine research—but the division was nonetheless central to early research ethics codes.

Like national medical societies in Europe, the WMA also began formulating principles for research conduct during the early 1950s, with the hope that its standards would have international impact. It released a brief preliminary set of standards in 1954. Then in 1964, after years of wrangling within its periodically reconstituted ethics committee, the WMA adopted research ethics guidelines widely known as the Declaration of Helsinki. The document would later undergo repeated revisions and arguably become more influential within medical circles than the Nuremberg Code.

Both the 1954 and 1964 WMA standards retained the distinction between therapeutic and nontherapeutic research and gave physicians greater flexibility when experimentation was aimed at alleviating the patient's medical condition. Initial drafts of the 1964 declaration were markedly different than the final product, particularly for studies unrelated to subjects' medical treatment. The WMA ethics committee came up with a draft code in 1960 that included explicit prohibitions against enrolling children or institutionalized persons in experiments conducted for the acquisition of knowledge. In 1962, the *British Medical Journal* published the proposed standards with their blunt proscriptions: "Persons retained in prisons, penitentiaries or reformatories—being 'captive groups'—should not be used as subjects of experiment; nor persons incapable of giving consent because of age, mental capacity or of being in a position in which they are incapable of exercising the power of choice. Persons retained in mental hospitals or hospitals for mental defectives should not be used for human experiment."

WMA members from the United States and Canada strongly objected to this wording, and the provisions were dropped from the final statement. Consistent with the wishes of American representatives, the 1964 WMA Helsinki Declaration included no proscriptions against nontherapeutic medical experiments with children or institutionalized persons. Instead, if an individual was not legally competent to freely give informed consent, the guidelines required consent from the individual's legal guardian. These standards were consistent with those Andrew Ivy had proposed more than a decade earlier.

Researchers in the United States traveled a different path than their European colleagues. After a very brief hiatus, they helped build a greatly expanded program of human experiments that included risk-laden, nontherapeutic medical studies with institutionalized populations. Scientists were buoyed by recent achievements in controlling infectious diseases: sulfa drugs introduced in the 1930s, new vaccines, and penicillin tested during the war. The legitimacy of American biomedicine seemed unassailable. Federal agencies were eager to proceed with further experimental work and, once again, the justification for hazardous human studies was that science would advance the national defense.

The war was barely over—and proceedings in Nuremberg subsequent to the Medical Trial still ongoing—when America began mobilizing against the threat of Soviet power. The Truman administration reorganized its military and foreign policy apparatus to counter the menace. The 1947 National Security Act created the Department of Defense, supplanting the Department of War and placing branches of the military under a single defense secretary. The act also established the Central Intelligence Agency, the National Security Resources Board, and the National Security Council.

In the international arena, nations worldwide were aligning into two opposing political systems. The U.S. Marshall Plan, designed to assist Europe's rebuilding, also strengthened America's influence in the region; the creation of the North Atlantic Treaty Organization in 1949 solidified Western defense alliances. Over the same period, Stalin moved to consolidate control over Eastern Europe.

America's resolve to fight Communism hardened with news in the fall of 1949 that the Soviet Union had successfully tested an atom bomb. The National Security Council's top-secret Report 68 advocated a massive buildup of weaponry to contain Soviet expansion. President Truman approved the development of a hydrogen bomb and fortified spending for both nuclear and conventional armaments. Defense budgets resumed World War II dimensions in 1950 and rose from there. The adversaries faced off in a proxy war on the Korean peninsula fought between 1950 and 1953.

With America's plunge into the Cold War, militarized features of the nation's economy, politics, and culture became entrenched. A pervasive rhetoric of peril warned of the need for continual civil vigilance and military preparedness. Officials declared that America was facing nothing less than a struggle for the survival of its way of life.

Federal agencies again turned to science to bolster national security. The Office of Scientific Research and Development disbanded, and the newly created Atomic Energy Commission took charge of research for the nuclear weapons program. The Research and Development Board within the Defense Department managed other military-related investigations. Biomedicine was very much part of the postwar national security agenda, with multiple agencies supporting risk-laden human interventions.

Defense imperatives spawned an array of dangerous and ethically problematic human experiments. Government-sponsored research during the early Cold War years included STD transmission studies with prison inmates in Guatemala (the Public Health Service); multiple studies exposing people to ionizing radiation, among them developmentally disabled children at Fernald State School (the Atomic Energy Commission); the testing of mind-altering drugs on unsuspecting subjects (the Central Intelligence Agency); and open-air release of microbial pathogens in American cities (the Defense Department's biological weapons program). Questions raised at the Nuremberg Medical Trial about consent for malaria transmission experiments with prisoners did not deter their continuation. The Army now assumed support for malaria infection studies, previously an OSRD project.

With the creation of the Department of Defense, the OTSG reconstituted its wartime AEB as the Armed Forces Epidemiology Board. Accompanying the board's revised title were modifications in personnel and organizational apparatus. Stanhope Bayne-Jones left the post of executive director, and a succession of military medical officers filled the position. The new appointees exercised less cohesive oversight than had Bayne-Jones, and the AFEB relied more heavily on committees of the National Research Council for scientific direction.

Defense officials added a new layer of administration to address medical issues in the armed forces: an assistant secretary of defense for health with his own medical policy council. The OTSG and AFEB were repositioned within the defense hierarchy, but the changes had little impact on the collaborations of medical corps officers and the university scientists who received Defense Department funds. Even with the extensive bureaucratic reshuffling, the military-biomedical elite remained fully intact.

The reorganized AFEB proceeded with an aggressive program of human research, and studies with hepatitis were a priority. In January 1947, William S. Stone at the OTSG announced, "The Army placed liver disease among the foremost problems to be solved." Investigators had uncovered basic features of hepatitis A and B in work completed during the war. Through human infection experiments, Stokes's team at the University of Pennsylvania and John Rodman Paul's group at Yale had shown the viruses to be distinct pathogens—immunity to one did not confer immunity to the other. Their studies had clarified the strains' typical routes of infection and incubation periods and the course of illnesses the viruses generate. Stokes's early trials of gamma globulin during hepatitis outbreaks suggested that the blood product created temporary immunity. Now scientists would set their sights on disease eradication.

In the postwar years, researchers pursued three major lines of inquiry. One concerned identifying and prolonging the duration of immunity generated by gamma globulin and involved the use of challenge procedures with both experimental and control groups. In a second line of research, scientists tried to neutralize hepatitis pathogens in stores of donated blood. A third focus was a preliminary step in vaccine development; here investigators tested the infectivity of viruses grown in laboratory media—initially in chick embryos and later in human tissue cultures. With all of these efforts, investigators transmitted hepatitis viruses to susceptible human subjects.

In March 1948, the AFEB created a dedicated Commission on Liver Disease and appointed University of Minnesota laboratory scientist Cecil Watson as its head. The three senior wartime hepatitis researchers stayed on as army medical consultants. Paul remained director of a renamed AFEB commission on viral diseases, which sponsored some hepatitis transmission research. Thomas Francis Jr. continued in AFEB leadership positions, but neither he nor Paul would have hands-on involvement in further hepatitis infection studies. Stokes was now a member of Watson's Liver Disease Commission and was again undertaking a large volume of hepatitis transmission experiments.

In the early 1950s, the AFEB enlarged its hepatitis infection research program to include additional scientists. Among the new investigators were Irving Gordon at the New York State Department of Health, George Mirick and Roger Herriott at Johns Hopkins University, and Robert McCollum at Yale. The board also funded a sizable project aimed at sterilizing hepatitis in blood, which was conducted by in-house researchers at NIH.

The Liver Disease Commission supported a good deal of research on the organ's metabolic functions that did not involve inducing illness in subjects. To accommodate the hepatitis infection researchers, the commission set up a Committee on Allocation of Human Volunteers and put Stokes in charge. Operative between 1951 and 1953, the Allocation Committee held quarterly meetings in which scientists coordinated research plans and discussed findings. Stokes's Allocation Committee—more than the broader commission headed by Watson—became the center of gravity for investigators conducting virus transmission experiments.

Stokes ran by far the most extensive postwar program of hepatitis infection experiments. Of the more than fourteen hundred subjects he estimated that his teams enrolled in virus transmission studies, in excess of twelve hundred participated after 1945. The army was no longer assigning medical corps physicians to university projects and Stokes made changes in his research staff. Many of his postwar collaborators would be young physicians holding short-term teaching and research positions at University of Pennsylvania hospitals after completing medical training at Penn. His research shop included Werner and Gertrude Henle, German émigré scientists who handled laboratory work for the team's virus transmission studies. The pair spent several years cultivating hepatitis A and B in chick embryos, a medium scientists had found supported a number of viruses, including those causing influenza and measles.

With CPS men no longer available for recruitment, Stokes needed to locate new sources of human subjects. He moved hurriedly to expand hepatitis infection research with mental patients. In September 1946, he made arrangements to continue experiments with adult inpatients at Trenton State Hospital. During the war, his team had conducted hepatitis studies there with residents classified as criminally insane; now he gained access to a wider array of the facility's patients. Between 1946 and 1953, the Penn group enrolled more than two hundred additional Trenton State patients in virus transmission studies. The vast majority of these participants received inoculations with serum that researchers believed contained hepatitis B.

Shortly after the war, Stokes embarked on a program of hepatitis research in New Jersey state correctional facilities. He initiated hepatitis infection experiments in institutions for disabled children, studies that some of his colleagues found morally problematic. A decade before researchers from New York University began hepatitis experiments at Willowbrook State School, Stokes was infecting impaired minors with live hepatitis viruses—primarily hepatitis A. This work built upon a

broader pattern of biomedical research, particularly vaccine trials, in facilities for the intellectually impaired. Stokes had been testing experimental vaccines—preparations against influenza, measles, and mumps—in
institutions for children since the late 1930s.

He and other vaccine researchers had multiple reasons for choosing
children as subjects. Because youngsters were less likely than adults to
have naturally acquired immunity to infectious diseases, they had more
to gain from vaccine interventions. Also, when research participants were
nonimmune, investigators could demonstrate vaccine effectiveness using
smaller samples of subjects. Institutions for children offered scientists
other practical advantages as well: residents were there on a long-term
basis, allowing investigators to easily follow subjects for months to evaluate outcomes or conduct additional procedures.

For their part, superintendents of these facilities, themselves physicians, were positively disposed to opening their doors to researchers.
University scientists, bringing with them expertise and resources, could
assist the institution in providing medical care. Outbreaks of infectious
diseases in the institutions were common and difficult to control. Vaccine
experiments held promise for preventing future epidemics of contagious
illnesses. In some instances, institutional managers had appealed to scientists for help in handling an ongoing outbreak.

Stokes was vigilant about shaping reports of experiments with institutionalized children that might reach public audiences. During the war,
his group conducted a variety of vaccine studies at Pennhurst State
School, a facility for the intellectually impaired in southeast Pennsylvania. Their interventions at the facility included injecting child subjects
with cultivated measles viruses and then exposing them and members of
a control group to unmodified measles pathogens; they were testing
whether the cultivated microbes conferred immunity. In December 1945,
the physician superintendent of Pennhurst, James Dean, wrote Stokes
asking for a list of journal articles resulting from the group's recent work
at the facility. Stokes forwarded the requested list and, in a cover letter,
noted that he had omitted the institution's name in the scientific publications. He advised Dean that information about the study site "should be
used with the greatest of caution, since this fact might be readily misun-
derstood if broadly publicized." Stokes continued: "If you use openly the
name of the institution in mentioning the work, emphasis should be
placed upon the fact that no study was ever conducted which would not
redound in the benefit of the inmates." Dean responded that he heartily

agreed that discussion of studies in state institutions like his should emphasize that the research was done "for the benefit of the patients," who would enjoy "the advantages of protection against infectious diseases." Stokes insisted that this research helped forestall illnesses and was beneficial for both the facility and its residents.

Stokes's initial hepatitis studies in institutions for children were, in fact, efforts at disease abatement. During the war, both he and Paul had provided assistance to children's facilities during hepatitis epidemics. Stokes's team had intervened in 1944 at a summer camp in Pennsylvania's Pocono Mountains where researchers had tracked the course of an outbreak, ultimately identifying contaminated well water as its source. During the investigation, they also administered gamma globulin, leaving a control group untreated to assess its effectiveness in curtailing new illnesses. Paul undertook a similar trial during two epidemics, one at a Catholic orphanage in New Haven and another at a girls' school in Providence, Rhode Island. His team also administered gamma globulin, leaving some residents untreated, in an effort to verify that immune serum generated at least temporary immunity to hepatitis infection.

Following the war, Stokes conducted additional research at institutions in response to hepatitis epidemics. During the late 1940s and early 1950s, he collaborated on investigations of hepatitis outbreaks and the administration of gamma globulin at St. Vincent's Orphanage in Chicago, Rosewood Training School in Maryland, and Vineland State School in New Jersey.

In short, Stokes's hepatitis transmission interventions with minors took place in the context of a wide-ranging agenda of research aimed at preventing infectious diseases, including hepatitis, in institutional settings. He would defend hepatitis transmission experiments with children by arguing that, like disease prevention procedures, these also were in the youngsters' best interests. But exposing human subjects to unmodified viruses is not the same as testing an immunizing agent composed of weakened microbes. Stokes's justification served to further blur an already permeable boundary between nontherapeutic and therapeutic research.

Stokes began hepatitis infection experiments with children in the spring and summer of 1947. The initial subjects were eighteen residents of Pennhurst School; there, members of his team injected children and youths with egg-passage virus from the Henles' laboratory. The purpose was to test whether the cultivated pathogens were viable; as it turned out, the materials did indeed generate symptoms of hepatitis. Later, in the spring of 1949, Stokes's researchers transmitted unmodified virus to fifty children at New Lisbon Colony in New Jersey, another institution for the developmentally disabled. Procedures there were challenge inoculations; the subjects had received gamma globulin nine months earlier, and the goal now was to determine whether the previously injected serum was still protective.

During the early 1950s, Stokes's team was administering an experimental skin test to hundreds of children in facilities where hepatitis outbreaks had occurred. The aim was to develop an easily obtainable indicator of the presence of antibodies against hepatitis. The skin test material was virus grown in chick embryos that was inactivated—or not—with ultraviolet irradiation. As these studies proceeded, Stokes acknowledged that the test material might contain live virus and proposed that it be conceived of as an experimental immunizing agent. Use of the skin test continued for months in the absence of a clear understanding of whether the pathogens were dead or alive; the test's sustained use amounted to seat-of-the-pants experimentation.

When introducing the prospect of procedures with live hepatitis viruses, Stokes built on relationships he had forged with institutional managers while helping them control hepatitis or other infectious diseases. His researchers had been at Pennhurst conducting vaccine trials before they began hepatitis infection procedures. And when Stokes sought approval for hepatitis transmission procedures at New Lisbon, the site had long been a locale for studies of both gamma globulin and experimental immunizing agents. When seeking approval from the facility to proceed with challenge inoculations with unmodified hepatitis, Stokes argued that the risks were low because he expected that the subjects would be immune.

He presented the following account to the New Lisbon director: "Since these patients are probably immune, we would expect none to develop hepatitis. If, by chance, any should contract the disease, it would probably be quite mild. There is no danger of spreading the disease in the institution, because the institution is now immune, or almost completely immune." Here, as elsewhere, Stokes normalized the transmission of unmodified hepatitis to children by arguing the impact on these subjects would be minimal—physicians agreed that symptoms of hepatitis were milder in youngsters than in adults—or even beneficial.

Stokes was able to avoid public criticism of experiments with institutionalized children by concealing some studies and depicting others as benign. But the hepatitis transmission studies generated discomfort among AFEB scientists. In February 1948, Stokes wrote AFEB president Colin MacLeod about "a point of ethics"—Stokes's term—that had been raised at a recent meeting in Washington. Stokes devoted the bulk of the letter to defending his hepatitis infection procedures with children. He began by saying that parents or guardians gave consent for all experiments with minors. He did not specify precisely who was providing consent; for children who were wards of the state, the manager of the custodial institution would be the legal guardian.

Stokes went on to present the core of his justification. He insisted that no experiment was undertaken "except under the provision that the study in our opinion could be of benefit to the individual himself." Hepatitis was like mumps, he stated, and with mumps it was "well recognized pediatric practice to plan exposure of children ... before puberty if the opportunity is presented to do so." Thus conceived, giving a youngster unmodified hepatitis virus was in the interests of the child.

Stokes elaborated: "Epidemic hepatitis may be a serious disease after puberty and is usually very mild in children. It appears also to be a disease to which most individuals are exposed and become immune before the age of 25 or 30 years.... It would be beneficial to the individual, therefore, to have a planned exposure to a known MILD virus under nursing care ... rather than to suffer an unplanned exposure to possibly a more virulent virus strain at a more dangerous age period after puberty." Stokes was claiming that exposing children to unmodified hepatitis was equivalent to administering an immunizing agent: the child subject was not the victim of a disease-inducing experiment but rather the recipient of enlightened preventive medicine. In advancing this position, Stokes was eviscerating the distinction between experiments for the benefit of subjects and those aimed at advancing medical knowledge.

Stokes distributed copies of his "point of ethics" letter not only to MacLeod, but also to Paul and other members of the AFEB's inner circle. Paul, unfailingly diplomatic in his communications with colleagues and also considerably more circumspect than Stokes on matters of research conduct, wrote Stokes urging that he exercise prudence. Paul said he agreed with Stokes in principle but wondered whether new standards might be applicable after the Nuremberg proceedings—the trial had ended just six months earlier. "During the war we more or less made our own policies on this," Paul remarked, "but I am not sure that that is possible today." However, no new rules were forthcoming as yet from the scientists' government sponsors.

At MacLeod's instruction, Cecil Watson, chair of the Liver Commission, sent Stokes's letter to officials in the OTSG. In his correspondence, Watson asked the OTSG for input on issues raised by Stokes's communication concerning "the advisability of immunizing children with hepatitis virus, presumably attenuated." (It was not at all clear that the virus was attenuated.) A determination on the matter from the chief of the Army's Research and Development Board accepted Stokes's argument that exposing children to mild hepatitis was preferable to a more serious case of the illness after puberty. For the time being, Stokes proceeded with further experiments exposing children to live hepatitis pathogens.

Unease among scientists about hazardous experiments with institutionalized children was not limited to that surrounding Stokes's hepatitis studies. Many European physicians felt that the principle of voluntary consent articulated in the Nuremberg Code precluded use of institutionalized persons in studies unrelated to the individuals' medical treatment. They found experiments with children and the cognitively impaired—even those testing new immunizing agents—particularly disquieting.

In the early 1950s, American investigators working with newly developed polio vaccines selected children's facilities to conduct human trials. Jonas Salk carried out initial human tests of his killed polio vaccine with children at Polk State School in Pennsylvania in 1952. But it was an earlier polio vaccine trial that stirred greater controversy. In 1950, Hilary Koprowski administered attenuated live polio strains to impaired children at Letchworth Village in New York's Hudson Valley and Sonoma State Hospital in California. Polio researchers considered Koprowski's experiments with live poliovirus especially hazardous; use of a vaccine of this type during the mid-1930s had caused multiple fatalities.

In March 1952, the British journal *Lancet* took Koprowski to task for testing an unproven live polio vaccine on twenty subjects widely known to be severely disabled children. As was customary, Koprowski referred to his subjects as *volunteers*. We "can only guess," *Lancet* remarked, "that the volunteers were very young and that the volunteering was done by their parents." The journal then offered satirical commentary on Koprowski's language and choice of subjects, noting that in a language as rich as English, the meaning of words continually changes: "Such a word is 'volunteer.' We may yet read in a scientific journal that an experiment was carried out with twenty volunteer mice, and that twenty other mice volunteered as controls."

In the United States, Rockefeller Institute virologist Thomas Rivers questioned Koprowski's claims about the inoculant's safety and rejected the use of impaired children for testing experimental live immunizing agents. He later remarked about Koprowski's selection of subjects: "I personally did not approve of using mentally defective children for such a test," but other investigators were using children for similar tests and "you might even say it was standard practice." Rivers was not averse to transmitting viruses to adults when it suited his scientific aims. For instance, he reported that he had tested live yellow fever vaccine on adult patients at Rockefeller Hospital in violation of New York City health code; he later said about the matter, "The law winks when a reputable man wants to do a scientific experiment.... Unless the law winks occasionally, you have no progress in medicine." But he was opposed to giving children hazardous experimental virus strains.

Rivers, who joined the AFEB's central oversight committee in 1948, would become a formidable critic of Stokes's hepatitis experiments with children. Nevertheless, through the early 1950s, Stokes would continue to expose children and youths to live hepatitis viruses. He did so with the knowledge of the AFEB and OTSG. His Defense Department sponsors set aside questions about the acceptability of transmitting unmodified hepatitis to minors and, for the present, Stokes's assertions that the interventions were acts of medical beneficence would stand. But pressure from Europe would grow and the social and political context of medical research with human participants would change. In the United States, reservations about enrolling minors and impaired persons in dangerous medical experiments were growing. It would only be a matter of time before hepatitis infection experiments with these groups would arouse more determined opposition.

CHAPTER FIVE

Tales of Redemption

E ARLY COLD WAR HEPATITIS researchers relied heavily on prisons
and reformatories for human subjects, with all of the investigators recruiting in whole or in part from inmate populations.
George Mirick at Johns Hopkins drew subjects from a reformatory and two prisons run by the Maryland Department of Corrections. Irving Gordon at the New York State Laboratory gained access to
the state reformatory at Coxsackie. Robert McCollum at Yale enrolled
subjects from Danbury Federal Prison in Connecticut. A team of NIH
investigators set up research units at three federal penitentiaries, facilities
in the states of Washington, Kentucky, and Pennsylvania. Joseph Stokes
Jr. not only drew subjects from a mental hospital and multiple institutions for children, he also enlisted inmates from five state correctional
facilities—a prison and four reformatories—in New Jersey.

The use of prisoners in hepatitis infection studies was one piece of a
much broader pattern. During the third quarter of the twentieth century,
American biomedical researchers maintained a well-organized and fully
entrenched system for conducting experiments in prisons and reformatories. The system's rise followed the course of biomedical research in the
United States more generally: growth during World War II, a marked
upswing during the initial postwar years, and meteoric expansion in the
1960s and early 1970s. According to one estimate, by 1975, twenty thousand inmates in federal and state facilities—10 percent of the total prison
population—were serving as subjects in biomedical studies.

Provisions in the Nuremberg Code concerning voluntary consent did not impede the growth of research in American prisons. Until the late 1960s, few commentators in the United States raised questions about the voluntariness of inmates' participation in medical studies. Controversies did arise, but coercion was almost never their focus; the debates centered instead on the early release of prisoners who had served as subjects.

The most hotly contested instance of early release was that of Nathan Leopold, convicted in 1924 along with his partner in crime, Richard Loeb, of kidnapping and murdering a teenager. At the end of a sensational trial, the court sentenced the men to life in prison. Leopold served time at Stateville Penitentiary, where he enrolled in malaria infection experiments and also performed laboratory and office tasks for project investigators. For his contributions to medical science, the Illinois governor commuted Leopold's sentence in 1949, making him eligible for parole in 1953. Leopold was released from prison in 1958. Meanwhile, in December 1952, a month before his first parole hearing, the House of Delegates of the American Medical Association passed a resolution condemning medical experiments with individuals convicted of "heinous crimes" and rejecting the practice of granting them "commendatory citations." At issue was not the voluntariness of inmates' consent, but rather that inmates' participation in medical research might pave the way for their expedited release.

Early parole for inmate-subjects would remain a sensitive matter, but the pace of experimentation in correctional facilities accelerated nonetheless, fueled by both governmental and commercial sponsorship. Federal regulations issued in 1962 required that, as a condition for product licensure, pharmaceutical firms obtain evidence of safety and efficacy through clinical trials. While these measures greatly increased the volume of research in prisons, the system's basic design had been established years earlier.

America's regime of medical experiments in correctional facilities had its origins in World War II and the early Cold War years. During this period, university scientists and their federal patrons regularized the system's normative foundations and operating procedures. The cooperation of wardens and state oversight agencies was essential. To secure buy-in from these officials, researchers argued that knowledge to be gained from prison research was necessary to the national defense. They also advanced claims that resonated with goals of the correctional community. Advocates for prison research insisted that, by serving as subjects in dangerous experiments, inmates would embark on a path toward redemptive transformation. Stokes, a true believer in human experimentation and a consummate strategist for securing institutional access, was at the forefront of implementing practices that would bolster the notion that a prisoner's participation in medical research was a route to rehabilitation.

Stokes began hepatitis infection experiments with prison inmates just as his Civilian Public Service camp in Philadelphia was closing. In his initial study with prisoners, Stokes's investigators ran into an unanticipated, even madcap complication. During the spring of 1946, his team recruited sixteen inmates from New Jersey State Prison at Trenton to participate in a virus transmission study. The aim was to determine whether subjects at the CPS camp who had lingering symptoms of hepatitis from earlier procedures were still harboring the viruses. For the new study, researchers harvested specimens from three unrecovered conscientious objectors and used the materials to inoculate prisoners. Stokes arranged for officials to transfer the sixteen inmate-subjects to Trenton State Hospital, the psychiatric facility where his program maintained a laboratory and an infirmary for hepatitis research. Sydney Gellis, one of the junior investigators on Stokes's team, was initially in charge of the study.

The complication arose on May 13: one of the prisoners exited a third-floor hospital window, scaled down the building wall, and fled. The escape triggered a manhunt and then an investigation by the New Jersey Department of Institutions and Agencies. During the inquiry, the director of inspections interviewed nurses and guards working on the research ward and submitted a six-page report to the commissioner. The inspector's account was filled with finger pointing from staff overseeing the prisoners. According to these informants, the problem arose because discipline on the ward was lax; Gellis had offered the inmates too many privileges and had "made promises to prisoners without consultation with custodial officers"—an account that Gellis disputed.

The incident did not seriously disrupt the study; John Neefe, who took over the project when Gellis left for another research post, reported on its results at a conference four months later. And Stokes's cordial relations with New Jersey officials continued without interruption. But he did learn from the episode that some prison populations would be easier to manage than others, and for subsequent experiments with prisoners he chose New Jersey correctional facilities housing younger and, likely, more pliable inmates. These included reformatories at Rahway (1947), Clinton (1949 through 1953), Bordentown (1951), and Annandale (1952). The Clinton facility, known as Clinton Farms, had the distinction of being an institution for women with a female superintendent and an all-women board of directors.

When seeking approvals from superintendents and state oversight agencies to recruit prisoners as subjects, postwar hepatitis researchers enlisted help from their Defense Department sponsors. In 1950, Mirick and Gordon were having difficulty gaining access to state prisons; at their request, the Armed Forces Epidemiology Board asked that the surgeons general of the army and navy write the governors of New York and Maryland urging cooperation—the task was eventually delegated to lower-level military personnel. Stokes, who began prison studies earlier, negotiated directly with the New Jersey Department of Institutions and Agencies but also provided that agency with letters of support from the Office of the Surgeon General–Army.

Even when appeals came from the Pentagon, gaining access to state facilities could be a hard sell, particularly during the years before Cold War ideology had fully taken hold. Stokes, for example, ran into obstacles during fall of 1946 when making arrangements for experiments at New Jersey Reformatory in Rahway. Officials at New Jersey's Department of Institutions and Agencies were receptive, but Stokes also needed the endorsement of the State Board of Control. He complained that the chairman of the board, businessman Reeve Schley, objected to continuing such studies "now that the war is over." Schley's misgivings about allowing risk-laden experiments during peacetime were a recurring hindrance that Stokes sought to circumvent.

Stokes had Colonel Stone at the OTSG dispatch letters to Schley and the state commissioner stressing the importance of the research for stemming a tremendous loss of military manpower caused by hepatitis. Stone wrote: "We have every reason to believe that in any war in the future we will experience infectious hepatitis and unless some means is found for the prevention and control of this important disease, it may adversely affect the outcome of any armed conflict we are forced to undertake. . . . You may rest assured that this work is being done in the best interest of both civilian and military personnel of our country and humanity in general."

Stokes did not rely solely on endorsements from the Defense Department. Of the hepatitis investigators, Stokes was the most adept at the politics of institutional access and devoted considerable effort to cultivating state officials and institutional managers. It helped that Stokes had social ties with people who ran New Jersey state agencies. He was on a first-name basis with the deputy commissioner in charge of corrections, F. Lovell Bixby, who signed letters to Stokes as "Bix"; and Stokes's older brother, Samuel Emlen Stokes, also a physician, held a seat on the State Board of Control.

Early in 1949, Schley was threatening to block hepatitis infection experiments at the Clinton Farms reformatory. Stone again wrote the commissioner emphasizing the importance of the experiments. Emlen Stokes appealed to Schley, urging that he abandon his opposition. With support from the commissioner's office and the influence of his brother's board position, Joseph Stokes was able to neutralize opposition from the board chairman.

Stokes also needed approval from Clinton Farms' managers before he could proceed with experiments at the facility. He energetically pursued Superintendent Edna Mahan and her board of directors, sending correspondence and joining the women for a luncheon meeting. In December 1948, he forwarded Mahan a statement about proposed studies for the board's consideration, describing the vital importance of the research. He declared that hepatitis was an enormous problem for the military and that, by assisting with the research, Clinton Farms would be doing "great service to the Armed Services—Army, Navy, and Air Force—and to civilians generally throughout the world." In a note to Mahan accompanying this narrative, Stokes remarked in a droll aside, "I trust it makes the eagle scream sufficiently." Evidently, Mahan had advised him beforehand that invoking patriotism would sway members of her board to allow medical experiments with Clinton Farm inmates.

Arrangements that scientists struck at different institutions varied, even among New Jersey correctional facilities. At Annandale, subjects accrued $1.50 per week in their canteen accounts while they were enrolled in a hepatitis study; those at other facilities received no financial compensation. At Bordentown and Clinton Farms, managers required parental consent for inmate-subjects younger than twenty-one. The agreement for Rahway prohibited inmates under twenty-one from participating. But two provisions were universal: the use of waiver and release documents—with wording approved by Defense Department lawyers—and the preclusion of any mechanism for compensating subjects in the event of research injuries.

Stokes made repeated attempts to persuade the OTSG to relent on the matter of compensation for research injuries. He began these efforts in 1947 while seeking access to inmates at Rahway reformatory. Stokes wrote the OTSG saying that the facility's superintendent wanted "assurances that if permanent disability developed we would be able to arrange financial assistance for the volunteers.... I believe the question is a proper one as to what arrangements, if any, might be made in case of disability." Stokes went on to say that while his virus strains were "apparently not virulent," there was "always, however, a bare chance" of permanent disability.

It was not the first time that investigators or institutional managers had raised this issue. Leaders of the OSRD's Committee on Medical Research had considered purchasing insurance for subjects in the agency's 1942 bovine-albumin study, but the insurer they approached viewed the risks involved as uncontrollable. Also during the war, both the American Friends Service Committee and state officials in Pennsylvania had pressed for a means to compensate hepatitis subjects in the event of long-term injury. The Defense Department had refused then and did so now. In approving experiments at Rahway, the New Jersey Board of Control accepted a statement that "medical authorities representing the Surgeon General's Office foresee no permanent ill effects to those inmates who volunteer." Cooperating state agencies yielded to the judgments of scientists and the conditions imposed by researchers' defense sponsors. Should long-term disabilities occur, waiver provisions were to protect scientists and government entities from legal responsibility.

Prison managers had reason to cooperate with medical scientists apart from patriotic entreaties and deference to scientists and their federal sponsors. Encouraging prisoners to participate in medical experiments was compatible with an ethos of rehabilitation widely embraced by members of the correctional community. A prominent socio-legal scholar describes a system of "penal welfarism" that prevailed among prison professionals between the 1890s and 1970s, reaching its most complete form during the 1950s and 1960s before a turn toward punishment took hold. While it flourished, penal welfarism supported innovative practices that gave prison officials a great deal of flexibility in handling inmates. It combined the goal of correction with a mission of social uplift. Accompanying practices included the use of reformatories and training centers as alternatives to conventional prisons; indeterminate sentences allowing early release and paroled supervision; and programs aimed at reeducation and social reintegration. Medical experimentation was one of the programs for remediating prisoners.

Sanford Bates, who served as the first director of the Federal Bureau of Prisons between 1930 and 1937, was a vocal advocate for medical research as a vehicle for inmate rehabilitation. Bates—Bixby's boss—headed the New Jersey Department of Institutions and Agencies from 1945 through 1954. He gave full expression to his belief in the transformative power of medical experiments in December 1952 when he learned that the AMA wanted to foreclose the participation of violent criminals. Bates dispatched a letter to the president of the New Jersey Medical Society expressing dismay at the AMA's position. He was adamant about the wisdom of encouraging prisoners to enroll as research subjects, insisting: "What must take place in a prison is some change in the individual's attitude toward the society, which he has wronged. And if he is willing to subject himself to personal danger . . . to the possibilities of disease, he . . . has taken a long step forward toward this rehabilitation. . . . I think the things that we have done here in New Jersey and in other states along this line are perhaps the most advanced, the most humanitarian and the most intelligent things that have been done in prison work in many, many years." The notion of participation in medical experiments as rehabilitation was, at its core, a belief that prisoners would be redeemed through service to others, particularly when their contributions were to the benefit of the nation.

Managers of Clinton Farms endorsed the goal of inmate transformation through humanitarian service and saw it as their mission to provide their charges with opportunities for patriotic altruism. In June 1949, Stokes arranged to have the army surgeon general, Major General Raymond W. Bliss, write Edna Mahan to thank her and her board for making possible the initial hepatitis studies at Clinton Farms. Bliss assured them that the research was of tremendous value to the military. The board secretary responded with a letter to the surgeon general conveying the group's appreciation for his "gracious and enthusiastic comments about the hepatitis study." She added: "It is a source of satisfaction to us as Board members to note the ready response of our girls to appeals such as yours where they feel they can be of some service to the community while they are undergoing their period of rehabilitation."

The idea of medical experiment as remediation received unreserved endorsement from defense officials, army-sponsored researchers, and many

working in the field of corrections. Both scientists and wardens urged inmates to embrace this ethos when researchers sought subjects from prison
populations. The process of recruitment was thus not only an effort to obtain participants for experiments, but also an inducement for prisoners to
adopt the notion of self as citizen-subject: a person whose value to society
could be restored through service to science and country.

Efforts to convey this ethos extended to parents whose consent was
needed when the prospective subject was a minor. A young inmate at
Bordentown named Danny expressed willingness to participate in a hepatitis infection experiment, but his mother, Mrs. G., was worried about
the health consequences for her son. In July 1951, Bordentown superintendent Albert Wagner wrote Mrs. G. to assure her that the study involved few dangers and that participants would receive the "utmost
medical attention." Danny would be contributing to scientists' efforts to
control an illness that was "a very real problem for our fighting men" in
Korea. Wagner went on to say that Danny would receive no rewards for
being a research subject except the "inmost knowledge that he is serving
the rest of humanity in an effort to stamp out this disease." Wagner continued, "Danny is doing a selfless good thing in participating in this
study and we would sincerely hope that you could find it possible to en-
courage him in it."

In addition to the pervasive language of rehabilitation, scientists and
wardens enacted ritualized procedures in an effort to shape inmates'
viewpoints and behaviors. The certificate of service, also called a commendation or award of appreciation, was a pivotal tool for encouraging
prisoners to see participation in experiments as a means of moral exoner-
ation. Scientists routinely promised these documents as an inducement
to enroll and dispensed them when a round of experiments was completed. Mirick even included the promise of a commendation letter in his
waiver and release form.

It is unclear when and how certificates of service originated, but an
abundance of records attests to their centrality in government-sponsored
experiments with prisoners in the wartime and early postwar years. Federal sponsors facilitated their adoption. Albert Sabin deployed one in
conjunction with human infection experiments with dengue and sand-fly
fever in 1944 at New Jersey State Prison at Trenton. Stanhope Bayne-
Jones, in his role as AEB director, sent Sabin's draft statement to the
agency's legal counsel for approval along with the project's waiver form.

The OTSG also permitted the AEB's name to appear on the document. A year later, Bayne-Jones arranged approval of a certificate for Thomas Francis's hepatitis subjects at Michigan's Jackson State Prison. Inmate-subject Herman Ford had died there weeks earlier and Bayne-Jones agreed with Francis that commendations "would be an aid to morale and willingness of the men to participate."

While the wording and official signatures appearing on postwar certificates varied, AFEB scientists went to considerable lengths to make the documents look official. Both Mirick and Gordon arranged to have theirs printed on special Defense Department letterhead. Stokes had his embossed with the seal of the University of Pennsylvania. The certificates included signatures of the lead researcher as well as AFEB or university officials. Gordon arranged for his subjects to receive two letters of commendation, one from the Defense Department and another from the New York State Department of Health.

If federal sponsors were amenable to commendations and assisted with their production, impetus for their use seems to have come from prison officials. The documents were a vital feature of a warden's program for rehabilitation. Because inmates knew that copies of these statements would be placed in their files, the certificates were a powerful incentive to enroll in medical experiments as a sign of good behavior. While prisoners seldom received promises of shortened sentences, they understood that correctional officers would take meritorious citations into consideration when making decisions about release and parole.

At many institutions, the distribution of the commendations was a celebratory occasion. Superintendents held events much like graduation ceremonies in honor of prisoners who had completed terms of service as subjects. Bordentown's superintendent held a special dinner in the fall of 1951 for inmates who had finished a round of experiments; he adjusted the date of the event so Stokes could attend. In May 1949, Mahan sent Stokes a list of twenty-four Clinton Farms inmates due to receive certificates of appreciation for their stint as research subjects. She was counting on him to be present at both a June luncheon with her board and the graduation exercise that followed. When Stokes would not be on hand to distribute certificates of merit at such events, he sent a team member in his place. In June 1951, Werner Henle, the project's senior laboratory scientist, was the honored guest at a Clinton Farms award ceremony.

The prison press was another instrument of persuasion. Many correctional institutions produced weekly, monthly, or quarterly newspapers or magazines for internal distribution. These publications carried recruitment announcements for upcoming medical experiments, stories about ongoing studies, and laudatory accounts of contributions made by inmate-subjects. Some also ran stories about government-sponsored research at other correctional facilities.

Jackson State Prison, where Thomas Francis Jr. conducted hepatitis studies during the war, had an expertly edited and printed weekly called the *Spectator*. In 1945, it carried four articles about hepatitis infection experiments at the prison. The headline for one read in part, "Volunteers Praised for Cooperative Spirit." A story appearing in December of that year extolled the inmates who had been subjects in virus transmission studies, even noting that some had become seriously ill and that one had died. It listed all participants by surname and prison number and declared the men "heroes—as brave as any who served in uniform." As described in the *Spectator*: "With no promises of leniency or reduction of sentences made, volunteers stepped forward. . . . Even after Doctors explained the dangers involved and how the disease might react, the men remained undaunted."

In July 1949, Clinton Farms' newsletter, *US Personified*, ran a story praising inmates who had taken part in initial rounds of hepatitis experiments at the reformatory. It quoted Stokes as saying the studies had yielded "splendid results," providing information with far-reaching implications for the armed forces and civilians "not only in the United States but also all over the world." His research team "had the fullest cooperation from the volunteers and from Miss Mahan and her staff." The article listed subjects by first name and last initial, in this way highlighting "the girls who are helping to write this page of medical history."

If the rehabilitative ethos portrayed the inmate-subject as a person undergoing social reintegration through public service, it also cast the researcher as steward of the prisoner's transformation. At Clinton Farms, Stokes enacted this role in ways other than distributing commendation certificates. In August 1949, residents of the facility's Wittpen Dorm, a cottage housing two rounds of hepatitis subjects, invited Stokes to attend an evening of entertainment. A mimeographed playbill accompanying the event—a document Stokes retained that became part of his collected papers—shows that the inmates were performing a series of skits they called "Jaundice Follies of 1949." The playbill listed Stokes and his onsite technicians as event patrons. Stokes sent regrets that he could not attend, but forwarded a donation. He also sent Wittpen residents a telegram:

"PLEASE ACCEPT OUR APPRECIATION AND BEST WISHES ON THIS OCCASION. HAVE FUN. Dr. Stokes and Staff." Stokes received two handwritten notes signed by "Jaundice Unit Members" thanking him for his contribution. Such good-natured interactions further normalized inmates' participation in disease-inducing studies.

Documentary sources provide scant information about the inmates who served as subjects in early postwar hepatitis experiments. Records are silent on the race of enrollees, although it is clear that the correctional facilities housed African American as well as white inmates. Available materials on Clinton Farms are more revealing than those for most of the study sites. A history of Clinton Farms notes that Mahan, who was superintendent between 1928 and 1968, desegregated the dormitories in 1947; it is likely that a good portion of the facility's hepatitis subjects were African American women.

Other particulars about research participation at Clinton Farms are also of interest. Records show that when Stokes began hepatitis studies there in 1949, the facility's average population was 435. Over the course of four years, 250 of the facility's inmates signed on to be subjects; Stokes's researchers transmitted viruses to 185 prisoners in a sequence of thirteen rounds of experiments. A document from one round of interventions during May 1951 indicates that the twenty participants in this study ranged in age from eighteen to thirty-eight, with the majority in their late teens or early twenties.

Although both researchers and Clinton Farms' overseers referred to their inmates as "girls," many of the prisoners had children of their own. One of the reformatory's distinctive features was its nursery. Managers allowed newborns to stay with their mothers for six months to a year before placement with relatives or foster care. In 1949, Clinton Farms had an average of thirty-five babies in the nursery. While Stokes included no infants—and presumably no mothers of in-house children—in his hepatitis transmission experiments, virtually all of Clinton Farms' subjects were of childbearing age. If researchers were transmitting blood-borne hepatitis to these women, consequences might have followed for their subsequent offspring.

Women who become carriers of hepatitis B can pass the virus to their infants in utero, during delivery, or through close contact after birth. In the postwar years, scientists were beginning to recognize maternal transmission. Early in 1952, Stokes noted that the virus of serum hepatitis "on rare occasions may remain in the blood of certain carriers." He recalled that "on one occasion, in a Trenton woman who was never a volunteer nor in any institution, we believe it traversed the placenta and caused the disease in her infant."

In correspondence, Stokes insisted that his team used only hepatitis A virus in studies at Clinton Farms. But an interim research report from the fall of 1950 suggests that his team considered inoculating subjects at that facility with serum from a blood donor they believed to be a long-time carrier of hepatitis B. While it is unclear whether they proceeded with such interventions at Clinton Farms, records of the team's work at Trenton State Hospital plainly show that, between 1949 and 1951, the group infected eleven female mental patients of childbearing age with serum hepatitis. Available records are mute as to whether there were long-term health consequences for these women or those close to them.

Archived documents provide only brief glimpses of the people whom prison investigators referred to as volunteers, or of what experiences these individuals had during or after their participation in hazardous research. By contrast, newspapers and magazines offered multiple descriptions of inmate-subjects, portrayals consistent with the notion of participation in experiments as rehabilitation. If these published accounts are to be believed, the outcomes for inmates were almost entirely favorable.

The mainstream press in postwar America catered to a communal fascination with medical experimentation by running numerous stories about research in prisons, including hepatitis infection studies. Scientists understood that sympathetic press coverage was critical to public acceptance of experiments in correctional facilities, and they devoted a great deal of attention to shaping these accounts. Through their efforts and those of prison officials, the rehabilitative ethos made its way into the media and public consciousness.

Stokes, among others, lobbied behind the scenes to influence depictions of hepatitis studies in news outlets. During the war, AEB executive director Stanhope Bayne-Jones had handled the oversight of press reports. Now Stokes and New Jersey correctional officials implemented strikingly similar strategies for influencing media coverage. Stokes accepted and even encouraged articles about his prison research in the popular press— so long as reporters and editors observed certain rules of conduct.

In January 1951, Bordentown's Superintendent Albert Wagner wrote Stokes saying that a local reporter wanted to do a story about hepatitis experiments at the reformatory. Stokes responded that he would be happy to cooperate, provided the reporter agreed to submit a draft for review; the article would need approval from Stokes, a collaborating investigator, and Wagner before publication. Stokes had been imposing requirements of this type for a number of years. The procedures applied not only to the popular press but also to publications like the *Welfare Reporter*, a monthly published by the New Jersey Department of Institutions and Agencies. In 1946, the *Reporter* sent Stokes the draft of an article on medical research in state facilities. The assistant editor noted in a cover letter that he had made an effort to use the word *studies* rather than *experiments* and added, "This is in keeping with your suggestion that we avoid anything which might be likely to arouse apprehension among parents of inmates in public institutions."

On at least one occasion, it was not the scientists but the state agency that sought the greatest control over depictions of prison research. The public relations director at Philadelphia children's hospital was eager to arrange for a story in the Sunday supplement of the *Philadelphia Inquirer* about hepatitis experiments in New Jersey correctional facilities. In 1952, Stokes wrote Deputy Commissioner Bixby suggesting that such an article would be mutually advantageous. Bixby agreed so long as Stokes oversaw its preparation and the commissioner and his board approved the piece before it appeared. But when a story did come Bixby's way, he and the State Board of Control rejected it. Bixby complained that the report failed to do justice to the seriousness of purpose behind the state's program of medical experiments with inmates. He elaborated: "The Board feels that the significance of the work to public health and military medicine has not been properly emphasized. . . . It was only the extreme importance of the research . . . that persuaded the Board to permit inmates to volunteer to render what to our minds is a very great public service." He added that his board would be willing to consider a different version of the article.

Many of the media reports that did appear were brief and apparently neutral. But even these pieces reinforced claims made by scientists and prison officials alike: that the goal of hepatitis infection studies was disease prevention, that the research was aiding the military, that the recruitment of subjects involved no coercion, and that participants were performing acts of public service. An article about hepatitis experiments at Clinton Farms appearing in the *New York Times* (September 1950), for instance, reported that over the course of two years, two hundred female prisoners had "been offering themselves . . . as volunteers" to help solve "one of the Army's biggest disease problems." Invaluable findings about the viability of hepatitis grown in laboratory media would not have been possible, the author wrote, without the courage of the women and the model program of the New Jersey Department of Institutions and Agencies.

The most elaborate of these accounts were human-interest stories in popular magazines. In 1948, *Reader's Digest* published a piece by John O'Hara, former warden of New Jersey State Prison at Trenton, who proudly espoused the rehabilitative ethos. The story featured James Duncan, an inmate sentenced to life for a mob-related murder. While incarcerated at the Trenton facility, he enrolled as a subject in five army-sponsored medical experiments—one of these was the hepatitis infection study in which a recalcitrant inmate made his dramatic escape. In O'Hara's extravagantly worded account, Duncan followed a path to redemptive transformation. The story quotes Duncan as saying that he sought out medical experiments because he "knew it was the greatest chance of all—a chance to [do] something not just for a few but for thousands. For the men fighting overseas . . . for generations to come." The changes O'Hara witnessed in Duncan and other inmate-subjects were "close to miraculous." According to O'Hara, Duncan declared, "If I were in charge of penal reform, I'd install a human guinea pig ward in every prison in the country. I honestly believe it would be the greatest force for rehabilitation of prisoners ever set up—to say nothing of what it might do for medical research."

Duncan secured parole in 1946 after persuading Stokes to write him a letter of support and submit it to the New Jersey Court of Probation. But his brush with hepatitis was not over. In 1952, after reading of the death of a prisoner in a hepatitis transmission experiment, Duncan sent a letter to the OTSG recounting his own experience: "Two weeks after I was paroled I was hit hard by a relapse of Yellow Jaundice. None of the local doctors knew anything about it, or what to do for it. Finally, a doctor was located at the University of Penna., who said he'd get me a bed. I stayed there for a couple of weeks." He went on to say that while he understood the importance of the human studies with hepatitis, "some method must be worked out to take care of a volunteer later if what he is suffering from is a direct result of past experiments." Duncan received a polite response from the AFEB's executive director thanking him for his continued interest in the problem of hepatitis in the armed forces and noting that although scientists still had no animal model for hepatitis, program researchers were able to recruit willing human subjects and to care for them appropriately. The letter did not address Duncan's returning illness.

The reality of prisoners' motivations was undoubtedly more complex than outlets like *Reader's Digest* depicted. Inmates likely had multiple reasons for participating in medical experiments, and whether altruism was typically preeminent among them is certainly open to question. While prospective subjects rarely received promises of shortened sentences, the system of commendations generated a reasonable expectation that enrolling in a medical study would hasten release.

Nathan Leopold and James Duncan were not the only subjects in government-sponsored studies to have their sentences reduced. In 1947, Governor Dwight Green of Illinois announced that 445 Stateville inmates would be given special consideration in decisions about parole or executive clemency for participating in wartime malaria experiments. That year, the *Chicago Daily Tribune* reported that parole boards were shortening prison sentences for participants in malaria experiments by an average of two years. Subjects in some studies also received at least modest financial compensation for their participation. Another dynamic may have been operating as well: becoming a research subject was a means for gaining attention, recognition, elevated standing, and enhanced privileges within the regime of many correctional institutions.

In a memoir, Leopold discussed his own motivations for enrolling in the malaria experiments at Stateville Penitentiary. While his reasons were mixed, central among them was that participation might open the door to parole. He also found his work on the project fascinating and satisfying. Leopold offered an assessment of why other Stateville inmates signed on. Some men, he observed, had relatives or friends in the military and wanted to help soldiers. He continued: "Many took part because they hoped that their sentences would be reduced; some few actually took malaria to earn the hundred dollars. And there were some few who . . . went into the thing entirely on an idealistic basis. . . . They saw it as a chance to do something decent and worth while for a change . . . to make their tiny contribution to humanity." Whatever their dominant motivation, quite a few prisoners—Duncan among them—became proficient at the language of rehabilitation.

By the late 1960s, critics would question the voluntariness of prisoners' participation and press accounts would become less favorable. But during the 1940s and 1950s, depictions of prison experiments in the U.S.

mainstream media were overwhelmingly positive. The popular media portrayed even risk-laden human experiments in correctional facilities as not only morally acceptable but exemplary of the nation's values.

America's hepatitis researchers succeeded in establishing the legitimacy of a moral framework that celebrated disease-inducing experiments. They won acceptance for this framework during the war by advancing accounts of draft objectors' altruistic patriotism, and further bolstered it in the postwar years by highlighting prisoners' rehabilitative service to the country. Scientists' success rested on deference from the press and their own skills at invoking institutionally embedded meanings and broader cultural symbols. If the prevailing narratives were to be believed, hepatitis transmission and other medical experiments in U.S. prisons were "as American as apple pie."

CHAPTER SIX

Cold War Calculations

A T THE START OF the Korean War, the Armed Forces Epidemiology Board sponsored a large-scale experiment that would become the deadliest of all the hepatitis infection studies. Its aim was to find a means of inactivating hepatitis B, which was polluting the U.S. supply of blood and blood products. Researchers applied ultraviolet rays and chemicals to contaminated serum and, to test whether they had succeeded in disarming the virus, injected subjects with the treated specimens. None of their methods prevented illnesses among study participants. In the course of the research, three inmate-subjects died of fulminant hepatitis B with a fourth nearly succumbing to the same ailment. The casualties confronted scientists as never before with the hazards of inducing blood-borne hepatitis.

Intra-agency and international Cold War politics came into play in planning for the study and again during its tumultuous aftermath. A new war and the perceived threat of a Soviet nuclear attack spurred federal officials to initiate the project, an effort they saw as imperative for nuclear preparedness. Then, while investigators were still reeling from the fatalities, the secretary of defense ruled that Nuremberg principles would govern department-sponsored medical research. The directive was an effort to reconcile the agency's burgeoning program of dangerous human experiments with the administration's policy on international human rights. But what the Nuremberg principles would mean for research practices was far from clear.

The new policy reignited tension between Department of Defense leaders and government-sponsored researchers over legal responsibility for research injuries, and among AFEB investigators over experimenting with children and disabled persons. A dispute emerged between Joseph Stokes Jr. and Thomas Rivers, the prominent Rockefeller Institute scientist, about exposing children to virus strains. Conflicts unleashed in the deaths' aftermath highlight major threads weaving through postwar human research policy: national security priorities, the Nuremberg Code, and approaches to research risks and legal liability. The blood sterilization project's failure to identify a means for inactivating hepatitis in blood triggered additional discord. A high-level military medical officer complained bitterly about this shortcoming, and about a more general lack of progress toward hepatitis prevention.

All of these conflicts took place behind closed doors; scientists and their federal sponsors were able to keep the upheaval from becoming visible to the press and the public. But the episode was a turning point for the hepatitis program. Faced with multiple divisive issues, the AFEB shut down not only the blood sterilization project, but also its entire roster of studies involving hepatitis transmission. The AFEB would later resume its program, but in the meantime, it quietly dismissed all of its hepatitis infection researchers. Neither Stokes nor any other World War II or early postwar investigator would conduct further studies that induced the illness in subjects.

In the late 1940s, the medical community found that recipients of donated blood and its derivatives were developing jaundice in alarming numbers. The condition was especially prevalent after the use of plasma, made from the liquid portion of blood. During World War II, plasma had become a mainstay of military treatment for battle casualties. It could be dried, and thus easily preserved and transported. However, when manufacturing plasma, laboratories pooled blood—typically combining more than a thousand donations—greatly increasing the likelihood of hepatitis contamination.

After the war, researchers had been confident that ultraviolet radiation inactivated the blood-borne virus. In a publication from his last experiment at Lynchburg Colony, John Oliphant had reported that irradiation was effective in disabling the pathogen, and other researchers confirmed his finding. In 1949, the NIH Laboratory of Biologics Control, the federal unit responsible for licensing vaccines and other biological products, began requiring that plasma be irradiated. But reports in the *Journal of the American Medical Association* (*JAMA*) during the fall of 1950 cast doubt on the effectiveness of ultraviolet radiation for neutralizing active hepatitis. As Korean War injuries began to mount, the military medical corps found that more than 20 percent of servicemen receiving plasma, even irradiated plasma, were contracting hepatitis. Soldiers were surviving combat wounds only to suffer from a serious illness caused by their treatment.

For the American military, hepatitis in the blood supply was not only an immediate problem, but also an impediment to long-term defense planning. On learning that the Soviet Union was building a nuclear arsenal, President Harry S. Truman directed federal agencies to formulate strategies for surviving a nuclear attack on the continental United States. According to the projections of defense planners, vastly increased supplies of blood and plasma would be critical.

The administration responded by revitalizing blood donation campaigns, relaxed during World War II disarmament, and by centralizing blood collection and distribution. The President's Office of Defense Mobilization set up a Subcommittee on Blood to coordinate voluntary donations, and to allocate blood products for military and civilian uses. The Truman administration ordered federal scientific agencies to find ways to enhance the supply and purity of blood products. At the government's behest, the medical division of the National Research Council convened a series of committees on blood-related issues.

By the time the blood sterilization project began, discussion of hepatitis contamination of the U.S. blood supply had reached the highest levels of government. In June 1951, just before investigators in the blood sterilization project started interventions with subjects, Secretary of Defense Robert A. Lovett informed President Truman that research was under way "to eliminate the causative agent of hepatitis (a liver disease) which has been found to contaminate all of our currently available stores of plasma." The Defense Department considered the situation a national emergency. Without a means for neutralizing the hepatitis B virus, America's entire blood program was in jeopardy.

The blood sterilization project was by design a collaboration of federal agencies. The AFEB funded the study and was one of several units exercising scientific oversight. Researchers at the NIH and its parent agency, the Public Health Service, prepared specimens and conducted the experimental interventions. The Bureau of Prisons provided access to inmates at three federal penitentiaries: facilities at McNeil Island, Washington; Lewisburg, Pennsylvania; and Ashland, Kentucky. The PHS had been delivering medical care to inmates at federal correctional facilities since the early 1930s; now it assigned a commissioned officer to each of the study sites to handle research-related activities and illnesses.

NIH's central role in the study was consistent with directives concerning its Cold War mission. The National Security Resources Board had charged the NIH with assisting in nuclear preparedness by serving as the research and development wing of the national blood program. The research agency oriented its intramural programs toward matters of national defense, particularly to the problem of hepatitis in blood. It allocated a large staff of NIH personnel and PHS commissioned officers to work on the blood sterilization project. Its Laboratory of Biologics Control and Laboratory of Infectious Diseases assumed responsibility for technical aspects of the study.

To lead the project, NIH officials chose John Oliphant, the PHS physician who had conducted virus transmission procedures for the agency's earlier hepatitis experiments at Lynchburg Colony. His role in those World War II studies had brought Oliphant notice and a meritorious promotion; but much of his subsequent service for the PHS was administrative. After the Lynchburg assignment, he served as associate director of the agency's Rocky Mountain Laboratory in Montana, and was then acting clinical director of a marine-service hospital in Seattle.

A broad swath of America's biomedical elite had input into the study's conduct through committees of the AFEB and NRC. Oliphant submitted progress reports to the AFEB, its Commission on Liver Disease, and the Commission's Committee on Allocation of Volunteers; he also provided regular research updates to the NRC Subcommittee on Sterilization of Blood and Plasma. These advisory panels allowed an array of government and university researchers to influence the project's direction.

Stokes was among the behind-the-scenes players. He headed an ad hoc NIH committee that, in December 1950, endorsed the study's conduct and recommended that Oliphant serve as lead investigator. Stokes also chaired the Committee on Allocation of Volunteers; Oliphant was a member and regularly attended its meetings.

The blood sterilization project took form during the winter of 1950–51. While the initial aim was to assess the effectiveness of ultraviolet rays for inactivating hepatitis virus in serum, over time the scope widened substantially. When irradiation failed to disable the pathogen, researchers tried other methods for sterilizing blood, such as heat and the application of chemicals, including sulfur-mustard compounds. And with a steady stream of subjects available for virus infection procedures, researchers piled on additional objectives beyond blood sterilization. In response to requests from university researchers, project scientists tested both serum from blood donors suspected of being hepatitis B carriers and hepatitis specimens grown in tissue media. The scale of the project made it difficult to manage, and the long distances between the NIH campus and the study sites were burdensome for investigators. Unwieldy from the outset, the study would soon become a debacle.

In February 1951, Oliphant relocated from Seattle to the NIH campus in Bethesda with a position on Biologics Control. He began full-time work on the project in May and within weeks was visiting research sites to enlist subjects. The McNeil Island Penitentiary newspaper, *Island Lantern*, recounted his recruitment pitch there.

According to the *Lantern*, Oliphant met with inmates to announce that PHS was seeking volunteers for a study that would involve being infected with hepatitis. He described the disease, its symptoms, and its risks. On the matter of hazards, he told inmates that recovery from hepatitis was usually complete within a month. But he "admitted frankly that fatalities *did* occur in two tenths of one percent of the cases." He added a statement that was new to hepatitis study recruitment narratives: "permanent disability as a result of infection occurs in one or two percent of infected cases."

The central terms of inmates' enrollment would be consistent with those in other hepatitis experiments with prisoners. Participating inmates would receive several types of compensation—the word used was "consideration." When the study was over, each would receive a Certificate of Merit and have a Statement of Testimony placed in his record. "There are definitely not any pardons," the *Lantern* reported, "but the Testimony *will* be considered in any parole action." Other provisions were more generous than was typical: for each week a prisoner was involved in the experiment, he would earn $2, and for each month, a five-day reduction in his sentence.

The *Lantern* story concluded with a bombastic appeal for recruits that combined an idealized depiction of medical research with a call for altruistic service. The recruits would be aiding in the defense of the country. Hepatitis was plaguing soldiers and the goal of the research was to find a way to control it. Participating prisoners would be medical heroes; the experiments would "advance the science of medicine another stride toward the ultimate goal of complete knowledge." Volunteers—Oliphant employed the routinely used term—would "contribute in a magnificent way toward that final goal. . . . Publicly honored or not, their reward will be the gratitude of generations to come." Subjects would be among the great warriors of medical science, "unsung heroes who allow themselves to be infected . . . to provide a clue for the baring of medical secrets."

Whether moved by the terms of participation or the accompanying rhetoric, inmates signed up in large numbers: NIH investigators reported enrolling 550 inmates from the three penitentiaries: 119 from Ashland, 217 from Lewisburg, and 214 from McNeil Island.

As was customary, subjects signed waiver and release statements. In documents for the blood sterilization project, enrollees attested that researchers had explained "the risks to my health of participation in this study" as well as "the potential benefits to humanity." The text continued: "I understand that I may become ill. I also understand that infectious hepatitis can in some cases cause fatal results. I hereby freely assume all such risks of participation in the investigation." A prison chaplain witnessed the consent process and affirmed that researchers had fully explained the study's procedures and risks. The witness statement read in part, "I am convinced of the applicant's complete understanding and willingness to participate in this study. I am confident that no duress of any kind was present in these proceedings."

Oliphant's team started human inoculations at the study sites in July 1951. The goal of the initial interventions was to specify the dosage of ultraviolet radiation needed to inactivate the virus. Researchers were hopeful that inconsistent results with use of irradiated blood and plasma were the result of differences in how irradiation was delivered. The inoculations were followed by a lengthy wait during the virus's months-long incubation period.

Outcomes from the initial inoculation procedures were available in late fall. When they arrived, the results were profoundly discouraging: large numbers of participants were contracting hepatitis and none of the irradiation methods protected subjects from illness.

In early December 1951, Oliphant presented a formal report of these inauspicious findings to the NRC's Subcommittee on Sterilization of Blood. NRC leaders sent word to the defense secretary's medical advi-

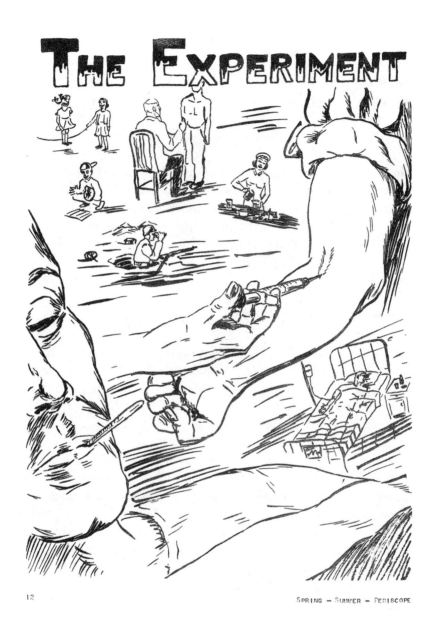

An inmate artist depicts the thoughts and experiences of hepatitis subjects at Lewisburg Federal Penitentiary. (Drawing by O. R. Tomlinson from the Lewisburg Prison publication, *Periscope.* Courtesy of Science, Industry & Business Library, The New York Public Library.)

sory committee stating that current methods of inactivating hepatitis in plasma were ineffective. The findings were deeply disheartening to military planners and a personal defeat for Oliphant. He had been the first to report that ultraviolet irradiation disabled blood-borne hepatitis. Now he was presiding over the upending of his earlier claims, with no alternative for controlling the blood-borne virus in sight. The failure had national consequences, and news of it was reaching the top echelons of government.

In late December, Oliphant began another round of experiments at Lewisburg, using materials irradiated with different equipment. He visited the West Coast study site in early January to oversee additional inoculations, some with specimens treated with sulfur-mustard compounds. He arrived back in Washington, DC, on January 10, 1952.

The next day, DC newspapers announced John Oliphant's unexpected and untimely death.

According to the *Washington Times-Herald*, the fifty-year-old researcher returned from McNeil Island in the late morning and told his wife he was going to his NIH office in Bethesda. That evening, family members found him asphyxiated in the garage of their home. The hood of the car was raised, and the garage doors were shut. According to press accounts, homicide detectives told reporters that Oliphant was apparently tinkering with the engine of his car when he was overcome by carbon monoxide gas.

From a distance, Oliphant's death certainly looks like a suicide; but the police ruled that it was an accident and the city coroner agreed. Records from a freedom-of-information inquiry to the PHS suggest that NIH personnel may have had a hand in how the incident was classified. When Oliphant's wife found her husband's body, she phoned his boss, the head of Biologics Control at NIH. He instructed her to call the police and an ambulance; he then went to the family's home and was the first physician to arrive. Correspondence reveals that among the concerns of Oliphant's superiors was the speedy allocation of death benefits for his widow and children. Two weeks later, the agency's newsletter, the *NIH Reporter*, published a brief notice of Oliphant's passing and expressed deep sorrow; it made no mention of the cause of death.

NIH officials moved swiftly to appoint a successor so that the blood sterilization project could proceed without interruption. Oliphant's replacement was Roderick Murray, assistant director of the Biologics Control Laboratory. Murray quickly assumed Oliphant's responsibilities and, on January 22, was meeting with members of Stokes's Committee on Allocation of Volunteers. By March, he was overseeing new rounds of inoculations. He would have the misfortune of being the responsible investigator when the deaths began among study participants—the first two resulting from inoculations performed while Oliphant was in charge.

Ruth Kirschstein worked as a research scientist under Murray's direction early in her career; she went on during the 1990s to become deputy director of the NIH. In an oral history interview from the later period, she described Murray as introverted, shy, and private. "He was a consummate South African gentleman," she recalled. "Everything you would expect of that apartheid society. He was elitist and very proud."

When faced with another emergency in 1955, NIH officials appointed Murray director of the Division of Biological Standards, a position he was reluctant to assume. Having that responsibility, Kirschstein said, was not something he had wished for or would enjoy; but "they told him he had to do it, and so he did." Murray may well have felt the same way about heading the blood sterilization project. There was certainly little to prepare him for what was about to unfold.

The fatalities among subjects began less than four months after Murray became lead investigator. The affected prisoners were white men between twenty-two and forty years of age. In each case, a penitentiary official announced the death, and one or more local newspapers reported the event, identifying the inmate by name. The first death occurred in May 1952 at McNeil Island Penitentiary. The deceased was Richard H. Higgins, thirty-three, who had less than six months left on a three-year sentence for interstate transfer of forged securities. The second death followed in early October: another McNeil Island inmate, thirty-nine-year-old Walter Harvey Wood, serving a four-year term for forged securities. Both men had recovered from what had been seen as a mild bout of hepatitis, but after some weeks' time had relapsed, with fatal results. Researchers biopsied the men's livers after their deaths; Murray described the results of Wood's procedure as a "picture of complete atrophy."

Prison officials expressed regret at the inmates' passing and praise for the men's contributions to medical science. The associate warden called Higgins "a real nice fellow ... we were all sorry to see him go." After Wood's death, Warden Fred Wilkinson voiced the opinion that prisoners of the nation were among its most patriotic groups. During the ongoing Korean War, more than thirty thousand American servicemen died from battle casualties. In Wilkinson's view, Wood had also "died in the service of his country."

Scientists addressed the fatalities at committees of the AFEB and the NRC, discussed the specimens used with Higgins and Wood, and detailed the course of their illnesses. At this point, the assembled researchers did not consider ending the experiments.

But in the second week of December, advisory panel members became alarmed on learning that two subjects at Lewisburg were comatose with fulminant hepatitis B. The two deaths at McNeil Island could be attributed to chance; with these additional life-threatening illnesses, scientists had to acknowledge a disturbing pattern. The AFEB sent Walter Havens and John Neefe to the Lewisburg prison to investigate the situation and provide additional medical support. Havens had been second-in-command at John Paul's wartime hepatitis infection program at Yale, and Neefe had served in a similar capacity at Stokes's program at the University of Pennsylvania. Both men had extensive experience treating patients with experimentally induced hepatitis. They examined the comatose inmates and conferred with Murray but could suggest no additional clinical interventions.

Several days later, one of the Lewisburg inmates pulled out of his coma. The other succumbed to multiple organ failure on December 15. His name was John F. Gavin, twenty-three years old, from Washington, DC. He had served one year of a sixteen-month to four-year sentence for breaking and entering.

Prison newspapers at McNeil Island and Lewisburg published page-long eulogies for the deceased inmates, informing the inmate populations that the men were heroes who had died making sacrifices for their country. The tribute to Gavin included a message from the research project's sponsors: "Officials of the Bureau of Prisons, the Public Health Service, and the Department of Defense express their sincere regrets on learning of John Gavin's death, and commend him for his courage and patriotism in that he has performed an outstanding service in aid of the defense effort and in helping further a defense project which holds promise for humanity." In a subsequent article, the Lewisburg prison newspaper, *Periscope*, declared, "John Gavin died as brave a death . . . as a soldier in Korea."

Prison papers also printed the roster of inmates who had served as subjects. The *Island Lantern* titled its acknowledgment of 214 research participants "Honor Roll." The *Periscope* listed the names of 175 men being recognized "in grateful appreciation of services as a volunteer in a research study of broad significance to the advancement of medical science and the ultimate benefit of mankind." At the bottom of this tribute were the signatures of four U.S. government officials, including the PHS surgeon general and the director of NIH.

With the third subject's death, scientists faced the fact that they had dramatically underestimated the experiment's hazards. The implications of their miscalculation reverberated through the biomedical community. Researchers had embarked on the blood sterilization project with a projected death rate; Murray disclosed these risk calculations at a meeting of the NRC's Blood Sterilization Subcommittee, stating: "The danger of possible fatalities was anticipated at the outset of these experiments and this possibility is always presented to the volunteer subjects. A fatality rate of 0.5% was considered to be the calculated risk. Thus far, there has been a fatality rate close to 3%."

Investigators had based their assessment of risk on past experience with commonly used hepatitis strains. They had sustained these strains by passing them serially through human subjects, procedures that may have attenuated the viruses. The inmates who died had received serum not typically used in hepatitis transmission studies. These men had been inoculated with serum from blood donors at the University of Pennsylvania that Neefe had identified as being what researchers were now calling "silent carriers": people with no history, signs, or symptoms of hepatitis, but whose donated blood generated the disease in recipients.

That unfamiliar specimens produced such deadly results underscored how little researchers understood about the full range of the hepatitis viruses. At professional meetings scientists voiced apprehension about a newly identified danger, which they referred to as "street viruses": blood-borne hepatitis strains of unknown pedigree and high virulence.

In the weeks following Gavin's death, multiple scientific committees considered the cause of the fatalities and addressed whether the blood sterilization project should be discontinued. Because the initial consensus was that the problem of hepatitis in blood was too urgent to abandon the research, none of the committees moved immediately to terminate the study.

They did, however, develop stricter guidelines for the project. In January 1953, Stokes's Committee on Allocation of Volunteers specified precautions for further transmission studies. Its members advised using only well-documented virus strains and limiting the age of subjects to under thirty. They also recommended upgrading medical facilities for treating severely ill subjects and requiring that participants be at locations close to scientists and medical emergency teams. Stokes's meeting minutes include the entry: "Even though no one likes to infect volunteers, the failure thus far to find a susceptible [animal] host and the importance of viral hepatitis make such action essential." However, the committee now wanted the express backing of the program's federal sponsors: "In order to proceed further, official approval should be obtained from the highest possible level."

A month later, the AFEB reaffirmed its support for virus transmission experiments. In early February 1953, board administrator Adam Rapalski said that, given the magnitude of the problem of hepatitis and the absence of other means of investigation, "well-considered studies on hepatitis using human subjects should be continued." But the board did mandate changes that downsized the project. It instructed NIH researchers to abandon work at McNeil Island and suspend experiments at the Ashland site, while still proceeding with additional blood sterilization studies at Lewisburg.

Yet another meeting took place on March 28, this one at the NIH and attended by military and PHS physicians. Murray prepared a packet of background material for the gathering. In mid-April he reported that a decision was pending about the future of the blood sterilization project from an unidentified high-level committee.

At this point, decision makers had a number of options; these included making further changes to the blood sterilization study, suspending it, or terminating it altogether. But in a dramatic change of course, the AFEB chose instead to terminate not only blood sterilization interventions but *all* human transmission experiments with hepatitis. During the late spring of 1953, the board informed researchers they would be permitted to complete human studies already under way, but a complete halt would go into effect as of June 30, 1954.

While available records provide no official rationale for the total retreat from human interventions, a great many documents speak to researchers' preoccupations in the months following the fatalities. Professional, intra-governmental, and international politics impinged on decisions about the program's future. Responses to the Nuremberg Medical Trial propelled some of the underlying dynamics.

On February 26, 1953, Charles Wilson, secretary of defense for the incoming Eisenhower administration, adopted the Nuremberg Code as a standard for department-sponsored human research. The issuing document became known as the Wilson Memo.

Planning for the policy had begun months earlier under Truman's defense secretary, Robert Lovett. In October 1952, Lovett's medical advisory committee, the Armed Forces Medical Policy Council (AFMPC), recommended that the department endorse Nuremberg principles. It did so at the urging of Stephen S. Jackson, assistant general counsel in the Office of the Secretary of Defense.

Historians have suggested that the new policy was an effort by a liberal wing within the Defense Department to bring its research practices in line with international legal standards, and to do so at a time when the agency was moving forward with an aggressive Cold War research agenda. Endorsing Nuremberg principles was compatible with the official U.S. position on human rights. The United Nations had released the Universal Declaration of Human Rights in 1948, and American representatives had promoted the measure. The declaration had no enforcement provisions; as one observer aptly noted, it was "intended to be a beacon, not a guide to actual behavior."

Human rights claims had become a feature of the contentious ideological struggle between the United States and its Soviet adversaries, and missteps in the arena of medical research could trigger comparisons to Nazi experimentation. As early as 1948, *Science News Letter* reported that a Soviet scientist had equated hazardous studies in American prisons with German concentration camp experiments; in this context, the Wilson Memo was an assertion of moral high ground directed toward potential detractors.

The Defense Department policy was likely also a response to recent developments in Europe, where medical associations were beginning to seriously address the matter of research ethics. An international medical congress meeting in Rome invited the pontiff to speak about ethical matters, and in September 1952, Pope Pius XII delivered an address on the boundaries of acceptable human experimentation. The crux of the pope's statement was that neither the interests of science nor of the community— and by extension, of the government—has unlimited moral precedence over the individual's best interests. Thomas Rivers later remarked of the pope's address, "That speech had a very broad impact on medical scientists both here and abroad."

The adoption of Nuremberg principles would have limited impact on the trajectory of government-sponsored research in the United States during the 1950s and 1960s. The Wilson Memo included significant caveats.

The final document contained explicit provisions allowing officials to approve human experiments with radioactive isotopes and with biological and chemical warfare agents—studies the Defense Department and other agencies were pursuing. And because the memo was classified "top secret," a good many university researchers receiving Defense Department funds were unaware that new rules were in operation. But AFEB leaders were well informed about the policy, and they were dismayed by its issuance. Given the recent hepatitis casualties, one provision in particular concerned them: "No experiment should be conducted where there is an a priori reason to believe that death or disabling injury will occur."

At a meeting in February 1953, AFEB president Colin MacLeod asked Defense Department attorney Stephen Jackson to clarify the implications of this provision. Jackson responded that a researcher had no right to conduct an experiment he knew would cause the death of a subject. However, if there was a chance but not a certainty that death would ensue, "the question of whether he proceeded with the experiment becomes a purely ethical and moral one—whether the end results he obtained would justify the means." It was a blunt and unembellished statement of the Defense Department's utilitarian views on the matter of human harm.

Defense leaders did not intend the Wilson Memo to impede human research with hepatitis. Indeed, officials were emphatic in their desire for the hepatitis transmission program to continue. Melvin Casberg, AFMPC administrator and assistant defense secretary for health affairs, "gave instructions that everything be done to insure that the hepatitis experiments proceed." But there was an important qualification: Jackson required that a statement be drawn up specifying that the scientific, ethical, and legal review and approval of such experiments be "firmly delegated to either the Armed Forces Medical Policy Council or the Armed Forces Epidemiology Board." This was to make sure "that the Secretary of Defense was not left 'holding the bag.'"

In short, the Defense Department urged investigators to continue with their research while at the same time insisting that medical scientists, not agency leaders, assume responsibility for the human consequences. If an experiment generated legal action or moral outrage, it was the researchers, and perhaps also advisory committee members, who would take the fall.

Casberg's instructions brought the matter of legal liability for experimental injuries into sharp focus. It was not the first time researchers had addressed this issue; in earlier discussions, liability was a subtext in questions about insurance for research participants. As elaborated earlier, in 1947, Stokes began lobbying the OTSG to allow AFEB researchers to purchase disability or life insurance for participants in hepatitis infection studies. Stokes argued that it was entirely proper that remuneration be available to injured subjects and urged that Congress allocate funds for this purpose. The topic was on the agenda for discussion at a 1948 AFEB meeting. Both scientists and Defense Department officials understood that the insurance under consideration would not only compensate injured subjects, it would also buffer researchers from lawsuits.

Government lawyers rejected investigators' requests for leeway to purchase life or disability insurance for research subjects, instead instructing scientists to rely on waiver clauses in consent documents and on their own liability insurance. The only exception to the rule of no compensation for research subjects was the coverage of burial costs for those who died in the course of experiments. The AFEB provided funds for Gavin's burial, with the payment deducted from Murray's research account.

The government's position on the use of waivers provided investigators little reassurance. In 1948, Cecil Watson, director of the Commission on Liver Disease, asked the law school dean at his University of Minnesota campus whether waiver clauses would protect scientists in the event of legal action. The dean's answer was that waiver provisions were unlikely to hold up in court, and that responsibility for injury to a research subject would fall on the individual scientist. If a subject died, it was even possible that the researcher could be charged with murder.

Watson shared this information with hepatitis researchers and the AFEB central board. The scientists were not happy with the Defense Department's refusal to allow the purchase of life or disability insurance for subjects; it left study investigators in legal jeopardy. But before the spate of inmate casualties, they thought it improbable that a hepatitis subject would be very seriously injured.

Scientists' legal vulnerability gained immediacy with events following the third hepatitis death, that of Lewisburg inmate John Gavin. An attorney in the NIH Office of Research Planning noted that "legal representatives were active" after that fatality. If a complaint was filed, it was apparently settled out of court, its terms undisclosed.

The threat of legal liability for injuries to human subjects clearly unnerved university researchers. Murray and his PHS colleagues were federal employees, so they could rely on government lawyers to handle litigation if it occurred. But the majority of hepatitis investigators were federal contractors, and would be on their own if sued. Given recent events, the possibility of legal action after a research casualty could no longer be dismissed as remote.

While scientists were troubled by their legal vulnerability, it was the use of children and disabled persons as human subjects that triggered outright dispute within their ranks. All participants in the blood steriliza-tion project were prison inmates; during the 1950s, neither American scientists nor their federal sponsors viewed incarceration as an obstacle to freely given consent. Jackson even proposed an amendment to the Wilson Memo stating that prisoners, except prisoners of war, could be used in human experiments. While this wording was not included in the final document, Jackson's proposal did reflect the biomedical elite's favorable views on the use of prisoners as research subjects.

But whether it was acceptable to enroll persons with diminished ca-pacity in dangerous experiments was a matter of open debate. The AFEB and OTSG had addressed these matters some years earlier with regard to Stokes's hepatitis infection studies with mental patients and institu-tionalized children. Neither body had restricted Stokes's recruitment from these subject pools. With the Defense Department's move to adopt Nuremberg principles, though, use of these groups in disease-inducing experiments would receive renewed attention.

In November 1952, a month after the AFMPC endorsed the forth-coming policy directive, AFEB president MacLeod wrote Stokes, saying that he wanted to be sure that "only those practices are being followed that would be agreed upon as not contravening ethical principles." Mac-Leod added: "I think it would be of greatest importance to discuss the use of the criminally insane, defectives, and other state wards." A month later, he urged Stokes to have the Committee on Allocation of Volun-teers go beyond discussion of scientific issues to critically evaluate each study's use of human subjects.

A blunt critic of Stokes now spoke up: Thomas Rivers, a member of the AFEB central board known for his stinging takedowns of other sci-entists. Rivers's reputation as a virologist and his position at the Rocke-feller Institute for Medical Research made him a formidable opponent. In early February 1953, Stokes wrote Watson (still chair of the Liver Disease Commission), complaining, "At a recent meeting he [Rivers] criticized privately our studies with children." Stokes did not specify the content of the criticism, but Rivers was a stickler on scientific matters and he disapproved of using disabled children in tests of virus strains. Elsewhere Rivers remarked that children were not free agents; the decision to be a research subject was made for them.

Stokes responded to Rivers's rebuke by dispatching an impassioned six-page statement to AFEB scientists defending the ethics of transmitting hepatitis to children. In it, he restated that he had obtained consent from the children's parents or guardians and insisted that the experiments were in the youngsters' best interests. He again argued that, like mumps and German measles, hepatitis was milder in children than adults. As he had done when facing pushback earlier, Stokes equated virus transmission with preventive medical treatment, and a bout of hepatitis with immunization. Stokes insisted it was common pediatric practice to arrange for youngsters to be exposed to illnesses like mumps and German measles at an early age to avoid complications that could arise if the illnesses occurred later. In short, Stokes was arguing that his hepatitis experiments with children were therapeutic in intent.

Stokes had a strong aversion to direct confrontations, and after Rivers had made him uncomfortable at AFEB meetings, Stokes asked Werner Henle, the Philadelphia project's senior laboratory scientist, to attend in his place. Henle stood his ground when Rivers interrupted him to dispute the team's research findings. About his encounters with Rivers, Henle observed: "As so often happens, bullies change their tune once one stands up to them."

Stokes's experiments with mental patients may have generated even greater consternation than his procedures with children. During and following the war, the OTSG had approved Stokes's program of virus transmission studies at Trenton State Hospital, knowing that the hospital director was testing whether inducing hepatitis alleviated patients' psychotic symptoms; hospital psychiatrists framed this as an alternative to infecting patients with malaria for therapeutic purposes. But the psychiatric community was moving on to new strategies for treating psychotic disorders. By 1953, mental hospitals were terminating use of malaria therapy and would soon be introducing psychotropic medications. The changes undercut any remaining medical justification for exposing psychotic patients to hepatitis.

The AFEB now asked Stokes to provide an accounting of his experimental procedures at Trenton State Hospital and their impact on subjects. A typescript in Stokes's archived papers reveals that 297 mental patients at the facility received hepatitis inoculations—nearly all of them hepatitis B—between 1944 and 1952. Not surprisingly, the outcomes failed to support the notion that contracting hepatitis improved a patient's psychiatric condition. The report also noted that 19 of the research participants developed tuberculosis after being inoculated with hepatitis and that the tuberculosis rate among subjects was substantially higher than in the institution as a whole.

Yet another consideration weighed on deliberations concerning the future of government-sponsored hepatitis research: judgments about the quality of the program's scientific work. Investigators projected a picture of medical progress when recruiting subjects and addressing lay audiences, but behind the scenes they told a different story. It was plain that the blood sterilization project had failed, and some within elite scientific circles judged the entire hepatitis program to be yielding unacceptably meager results.

Early in 1952—when it was clear that blood sterilization interventions were unproductive—a general in the Air Force Medical Corps who was an AFMPC member submitted a memo for the record exemplifying this stance. He pointed to the paltry gains despite the "great amount of time, money and research skill . . . applied to the problem of hepatitis." The recently discovered ineffectiveness of ultraviolet radiation only highlighted ongoing shortcomings of the AFEB's program. The general's memo concluded with the suggestion that perhaps it was time for a different group of scientists to pursue the research.

Several years later, investigators involved with the hepatitis program would express their own frustrations. Writing as the AFEB was about to resume hepatitis experiments, Yale researcher John Paul, who was still serving as director of the board's Virus Commission, lamented the postwar research trajectory. He noted that, after a rapid growth of information about the viruses during World War II, advances had ground to a halt, leaving basic questions as unanswered as they had been in 1942. Researchers had repeatedly tried to identify an animal model for hepatitis, isolate the viruses, find a stable growth medium, inactivate the pathogens, and introduce a viable immunizing agent; all these attempts had failed.

The critiques did not mention that significant strides were being made in preventing other major infectious diseases, but the research community was well aware of the comparisons. In combating polio, scientists had a long-standing animal model, a tissue culture medium introduced in 1948, and an effective immunizing agent: Jonas Salk's vaccine, successfully tested—initially on institutionalized children—during the early 1950s. In sharp contrast, researchers working with hepatitis had none of the basic tools needed to control these viruses.

In 1954, the board officially disbanded its Commission on Liver Disease and Stokes's Committee on Allocation of Volunteers. The Commission on Viral Infections under Paul's management was given oversight of remaining laboratory studies, which were to focus on propagating hepatitis in animals and tissue media. Murray stated later that no formal decision forbidding further virus transmission experiments had been made, but given past experience with deaths and injuries with hepatitis B, "any future study would have to be very carefully considered, and the results that one might hope to obtain would very clearly have to justify the risk." The failure of the blood sterilization project had damaged the Epidemiology Board's standing within the Department of Defense. And while the board would resume hepatitis infection experiments, it would never regain its previous cachet.

Stokes withdrew from hepatitis research a year before other AFEB researchers, and was uncharacteristically subdued about his departure. In late February 1953, within weeks of his last run-in with Rivers, Stokes shut down his research unit at Trenton State Hospital. Three months later, he informed the Trenton hospital director that he was leaving hepatitis transmission research; future work on hepatitis would focus on laboratory cultivation of the virus. For a decade, Stokes had managed the largest hepatitis infection project in the country; several times he had stated proudly that no deaths had resulted from his experiments. With the closure of the AFEB's entire hepatitis transmission program impending, Stokes walked away from what had been a major professional commitment, and turned his attention to other projects. He remained an active infectious-disease researcher through the late 1960s, collaborating next with Koprowski on testing strains of live polio vaccine.

Henle became lead investigator on a contract Stokes vacated, and for a time continued efforts to grow hepatitis in egg embryos and tissue cultures. Neefe, who supplied the serum that generated cases of fulminant hepatitis B, had been supporting himself with government contracts. But now the specimens he worked with were understood to contain dangerous "street viruses." Even if the AFEB had continued support for virus transmission procedures, human studies with these materials were now seen as too hazardous to continue. In 1955, Neefe left academic medicine.

Murray moved on to his position as director of the newly renamed Division of Biologics Standards, a post he held until 1972. According to Ruth Kirschstein, Murray's role in the biologics unit was largely that of a figurehead; the NIH director relied on the division's laboratory chiefs to make consequential decisions. Kirschstein referred to Murray's participation in the deadly hepatitis experiment as "an unfortunate experience."

Astonishingly, hepatitis researchers and their government sponsors weathered the turmoil without facing a public relations crisis. During the entire chaotic aftermath of the blood sterilization project, they were able to keep disputes in scientific circles hidden from the outside. The deaths of prisoners did attract attention from the press. In the early 1950s, media reports of casualties among healthy subjects participating in a variety of medical studies became more common. This coverage was remarkable for its absence of critical commentary; journalists were careful to provide depictions consistent with public support for the research enterprise.

In September 1953, the *Washington Post* ran a three-part series on government-sponsored human experiments in prisons, highlighting recent events in the hepatitis infection study. The series' author, science reporter Nate Haseltine, had spoken with senior PHS officials; they told him that more than two thousand prisoners were enrolled in government-sponsored medical experiments, sixteen hundred of them "in admittedly hazardous research." Publicity about the program, they worried, would "be twisted by the Communists for propaganda purposes. . . . Communists would like to picture American physicians as no better than the Nazi doctors who performed atrocities on unwilling subjects."

The *Post*'s coverage repeatedly emphasized that inmates had enrolled voluntarily and with full knowledge of the risks. Reporting on Gavin's death in December 1952, the paper's headline read, "Convict Told of Dangers in Fatal Tests." The article quoted his mother as saying, "I'm very proud of my boy, even if he was in the penitentiary. I think it was a very fine thing he did. It might help save some of our boys on the other side"—referring to soldiers in Korea. An editorial in the same issue of the *Post* lauded Gavin, who, "of his own free will . . . gave his life for the benefit of others."

Haseltine's more comprehensive articles returned to the theme of free will. Officials gave him access to Lewisburg inmates who had participated in hepatitis studies, and he reported that the prisoners resented any suggestion that they had been coerced or compelled to participate in the research. "All insisted unequivocally that the Public Health Service 'bent over backwards' to keep compulsion out of the program," he wrote. Inmates told him that patriotism was a reason they decided to be subjects. During World War II, conscientious objectors had been the public face of hepatitis infection research; now it was inmates depicted as willing subjects in dangerous experiments with viruses who embodied the ideal of service to country.

News outlets well beyond the capital covered the hepatitis fatalities, also describing the deceased men as making voluntary sacrifices motivated by patriotism. The accounts were public eulogies. Lewisburg's town paper, the *Union County Standard*, reported that Defense Department and PHS officials commended Gavin "for his courage and patriotism." The *Harrisburg Patriot-News* declared, "These men, ineligible for military duty, are doing their own kind of fighting for their country." The national magazine *American Mercury* commented on the hepatitis deaths, extolling inmates' voluntary service in the face of grave dangers.

This press coverage both reflected and helped shape public sentiment. Drawing from narratives provided by scientists and prison wardens, journalists wove accounts of medical research practices compatible with core American values of service, patriotism, and freedom of choice. And with the assistance of these celebratory press accounts, the research elite navigated the hepatitis deaths with its legitimacy fully intact. Haseltine quoted PHS officials as saying that "whether or not the use of prisoner volunteers in medical research will continue depends largely on public reaction." Human infection experiments with hepatitis had stopped for now. When the AFEB was ready to restart such studies, public sentiment about dangerous experiments with prisoner inmates would be no obstacle.

1956–1972 AND BEYOND

The whirlwinds of revolt will continue to shake the foundations of our nation until the bright day of justice emerges.

—MARTIN LUTHER KING JR., "I Have a Dream," August 28, 1963

There are no civil rights for young retarded adults when they are denied the protection of the state. . . . There are no civil liberties for those put in the cells of Willowbrook living amidst brutality. . . . Nobody who has ever raised a child would want him to live for a moment as thousands of mentally retarded now live.

—ROBERT F. KENNEDY, statement to the New York Legislative Committee on Mental Retardation, September 9, 1965

CHAPTER SEVEN

Science on the Cusp

T
HE HALT TO HUMAN experiments with hepatitis under way as
of June 1954 lasted only eighteen months. In the fall of
1956, the Armed Forces Epidemiology Board's new executive secretary, R. W. Babione, wrote a senior medical officer
in the navy saying that research aimed at preventing hepatitis was again
under way. It was "a fresh start" in addressing "one of the largest and
most frustrating communicable disease problems in the military." Researchers still had no animal model for hepatitis, so the fresh start meant
additional experiments with human subjects.

Two long-term hepatitis transmission projects began in 1956. One became notorious; the other remained largely unknown. Babione was referring to studies at Willowbrook State School, where scientists from New
York University conducted hepatitis infection experiments for seventeen
years, all with AFEB support. The investigators' focus was testing serum-
based preparations for generating immunity. Their subjects were disabled
children, including eight hundred youngsters admitted to a special research unit and then discharged into the institution's general population.
The research community would hail the experiments for yielding important scientific results. But the project was controversial from the outset,
with critics reviling the use of impaired children as human subjects.

The other project took place at Joliet Penitentiary, an Illinois state
correctional institution near Stateville prison. The pharmaceutical firm
Parke-Davis Co. initiated human studies at the Joliet facility with the

goal of developing a commercially viable vaccine. Its researchers grew viruses for the experimental immunizing agent in a potentially hazardous
tissue culture derived from human cancer cells. In 1962, a recently constituted liver disease advisory committee for the army surgeon general
allocated funds for the effort and, in 1966, that committee exerted control over the project. The growth medium Parke-Davis scientists were
using did not reliably sustain hepatitis virus and no vaccine materialized.
But before researchers abandoned testing, hundreds of prison inmates
had served as subjects for dangerous experimental interventions.

The two projects involved different technologies, had competing
oversight panels, and diverged in their success at meeting scientific goals.
They had in common that both were collective efforts. At Willowbrook
from the start and at Joliet after 1966, scientific advisory committees
made key decisions about what interventions would take place and at
what level of risk to research subjects. At both locations, researchers provided hepatitis specimens to other laboratories when asked, and tested
experimental materials with human subjects at the request of outside investigators. Willowbrook was a collective effort in another way as well:
when experiments there became the target of condemnation, AFEB scientists took measures to mobilize support for the research from leaders
of academic medicine. In response to criticism of the Willowbrook experiments, America's biomedical elite circled the wagons.

Research efforts during the late 1950s and early 1960s were a prelude
to profound change in both the science and the social context of experiments with hepatitis. In the late 1960s, an investigator from outside the
field of virology discovered an antigen of hepatitis B—a microbial particle that signals the virus's presence. It was a breakthrough that yielded
tools for controlling that pathogen's spread and also transformed hepatitis research. Studies at Willowbrook helped consolidate these gains. But
just as the science was leaping forward, resistance to the use of children in
virus transmission research redoubled. The failed experiments at Joliet
would be forgotten. Studies at Willowbrook would be remembered:
sharply divided sentiments about the use of child subjects would be their
contradictory legacy.

Studies at Willowbrook began like many earlier research efforts at
facilities housing intellectually disabled children. The institution's physician manager, Harold Berman, invited NYU researchers in to assist in
controlling infectious illnesses. At the time, Willowbrook was on its way

to becoming the facility in the United States with the largest population of persons with cognitive impairments. Admissions were soaring and many of the new entrants were young children. The postwar baby boom contributed to this trend, as did recommendations from medical practitioners. The advice many physicians gave to parents of children with developmental disabilities was that institutionalization was the best option for both the child and the family.

Willowbrook School was home to some of the New York State hospital system's most disabled patients: 39 percent were not ambulatory; 64 percent could not feed themselves; and 60 percent were not toilet-trained. Conditions at the institution deteriorated significantly during the 1960s, but even in the early 1950s, Willowbrook was plagued with over-crowding, staff shortages, and poor sanitation. Outbreaks of contagious illnesses were common.

When the research project started, Robert Ward, chair of pediatrics at NYU, was lead investigator and Saul Krugman, associate professor of pediatrics, was principal assistant. The two joined the Willowbrook staff as medical consultants and began their work by surveying infectious diseases in the sprawling institution's more than two dozen buildings. They found evidence of numerous contagious illnesses, including hepatitis, but their initial research concerned rubella (German measles). Then in 1956, at the urging of the AFEB's Commission on Viral Infections, they made hepatitis their primary focus and set up a dedicated hepatitis research unit. They added pediatrician Joan Giles to the team to serve as on-site investigator.

Midway through 1958, Ward left NYU for a job in Los Angeles and Krugman became senior scientist on the project, a position he held for the next fifteen years. Krugman's origins were modest. Born in the Bronx to Russian Jewish immigrants, he had completed his bachelor's degree—with time off to earn money for his education—at the University of Richmond; obtained his MD degree at the Medical College of Virginia; and completed an internship at a hospital in Brooklyn. After serving as an Air Corps flight surgeon during World War II, he had returned to New York City, where he joined the medical staff of Bellevue Hospital and worked his way up at NYU from instructor of pediatrics to professor to department chair in 1960. In the process, he earned a reputation among colleagues as a dedicated clinician and, as his hepatitis studies proceeded, an accomplished researcher. But condemnation of his experiments at Willowbrook would mark his career.

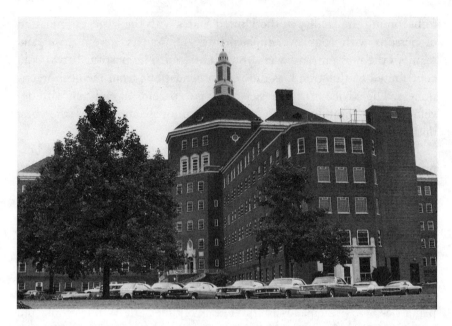

Willowbrook State School's administration building housed the hepatitis research unit on its fifth floor. (Photo by John Senzer. Courtesy of McGovern Historical Center, Texas Medical Center Library, *Medical World News* Photograph Collection.)

For the project's duration, Krugman and Giles admitted approximately forty-eight youngsters into the hepatitis unit each year—four groups of twelve. All of the child subjects entered Willowbrook through admission into the research unit and thus had no prior exposure to the hepatitis endemic at the facility. Over the course of the project, the NYU team conducted studies on nearly seventy groups of subjects composed of children between three and ten years of age. The NYU hepatitis research unit was located on the fifth floor of Willowbrook's immense, multi-winged Building 2, the facility's administration building. When a youngster's participation as a research subject ended, she or he transferred to one of the institution's units for children. Many of these were located in freestanding redbrick buildings with rooms containing large numbers of cribs or beds. Staff called these the "babies' wards." It was in one of these units where Diana McCourt—one of my interviewees—sought to have her daughter placed.

Available sources bearing on the experiments include scientific publications, investigators' progress reports, and minutes of the AFEB and its

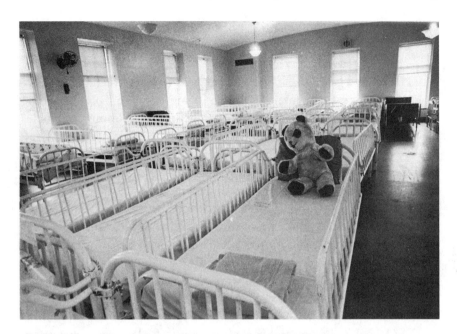

A babies' ward at Willowbrook State School in 1972.
(Courtesy of photographer Eric Aerts.)

Commission on Viral Infections (also called the Virus Commission). A
lone correspondence among the archived records offers a glimpse of one
small segment of Willowbrook subjects. In the 1960s, Krugman sent a
colleague blood test readings for ten enrollees along with descriptions of
the children. This group, whose median age was five and a half, com-
prised two girls and eight boys. Two of the boys were identified as
"Negro"; seven of the children, one girl and six boys, had Hispanic sur-
names—they were likely from Puerto Rican or Dominican families. Surviving materials provide very few details about Willowbrook's young
subjects more broadly—their race or ethnicity, exact ages, or the nature
of their impairments—and they are silent about what the children experienced as participants in the research.

The hepatitis studies at Willowbrook unfolded in three phases. Initially, the goal of NYU researchers was control of hepatitis A. They administered gamma globulin to patients and then released them, along
with uninoculated subjects, into the facility's general wards where hepatitis was widespread. The investigators found that a good number of inoculated enrollees later had subclinical cases of hepatitis, and that the
overall effectiveness of the procedure in suppressing disease varied with

the recipient's age, and the dosage and quality of the gamma globulin. The group's work on this approach produced a steady stream of scientific publications between 1957 and 1962.

The second phase expanded the group's purview to include transmission of hepatitis B. In interventions ongoing between 1964 and 1966, Krugman and Giles conducted nontherapeutic cross-immunity studies, exposing subjects to unmodified virus of both hepatitis A and B. These studies confirmed the findings of wartime researchers that two distinct strains of hepatitis existed. In the project's third phase, begun in the late 1960s, the team focused on generating immunity to hepatitis B. They tested the efficacy of both a specially produced hepatitis B immune globulin and heat-treated preparations of virus-containing serum.

Throughout the project, NYU researchers used hepatitis viruses endemic to Willowbrook that they judged to be mild. They transmitted hepatitis pathogens in one of two ways: they had subjects ingest material derived from the stool of sickened patients or they administered injections of virus-containing serum.

Their goal in the first and final phases was to find ways to generate immunity to hepatitis; a good number of their subjects did acquire at least temporary immunity. But to test the efficacy of their preventive measure, the researchers used one of two strategies: at first they released both treated and untreated children into Willowbrook wards where the youngsters would be exposed to endemic hepatitis; later, the investigators employed challenge inoculations, administering unmodified viruses to children who had received a protective measure (subjects in experimental groups) as well as those who had not (unprotected controls). In all phases of the project, the investigators either arranged to have susceptible subjects exposed to natural hepatitis or deliberately administered unmodified live virus to such children.

Critics of the Willowbrook experiments typically portray Krugman as the project's sole architect, targeting him for castigation. But AFEB records reveal a much more complex picture. The project's sponsors not only provided funding for the studies, they were also deeply involved in decisions about research procedures. Both the board's central committee and its Commission on Viral Infections reviewed and then approved or rejected plans for human interventions.

The Virus Commission had extensive discussions about the risks of the experimental procedures proposed for Willowbrook. When the project started, John Rodman Paul was chair of the Virus Commission. During the war, Paul had overseen hepatitis infection studies at Yale; at that time he also headed a polio research unit at Yale, where Robert Ward was an investigator. In the mid-1950s, the army repeatedly asked the AFEB to resume human experiments with hepatitis B. But after three deaths in the blood sterilization project, commission scientists, including Paul, were wary, and during the 1950s, a majority of the body's members opposed the use of this strain at Willowbrook. NYU investigators refrained from conducting experiments with hepatitis B during the first eight years of the project.

What the Virus Commission did permit at the outset was human studies with hepatitis A virus extracted from Willowbrook residents that researchers had determined generated only mild illnesses. The NYU investigators began transmission procedures with hepatitis A only after the commission had given its unanimous approval and the AFEB's central committee had concurred.

The commission was also willing to make Willowbrook subjects available for interventions with specimens from outside researchers that it viewed as having low risk and high scientific value, particularly those originating from trusted investigators. In 1959, William McD. Hammon—who had replaced Paul as Virus Commission director—pointed to "a back-log of high priority [hepatitis] projects" needing human subjects for testing. One of these involved a human embryonic liver culture developed by the highly regarded scientist John Enders. Hammon noted that the tests, involving the same virus strain already in use, fell "within the scope of other work now in progress at Willowbrook." The Virus Commission approved the proposed studies and forwarded its recommendation to the central committee, which agreed; these would be studies employing "a benign strain of the virus to which the population is already being naturally exposed."

But the commission rejected other proposed interventions it judged to be unduly hazardous. In the spring of 1958, its members discussed allowing experiments with hepatitis virus grown in a tissue culture called Detroit-6, which was made from human bone marrow that was likely cancerous. Scientists at Parke-Davis were claiming success in transmitting hepatitis grown in this medium to subjects at Joliet. At least one Defense Department scientific consultant wanted the NYU researchers to undertake tests at Willowbrook of virus endemic to the institution that had been cultivated in the Detroit-6 cell line.

The AFEB refused to grant approval for use of the new medium at Willowbrook. Its members knew that Robert McCollum, a researcher in

Paul's department at Yale, had tried repeatedly without success to replicate Parke-Davis's work with the Detroit-6 cells. It remained to be seen
whether other laboratories could reproduce Parke-Davis's work. AFEB
scientists had other misgivings. Investigators who introduced the De-
troit-6 line reported that it likely contained metastasized cancer cells.
While cell lines harvested from human tumors could be very useful in
laboratory work with viruses, many researchers considered them unsuit-
able as a medium to grow viruses for vaccine production. Among other
dangers, growth materials of this type might contain unidentified cancer-
causing pathogens that could be transferred to recipients through the
immunizing agent.

Minutes of the Virus Commission record the outcome of the panel's
deliberations: "The use of Detroit-6 cells even with Willowbrook viruses
was not to be sponsored by the Commission. The promise did not match
the possible risk." Thomas Francis Jr., at that time AFEB president, was
among those rejecting the proposal. On the matter of human experiments with the Detroit-6 cell line at Willowbrook, Francis made his
opinion plain: "The probable risk is too great to be ignored."

The involvement of AFEB scientists in experiments at Willowbrook
went beyond determining allowable procedures. The board also actively
defended the project against detractors. The studies generated dissention
from the start, with members of the medical profession, particularly
practicing clinicians, voicing most of the early complaints. The AFEB
moved repeatedly to counteract objections raised by critics and also to
anticipate further opposition.

The initial grievance was a letter in the *New England Journal of Medicine*
appearing in August 1957, even before the project's first full journal publication. In June of that year, Ward and Krugman delivered a presentation on
studies with gamma globulin and live virus at the annual pediatrics meetings. *Scope Weekly*, a newsletter for physicians distributed by Upjohn Co.,
carried a brief description of their conference report. A Baltimore internist,
John De Hoff, read the notice in *Scope* and wrote in protest to the *New England Journal*. De Hoff insisted that "the feeding of living virus to nonimmune children in an institution" showed "lack of feeling for them as people
to be cared for." He went further, declaring that "work with live viruses on
'mental defectives' smacks of similar work in Nazi Germany."

AFEB scientists, offended that the prestigious medical journal had
printed a condemnation of studies at Willowbrook, responded by orga-

nizing a show of support for the experiments. The Virus Commission instructed Ward and Krugman to immediately submit a scientific paper to the *New England Journal*, which they did in short order. Meanwhile, Paul had two AFEB-affiliated scientists contact the *Journal*'s editor. According to Paul, "The suggestion was made, with which their Board of Editors agreed, that an Editorial be written to appear in the same issue of the journal in which the paper by Dr. Ward and his colleagues appeared."

In February 1958, the *New England Journal* published the scientific article from Willowbrook investigators and the accompanying editorial. The research paper had a feature not typical in journal articles: Ward, Krugman, and Giles included a seven-paragraph justification for the study's conduct. They stated that parents had consented to their children's participation; the pathogens transmitted were a local, benign strain of virus; experimentally induced illnesses were mild; the subjects received excellent medical and nursing care; and the studies were approved by the AFEB and New York State Department of Mental Hygiene. Furthermore, the interventions were aimed at controlling a disease widespread at the institution. Commentary from the *Journal*'s editors emphasized the study's scientific contributions. The editors commended the researchers for giving careful thought to the ethics of conducting illness-inducing experiments and for providing a frank discussion of their reasons for proceeding.

The *Journal*'s handling of the Willowbrook team's 1958 publication inaugurated a pattern. Editorial commentary praising the project's scientific work would accompany many of the group's major publications. And with encouragement from the Virus Commission, Krugman would expand discussion in research papers of rationales for conducting virus transmission studies at Willowbrook. Some of these would feature lengthy accounts of the process for obtaining parental consent.

Meanwhile, additional complaints followed De Hoff's: these were delivered as letters to Willowbrook researchers or to the facility's manager. In July 1959, Augusta McCoord, a researcher in pediatrics at the University of Rochester, raised questions about the ethics of experiments at Willowbrook. In January 1960, in response to the *Journal* article, J. H. Hutchinson, an internist in St. Louis, sent a letter of protest to Willowbrook's director. Hutchinson declared that deliberately inducing hepatitis in institutionalized children was wrong. He also described the studies as little more than a repetition of work done thirteen years earlier. Even if the disease was mild, "the incidence . . . of post-hepatitic cirrhosis as a long-term sequela of childhood hepatitis is not known. . . . We have a moral responsibility as to the type of research we do on human beings." The early objections to hepatitis studies at Willowbrook came from outside prestigious research circles, particularly from practicing physicians who as a group were becoming more willing to push back against the profession's academic elite.

Krugman responded to Hutchinson in a letter to Willowbrook's director emphasizing the scientific importance of the project and the unanimous endorsement of the AFEB, which was, he reminded the reader, composed of internationally recognized scientists. "We too," he retorted, "are keenly aware of our moral responsibilities. This study was not undertaken lightly."

The commission sent the letters of protest and Krugman's defense up the organizational ladder to the Office of the Surgeon General–Army and higher echelons within the Department of Defense. At the commission's recommendation, Krugman included ethical justifications for studies with disabled children at Willowbrook in grant renewal narratives submitted to the Army Medical Department. In March 1960, after the arrival of Hutchinson's letter, Virus Commission director Hammon made it clear that AFEB support for the studies at Willowbrook was unequivocal. Hammon wrote: "This matter of carrying on hepatitis experiments at Willowbrook has received most careful consideration on repeated instances by the Commission and by the Board, and none of us has any misgivings regarding the ethical aspects. We feel that the gains to the institution itself alone in cases already prevented have established its value and the potential gains in [the] future there and elsewhere are even further justification."

The AFEB also took steps to ensure that protests did not undermine cooperation from New York State officials. In May 1963, when Harold Berman was about to retire as Willowbrook director, the Virus Commission arranged for the board to write the New York State Commission on Mental Health underscoring the significance of the project and its achievements. "This is to counteract any complaints, or letters the Commissioner may have received in the past against the studies, so that he will be aware of the benefits and hopefully, will allow the program to continue under the new Director."

The extensive ethical justifications in Willowbrook publications were unprecedented; they stood in sharp contrast to how Stokes had handled experiments with mental patients and developmentally disabled children during the late 1940s and early 1950s. In scientific papers, Stokes with-held information about potentially controversial experiments, typically concealing the use of impaired subjects in disease-inducing procedures. Institutional managers helped suppress reports of controversial experiments, and members of the mainstream press did not attend scientific meetings in an effort to gather information on ongoing research. Only leaders in the AFEB and OTSG knew the extent of Stokes's use of disabled children and adults in his hepatitis infection research.

With experiments at Willowbrook, concealment may not have been an option. By the early 1960s, medical press outlets were more numerous and diverse. They included pharmaceutical newsletters—*Scope Weekly* among them—and independent news magazines for practicing clinicians. These publications obtained information about research developments from professional and scientific sources without consulting the parties being covered. Among the Willowbrook investigators' intentions in their scientific papers was to highlight the positive effects their interventions had for controlling hepatitis at the institution. But the team's elaborate justifications did not always have their intended impact. Indeed, these statements may have served to inflame critics rather than mollify them.

No comparable ethical controversy accompanied hepatitis infection studies at Joliet. Parke-Davis hoped to patent an immunizing agent against hepatitis and, in part for this reason, early studies at the Illinois prison proceeded in secrecy. According to the Joliet-Stateville warden (one warden directed both correctional facilities), the project took place in such "a hush-hush atmosphere" that only the researchers and prison personnel knew of its existence.

Parke-Davis Co. was a well-established producer of pharmaceuticals and biologics at the time it launched the human testing of hepatitis strains. Based in Detroit, it was one of two firms that supplied virus preparations for field trials of Salk's polio vaccine in 1954, and one of five that produced the immunizing agent for general use after its formal approval in 1955. The Salk vaccine was made from poliovirus grown in an animal-based tissue culture and then inactivated. The proliferation of new cell lines in the mid-1950s raised hopes that culture-based vaccines for other viral diseases were on the horizon.

Initial laboratory studies suggested that the Detroit-6 cell line sup-ported growth of several virus strains. W. A. Rightsel and I. W. McLean, in the Parke-Davis microbiology division, spearheaded efforts to cultivate hepatitis in the new medium. In 1956, they reported in *Science* that hepatitis viruses produced morphological changes in the Detroit-6 cell line that suggested an invasion of pathogens.

The next step was to see if the cultivated viruses generated clinical symptoms of hepatitis when administered to human subjects. For this, Parke-Davis scientists collaborated with Joseph Boggs, a pathologist at Chicago Children's Hospital and Northwestern University Medical School. It was Boggs who arranged with Illinois prison officials to conduct transmission studies at Joliet with hepatitis grown in the Detroit-6 culture. While it is unclear precisely when Boggs began studies at the prison, they were well under way in June 1959.

Boggs later shared with army-sponsored scientists a very brief account of subject recruitment at Joliet. He wrote that participants were told both verbally and in writing about the risks of acute and chronic hepatitis. They received financial remuneration similar to what an inmate could earn over an equivalent period of time working in a prison shop. The men ranged from twenty-one to thirty-eight years of age. Several listings of enrollees for particular interventions classified between 25 and 44 percent of the participants as "N" for Negro; the rest were categorized as "W."

During the summer and fall of 1961, the Parke-Davis group broke from its pattern of concealment, making its work public—briefly but with great fanfare. The researchers announced—incorrectly, it turned out—that they were on the verge of introducing a hepatitis vaccine. According to their statements, Joliet inmates receiving tissue culture–grown hepatitis A virus developed symptoms of the disease; then, when investigators passed the virus serially through Detroit-6 culture before inoculating participants, subjects developed immunity without clinical symptoms.

Boggs divulged his auspicious findings at the American Medical Association meetings in June, and McLean presented laboratory results at meetings of the American Public Health Association (APHA) in November. A scientific paper appeared in the *Journal of the American Medical Association* in September. Meanwhile, major newspapers declared that the Parke-Davis group had isolated and attenuated the hepatitis virus and that a vaccine for the disease was imminent. *Life* magazine ran a story about hepatitis that included a depiction of Boggs's work at Joliet as groundbreaking.

AFEB Virus Commission scientists reacted to these events with chagrin and more than a little skepticism. They had not forgotten that five years earlier, Robert McCollum had tried without success to replicate the group's laboratory work. Now he was a commentator on McLean's APHA paper. In a letter forwarded to Hammon at the Virus Commission after the meetings, McCollum described McLean's presentation as disjointed, piecemeal, and illogical. McCollum added that Parke-Davis researchers had been withholding distribution of their current cell line for close to a year.

But if AFEB researchers were unconvinced that the group's claims were reliable, military officials considered a possible route for preventing hepatitis as too urgent to forgo. For army medical officers, the problem of hepatitis remained front and center, and they were eager to expedite the introduction of a new immunizing agent.

The Army Research and Development (R & D) Command moved to press forward on developing a hepatitis vaccine. This effort would have two components. One was work on cell lines for growing the viruses for vaccine production. The other was evaluating etiological agents of hepatitis—what scientists called "candidate viruses"—that might be included in an immunizing agent. The strategy had been effective in developing multi-strained polio vaccines, and army scientists were hopeful it would speed progress on a hepatitis vaccine. Many of the pathogens proposed for use in a liver disease vaccine were strains of hepatitis A; others were apparently hepatitis B.

The army now set up a new administrative structure to coordinate hepatitis research efforts. An Advisory Committee on Liver Disease, reporting to the army surgeon general, was to manage research protocols and make recommendations to the R & D Command concerning research funding. The chair of the advisory committee was Hans Popper, chief pathologist at New York City's Mount Sinai Hospital. Developing a tissue culture–based hepatitis vaccine would be one of the committee's primary objectives.

Popper's committee was more aggressive than the AFEB Virus Commission in pursuing Defense Department goals; the new panel quickly became the center of gravity for government-sponsored hepatitis research. During the 1960s, the Liver Disease Committee would have grant-approval power over a growing budget and an expanding roster of projects. Ongoing AFEB projects would continue, but the long-existing board was becoming increasingly marginalized.

The army's determined push for a hepatitis vaccine took place against the backdrop of escalating international Cold War conflict. East Germany constructed the Berlin Wall in 1961, the Cuban missile crisis unfolded in 1962; in 1965, U.S. troops were on the ground in Vietnam and would remain there until 1973. Under the presidencies of John F. Kennedy and Lyndon Johnson—1961 through 1968—the United States implemented targeted increases in defense spending. Government-sponsored medical science benefited immensely from this trend. Between 1958 and 1968, army funding for medical research multiplied five-fold.

If budgetary allocations provided resources, America's involvement in yet another war heightened pressure for a solution to the problem of hepatitis among soldiers. In the mid-1960s American service personnel in Vietnam were contracting hepatitis, mostly hepatitis A. But by then, the move to accelerate hepatitis vaccine development was already under way; it began with the 1961 announcement of Parke-Davis researchers that they were on a sure path for producing an immunizing agent.

In 1962, the R & D Command awarded a three-year renewable contract to the Parke-Davis microbiology division to expand work on candidate viruses and cell lines for growing hepatitis pathogens. The company negotiated a provision allowing it to retain ownership of a resulting vaccine patent. Meanwhile, the Liver Committee arranged for subjects at Joliet to be available for other interventions. Marcel Conrad, a colonel and career scientist at the Walter Reed Army Institute of Pathology, collected serum from soldiers still stationed in Korea who had contracted hepatitis and brought the specimens back to the United States for testing as candidate viruses. Boggs agreed to conduct experiments with these materials on prisoners at Joliet and, in 1964, he received a separate research contract for that purpose.

With the Army Medical Department now supporting research at Joliet, Conrad and the Liver Committee got a close look at Boggs's research methods—or, more accurately, the lack of them. Army scientists were dismayed to find that Boggs was performing no safety tests on viral specimens and was allowing inoculated subjects to mingle with the general prison population; this meant that inoculated subjects might have been infecting inmates who were not involved in the research, and also that endemic hepatitis at the facility might have been influencing study outcomes.

When Boggs's contract came up for yearly renewals beginning in 1965, the R & D Command was in a quandary. The Liver Committee was increasingly dissatisfied with his work. One member complained that, after more than a decade of human experiments, the Joliet project had "failed thus far to be productive of anything other than confusion and doubt." But military medical officials considered the research too important to abandon. So long as there was a chance the project might lead to an immunizing agent, the Liver Committee saw "no way out" of further renewals.

In 1966, the Liver Committee took over research efforts at Joliet. It set up a steering committee to design and oversee research interventions at the prison. That committee imposed experimental controls and required an army medical officer to be at the prison when studies were under way. It instituted safety tests and procedures for isolating subjects. The army began analyzing biopsy specimens taken from inmates who developed symptoms. Meanwhile, the Liver Committee brought in Joseph Melnick, a Yale-trained PhD virologist, to raise the level of the project's scientific conduct. He undertook laboratory work aimed at renewing the Detroit-6 cell line. Conrad, Melnick, and Boggs proceeded with the testing of candidate viruses, including specimens from Willowbrook, with inmates at Joliet. But even with improved research methods and the involvement of trusted investigators, basic problems with the Parke-Davis cultures could not be overcome.

A hepatitis vaccine was not in the offing. The Detroit-6 cell line did not perform as researchers had hoped; after repeated passages, the viruses became unstable and research results unpredictable. Biopsy results from prisoners inoculated with the cultivated pathogens indicated that the microbes being grown were not hepatitis. Parke-Davis scientists achieved no better outcomes with other cell lines. Like chick embryo cultures and blood sterilization efforts in the early postwar years, human tissue cultures of the late 1950s and early 1960s turned out to be yet another blind alley. Meanwhile, fifteen Joliet inmates had undergone invasive liver biopsies and the researchers had exposed hundreds of prisoners not only to live viruses but also to a potentially cancer-inducing growth culture. A cumulative record of Joliet subjects that Boggs compiled in 1969 listed more than three hundred participating inmates. No effort was made to determine long-term health outcomes for these research participants.

At Willowbrook during the mid-1960s, Krugman and Giles undertook a major change in focus: their future work would involve human experiments with hepatitis B. Scientists understood human studies with this strain to be more hazardous than those with hepatitis A. The scientific community had not forgotten the fatalities that had occurred a decade earlier from the blood sterilization project. Nonetheless, sentiment favoring the resumption of human experiments with the blood-borne virus was growing. Hepatitis B in the U.S. blood supply remained a serious and intractable public health problem, with as many as thirty thousand Americans per year developing jaundice from donated blood. In the fall of 1964, the Committee on Plasma and Plasma Substitutes of the National Research Council discussed restarting experiments with hepatitis B. The NRC's Division of Medical Sciences reported that the OTSG was open to considering research proposals involving human transmission of hepatitis B. Scientists were now looking for low-risk openings to begin such experiments anew; significantly, pediatric specialists believed hepatitis B to be a less severe disease in children than in adults.

The NYU team's work with the B strain at Willowbrook started with the observation that some children known to have had hepatitis A were getting second attacks of hepatitis. Krugman and Giles collected "second-attack serum" and began inoculation studies with what they assessed to be a mild strain of serum hepatitis present at Willowbrook. Their experiments were similar to the cross-immunity studies Army Epidemiology Board researchers had conducted during World War II. NYU investigators inoculated child subjects multiple times with two varieties of hepatitis—MS-1 (hepatitis A) and MS-2 (hepatitis B)—both endemic to Willowbrook residents. Their findings confirmed the existence of two immunologically distinct virus strains.

Krugman and his AFEB sponsors anticipated that the experiments would provoke objections and took measures to affect the work's reception. With their previous studies of gamma globulin, the NYU investigators had published results of early experiments, generating a series of interrelated articles. Now they delayed publication until they had completed a sequence of seven studies and the full scientific implications of the research were clear.

A report detailing two years of experimental interventions appeared in *JAMA* in 1967. The authors included extensive justification for the studies' conduct in the *JAMA* paper, stating that they had used only children "whose parents gave written consent after being informed of the details, potential risks, and potential benefits of the investigation." They listed multiple entities that had approved the experiments: the NYU Committee on Human Experimentation, the New York State Department of Mental Hygiene, and the AFEB. They insisted the work was consistent with the 1964 Declaration of Helsinki. An editorial appeared in *JAMA* accompanying the scientific paper that praised the work for providing definitive proof of two different strains of hepatitis; this was a contribution "that would have been impossible without the judicious use of human beings in carefully controlled experimental studies."

Willowbrook researchers were not the first to differentiate hepatitis A and B; World War II investigators had done so before them. But because Krugman and Giles drew their specimens from the same institution—indeed, from the same patient—their studies eliminated any doubt that the two virus strains were distinct entities. Their work also had practical importance for the research community in that Willowbrook investigators could now provide other laboratories with serum containing identified hepatitis strains (MS-1 or MS-2) of known virulence. Scientists considered the Willowbrook strains to be "pedigreed" specimens.

Krugman and Giles moved on to studies aimed at creating immunity to hepatitis B. Their strategies included administering heat-treated or boiled serum known to contain the B pathogen. After inoculating child subjects with the altered serum, they exposed children in both experimental and control groups to the unmodified MS-2 virus. In work published during 1970 and 1971, they were the first to report consistent success in immunizing against hepatitis B.

In the late 1960s, scientific developments outside the community of virus researchers fundamentally altered the study of hepatitis. In 1965, Baruch Blumberg, a geneticist studying variations in serum proteins across populations, reported the discovery of a blood-borne particle he called Australia antigen. Several research teams identified the particle as a component of the hepatitis B virus. Krugman and Giles confirmed its presence in MS-2 but not MS-1 serum. Scientists would soon understand Australia antigen to be the hepatitis B surface antigen, a noninfectious particle accompanying the highly infective virus core.

Investigators had tried for years to find a means to eliminate hepatitis B from the blood supply. Now bioassay techniques for identifying B surface antigen provided such a tool. By 1971, blood banks were using screening tests to identify hepatitis B carriers, permitting removal of that virus from stores of blood and plasma.

Researchers had long assumed that virus grown in cell lines would be the basis for hepatitis vaccines. This would be the case for immunizing agents against hepatitis A. Initial progress on this front came with the creation of an animal model (marmoset monkeys) for hepatitis A in 1967, and a reliable growth medium (fetal-monkey kidney cells) in 1979. In the early 1990s, Merck, Sharp & Dohme obtained a license for an inactivated hepatitis A vaccine made from tissue culture–grown virus.

With no available cell line for sustaining hepatitis B, scientists employed a novel approach in designing the first hepatitis B vaccine. It was composed of hepatitis B surface antigens harvested from human carriers and then sterilized. Blumberg envisioned this vaccine strategy, and Maurice Hilleman at Merck Laboratories navigated the technical procedures involved in production. Licensed in 1981, the immunizing agent was in use until the late 1980s, when a recombinant-DNA vaccine supplanted it. The original preparation was unique; it was the only vaccine to have been produced from the blood of individuals who were infected with a virus.

While Krugman and Giles's preparations were not the basis for a commercially distributed immunizing agent, their work demonstrated that it would be possible to make a vaccine from the serum of hepatitis carriers. Krugman later described his heated serum as "the first prototype inactivated hepatitis B vaccine." Colleagues called it "proof of principle." Hilleman and Krugman both received a prestigious Lasker Public Service Award in 1983 for contributions toward a hepatitis B vaccine. Blumberg won a Nobel Prize in medicine in 1976 for discovering Australia antigen.

During the 1970s, research on blood-borne hepatitis took a new direction. With hepatitis B no longer in the blood supply, the incidence of hepatitis from donated blood declined significantly; but a level of post-transfusion hepatitis persisted. This led to the recognition of yet another strain of hepatitis, non-A, non-B—what scientists would later call hepatitis C.

Meanwhile, increasingly sophisticated bioassay techniques yielded new insights into immunological processes underlying hepatitis B infections and the carrier status. Researchers would soon learn that children are considerably more likely than adults to become hepatitis B carriers; this would apply to the child subjects of Willowbrook. But in the heady years after the discovery of Australia antigen, investigators were focused on scientific openings, not on long-term harms from earlier transmission studies.

Identification of the B antigen infused the research community with a sense of possibility. John Enders spoke elegantly about the impact of Blumberg's work: "After a long and arid period, a new and exhilarating phase in the study of hepatitis has begun. The discovery of Australia antigen came like an unexpected shower on desert soil." The enthusiasm was palpable. Addressing an NRC committee in September 1971, McCollum

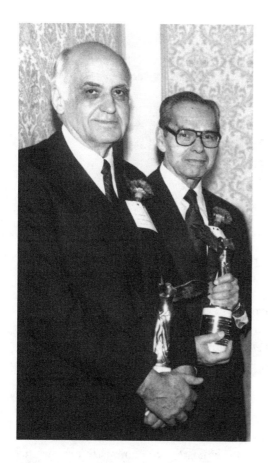

Maurice Hilleman and Saul Krugman (*right*) hold their 1983 Albert Lasker Public Service Awards for work on vaccines for hepatitis B. (Courtesy of the Lasker Foundation.)

described an explosion of interest in work with hepatitis pathogens: "In summer of 1969 we held a small meeting that brought together some 25 to 30 people who could be identified as having even put hands on the Australia antigen, and today if we tried to form such a meeting, I guess we would not be able to get them in any auditorium available to us." Hepatitis viruses had confounded scientists for decades; now researchers were mining the pathogens' secrets, and a new wave of investigators wanted in on the action.

The brief span from the late 1960s to the early 1970s was a watershed moment for the science of hepatitis; it was also a turning point in moral sentiment about human experimentation. The research field was becoming productive and exciting just as protests against studies at Willowbrook were turning vitriolic—and the two streams of events were about to collide.

CHAPTER EIGHT
Backlash

DRAMATIC CONFLICT OVER THE Willowbrook experiments erupted in April 1972 at the American College of Physicians (ACP) annual meetings in Atlantic City. The ACP was bestowing Krugman with an award for distinguished contributions to preventive medicine, citing his work with gamma globulin for controlling hepatitis A and his contributions toward a hepatitis B vaccine. But the honorary convocation was far from celebratory. The Medical Committee on Human Rights (MCHR) had organized a protest; as Krugman rose to receive his award certificate, 150 demonstrators shouted charges against him and some pressed forward, intent on storming the stage. The proceedings came to a halt as police dragged the intruders away.

Krugman and his wife had had an unnerving brush with dissidents earlier in the day. In the hallway outside their hotel room, a scuffle had broken out between protesters and security officers. When it was time to leave for the award ceremony, hotel personnel escorted the Krugmans out of the building through the basement; a police car drove them to the conference venue.

Demonstrators hounded Krugman for the better part of that year. In March, the MCHR installed daily picket lines outside the entrance to Bellevue Hospital, where the NYU Pediatrics Department had its offices. In October, dissidents organized a protest session at the New York meetings of the American Academy of Pediatrics. On his way to deliver an address to a conference in San Francisco, Krugman had to walk through a double line of picketers condemning his work. About this time in his life, he later remarked, "It was a very traumatic period, to put it mildly."

The clash at the ACP award ceremony was emblematic of unprecedented upheaval within American medicine over conducting risk-laden human experiments. Members of the biomedical elite continued to staunchly defend Krugman's work. Expert advisory committees had approved his experimental procedures, and the studies had yielded important results. His successes represented the research community's aspirations and hard-won achievements. But his detractors were adamant that Krugman's use of child subjects was unethical. It was a clash between the old guard of biomedicine and a new breed of progressively minded physicians, between long-standing research practices and emerging standards of conduct.

Hepatitis infection studies at Willowbrook ended in 1972. By that time, dissidents had defined these and other now-contested experiments as research abuses, and the press was covering and amplifying that message. Explosive conflict internal to biomedicine was a central feature of the complex events that changed public discourse about human experimentation and ushered in new rules for its governance. Underlying these developments were both pressures from outside medicine and altered dynamics within.

For a quarter century, America's biomedical elite had sustained a narrative that legitimized even highly injurious human experiments. Its members crafted accounts that resonated with wartime and Cold War ideologies and with the viewpoints of leaders of the multiple institutions that opened their doors to medical researchers. In these portrayals, risk-laden studies were crucial for advancing disease eradication and bolstering national defense; conscientious objectors and prisoners who participated in these studies were willing volunteers making heroic sacrifices for the common good. Mainstream newspapers and magazines disseminated stories about the altruism and patriotism of these subjects, while scientists kept disease-inducing interventions with impaired persons largely out of sight. With help from a deferential press, the biomedical elite controlled the public conversation about human experimentation and sustained widespread support for the research.

But the world around biomedicine had changed. In the 1960s and early 1970s, America underwent major cultural realignments. Activists challenged the authority of government and of established institutions and professions. Growing disaffection with the war in Vietnam eroded support for Cold War defense policies. Campaigns for minority rights in the 1950s spawned a surge of social movements in the 1960s addressing the plight of marginalized and disempowered groups. This "generalization of rights" extended to the rights of patients in relation to doctors and medical institutions. Activism promoting the welfare of disadvantaged groups heightened sensitivity to the choice of subjects for human research.

During the mid-1960s, social activism entered biomedicine itself. Young physicians and other health professionals adopted rights frameworks and promoted left-wing causes. The MCHR consolidated in 1964 around the voting rights campaign called Mississippi Freedom Summer. The group's initial focus was inequalities in access to health care. By the 1970s, the organization was recruiting medical students, and its local chapters were launching actions like those targeting Krugman.

Objections from physicians were not coming only from young radical activists. Established clinicians and even some elite investigators were now openly expressing disapproval of research conduct they found repugnant. They had come to reject the calculus that placed greater value on scientific gain and the common good than the rights and well-being of individual subjects.

Developments in institutional arenas outside U.S. medicine both fostered and gave shape to these expressions of moral discomfort. The priority of rights was ascendant within major institutions, including American jurisprudence. U.S. court rulings of the late 1950s and early 1960s used and defined the term *informed consent* for medical procedures. The requirement that subjects consent to medical interventions had long been embedded in legal theory. However, the notion of consent operative in previous decades rested on a belief in medical beneficence; the individual's consent gave the physician latitude to intervene in the patient's interests. In contrast, *informed* consent had roots in the notion of individual autonomy, the patient's right to self-determination. A medical battery case in 1957 (*Salvo v. Leland Stanford Jr. University Board of Trustees*) and a medical negligence case in 1960 (*Natanson v. Kline*) fundamentally altered judicial precedent. These rulings and subsequent legal judgments required physicians to inform the patient about both the risks a medical intervention entailed and what alternatives were available.

Concern with the implications of physician prerogatives for patient rights helped spur the emergence of a new profession: bioethics.

Contributors to this fledgling field found inspiration in contemporaneous social movements. As one early bioethicist put it, "I moved easily from civil rights to patients' rights." Ethical boundaries in human experimentation were among the field's earliest concerns.

Meanwhile, sentiments emanating from Europe about experimentation with hospital patients, children, and institutionalized persons were being felt in the United States. In the fall of 1962, British medical practitioner Maurice Pappworth published "Human Guinea Pigs: A Warning" in the popular magazine *Twentieth Century*. He argued that researchers were conducting nontherapeutic experiments on unsuspecting hospital patients unrelated to their treatment; Pappworth gave twenty examples. He also described experiments with children, some of whom were developmentally disabled. On the issue of consent for research with minors, Pappworth declared, "Parents may have the right, but have they the *moral* right, to allow their children—be they mental defective or not—to be used as human guinea-pigs?"

In 1964, the British Medical Research Council, unhappy with limitations in the Helsinki Declaration approved that year, released its own statement regarding the responsibility of clinical researchers. The council rejected nontherapeutic experiments with minors and persons with mental disabilities and questioned whether, in the strict view of the law, parents and guardians had the prerogative to give consent on a child's behalf for procedures that carried risk but no benefit. This interpretation of law would be contested but, in the meantime, objections in Britain to experimenting with vulnerable persons sent ripples across the Atlantic.

For progressive-leaning American physicians with qualms about how ongoing research was being conducted, conceptual tools for framing their objections were readily available. Dissidents repudiating research excesses mounted several arguments: that the experiments involved excessive and unjustified risk; that investigators failed to obtain informed and voluntary consent; and that scientists were exploiting vulnerable persons by enrolling members of institutionalized or otherwise marginalized groups. Studies that triggered the fiercest protests involved the obviously disempowered: enfeebled elderly patients, impaired children, and impoverished African Americans.

In previous decades, researchers had been able to control information about potentially controversial experiments. Now magazines for practicing physicians created in the early 1960s circulated reports of ongoing medical studies as well as the debates that surrounded them.

Medical investigators had long observed a code of conduct whereby ethical disagreements remained internal to the research community. But from the early 1960s forward, scientific leaders were unable to constrain members of the profession from openly declaring their moral grievances.

With disaffected physicians making their complaints highly visible, intra-professional disputes spilled into arenas outside biomedicine. The mainstream media, long purveyors of legitimizing accounts, were now spreading reports of feuding doctors and critical commentaries about human experimentation. A fundamental shift took place in discourse about the use of human subjects: accounts of research abuse supplanted depictions of willing volunteers making sacrifices for the collective good. The biomedical elite had lost control of the public narrative.

The altered depictions of human research went far beyond objections to hepatitis infection studies; yet unfolding disputes about the experiments at Willowbrook were inarguably a core feature of that larger transformation. The conflict surrounding Krugman's experiments was distinctive in several ways. More than any other research controversy of the 1960s and early 1970s, it mobilized sentiment and rationales against experiments with children and impaired persons; and more than any other controversy, it revealed how bitterly divided the medical community had become about standards for conducting human research.

Between 1964 and 1974, the American mainstream media covered a series of episodes involving allegations of research abuse. The first of these concerned an experiment at the Jewish Chronic Disease Hospital (JCDH) in Brooklyn, where the issues in contention centered on informed consent. In 1963, Chester Southam, a researcher from Memorial Sloan Kettering Cancer Center with NIH funding, injected elderly patients at JCDH with cancer cells to determine how long it would take their immune systems to reject the foreign material. He had previously conducted the procedures with both inmates at an Ohio prison (healthy adults) and cancer patients and had found the immunological responses of cancer patients to be relatively slow; he now wanted to test the responses of patients with debilitating conditions other than cancer.

The hospital's new medical director, Emanuel Mandel, a research-oriented physician, approved the study. Southam proceeded—without obtaining written consent and without many of the patients even realizing they were participating in a medical experiment. A number of JCDH physicians were outraged to learn that patients with diseases like Parkinson's and multiple sclerosis had been subjected to procedures without understanding that the experimental interventions were not part of their treatment.

JCDH was a community hospital whose patient base included Holocaust survivors; members of its medical staff were undoubtedly more knowledgeable about the Nuremberg Code than most American doctors. The incensed physicians filed a formal grievance with the hospital board. Some of their statements invoked Nazi medical experiments; one physician declared that Southam's procedures were "acts which belong more properly in Dachau."

When the hospital grievance committee failed to take disciplinary action, the physicians, together with a progressive lawyer on the hospital board, took the matter to the press, the courts, and the medical licensing board. They sued to get access to patient records and filed a complaint with the state agency responsible for professional conduct. After lengthy proceedings, the state oversight board censured Southam and Mandel for neglecting to secure informed consent for experiments with patients; the failure amounted to "fraud and deceit in the conduct of medicine." In 1964, when JCDH dissidents began legal actions, their allegations repeatedly made headlines in New York City newspapers. A clash that began as an intra-professional feud had overflowed into the public arena.

Within two years, the same underlying sequence—conflict internal to medicine reverberating outside professional circles—unfolded again. This time it was an exposé from an insider whistleblower, Harvard anesthesiologist Henry K. Beecher, that triggered the process. Beecher presented a damning critique of human research practices in March 1965 at a symposium in Michigan sponsored by Upjohn Co., and during June of the following year, a published version, "Ethics and Clinical Research," appeared in the *New England Journal of Medicine*. The paper described twenty-two experiments—studies at JCDH and Willowbrook among them—that, in Beecher's judgment, involved undue risk to subjects without benefit to them and without adequate consent. He argued that, with the vast expansion of medical research during the postwar years, experiments of this type had become routine and widespread.

Like many research-oriented academic physicians, Beecher had conducted defense-related clinical research under contract with the military. This included studies he and several colleagues pursued in the early 1950s testing hallucinatory drugs that might assist in mind control during interrogations; the human subjects in these experiments were naïve and unwitting. By the decade's end, however, Beecher had become disillusioned with standards for human experimentation. Now he wanted the scientific community to undertake reform.

Beecher exchanged letters with Pappworth before releasing his exposé and, like Pappworth, he described multiple cases of ethically problematic research. But reactions to the two authors from within medical circles were quite different. Pappworth was a British clinician without ties to the country's medical establishment. Beecher was a well-respected member of America's biomedical elite. He did not identify the investigators he was disparaging in his conference presentation or *Journal* article, but by openly faulting the research conduct of colleagues, he was breaking with a long-standing norm whereby members criticized fellow scientists only in private. Beecher's was the first highly visible condemnation of research practices from within the top echelon of academic medicine. His declarations generated consternation inside the U.S. research community. Several members of the Harvard medical faculty attacked his conference paper, arguing that his examples were not representative and that he had made unverified assumptions about the researchers' consent practices. Scientists continued to take issue with Beecher's claims in the wake of his *Journal* publication.

Beecher had given copies of his conference presentation to reporters at major newspapers and had also provided some with advance copies of his forthcoming publication. The result was a surge of attention from mainstream media, with outlets across the country reporting allegations of widespread investigatory misconduct. While Beecher had refrained from naming the investigators or the studies he repudiated, it was not long before the press identified experiments at Willowbrook as one of Beecher's twenty-two cases. His revelations spurred a subsequent round of media coverage, this one focused on Krugman's hepatitis program.

The first public condemnations of the Willowbrook experiments appeared in the wake of Beecher's *New England Journal* paper. On January 11, 1967, the *New York Times* reported that legislator Seymour R. Thaler had declared on the floor of the state senate that "thousands of patients" in the city's public hospitals were "being used daily as medical guinea pigs ... without their knowledge and consent." He pointed to hepatitis studies at Willowbrook as a primary example. Two days later, Thaler made renewed charges, again reported by the *Times*, explicitly citing Beecher's paper and declaring that studies at Willowbrook were "unethical, immoral and illegal."

Thaler argued that researchers had no right to use children in risky experiments unrelated to their medical treatment. He insisted as well that parents had no right to volunteer their children for medical experiments of this type. These were positions that Pappworth and the British Medical Research Council had advanced several years earlier.

Opponents of the Willowbrook studies then voiced another objection to the NYU team's consent procedures: they argued that parents of children on the research unit had agreed to the experiments under duress. In an effort to alleviate overcrowding late in 1964, Willowbrook's director Jack Hammond had imposed a delay on new admissions. Parents seeking a placement for their child received a form letter saying their youngster's name would be put on a waiting list. Some then received a second letter saying that there were vacancies in the hepatitis research unit. Complaints at the time prompted Hammond to discontinue the dual letters. But after Thaler's public statements, disability activist Jack M. Gootzeit charged on local television that researchers at Willowbrook were using a "high-pressure method" to obtain consent from parents who were "desperate to institutionalize their child." Hammond insisted the whole thing was "a complete misinterpretation . . . of an unfortunate coincidence."

For his part, Krugman responded that the dual letters had affected only a handful of parents and that waiting times for openings on the research unit were typically longer than those for admission to Willowbrook's general population. He insisted that his team was scrupulous in fully informing parents about the experiments and in securing freely given consent. Parents had signed consent statements and his team had used no wards of the state, a choice Krugman highlighted: "We decided at the start to use no wards of the state, although by law the administrator of Willowbrook could have signed for them."

Before the controversy had became heated, Krugman attempted to present his case for the NYU research program directly to Beecher. According to minutes of the Armed Forces Epidemiology Board, when Beecher's damning depictions of Willowbrook studies had been circulated, Krugman contacted the author personally. "Krugman invited Beecher to Willowbrook, talked to him on the telephone, but Beecher was curt and did not accept the invitation."

Krugman had a number of supporters among Willowbrook parents. A board member of the Willowbrook chapter of the Benevolent Society for Retarded Children—composed of concerned parents—rejected accusations of coercion in the recruitment of subjects. She said that, if parents did not want their child to participate in the research, the youngster was simply admitted to the facility's general population. In May 1967, the Willowbrook chapter presented Krugman with a plaque that read, "In recognition of ... distinguished, pioneering, humanitarian research on the prevention of infectious diseases and their complications in children everywhere, born and unborn." Several months earlier, the executive director of the Association for the Help of Retarded Children in New York accepted an invitation to visit the Willowbrook research unit. He spoke in person with Krugman and his co-investigator Joan Giles, and reviewed materials on admissions to the program. He then wrote a letter saying he was impressed with how well patients on the unit were treated, emphasizing "the individual love, care, and attention" each was receiving.

Prominent members of the biomedical elite were unwavering in their support for Krugman's work. In 1968, Franz Ingelfinger, editor of the *New England Journal*, wrote in the *Yearbook of Medicine* that the studies at Willowbrook not only yielded "medical knowledge in an abstract sense," but benefited the child subjects as well. In a 1969 special issue of the journal *Daedalus* devoted to the ethics of human research, two well-placed medical researchers argued in separate essays that the Willowbrook studies were justified. One of the authors, Geoffrey Edsall, who was affiliated with the Harvard School of Public Health, wrote that it was proper and ethical to conduct experiments with minors that exposed them to "no greater risk than the children were likely to run by nature"—meaning through "natural" exposure to other patients.

But in the aftermath of Beecher's accusations and the JCDH debacle, the tenor of media coverage of medical experiments, including those at Willowbrook, changed markedly. The press was reporting ongoing disputes and was publishing probing commentaries. The *Saturday Review* ran a series of articles about the appropriateness of existing human research practices. Mainstream American journalists were now asking whether there was a need for new rules governing human experimentation.

In the early 1970s, critics of hepatitis experiments at Willowbrook doubled down on questions concerning risks the studies posed and the benefits child subjects gained. From the outset, Krugman and his supporters argued that harms to children were minimal. In their accounts, hepatitis was milder in children than in adults; the virus strains used in experimental interventions were especially mild; and children in the research unit received expert medical attention—better than the care provided to Willowbrook's general population. They emphasized that the project's overall purpose was prevention: to induce immunity to hepatitis. And in an often-repeated assertion, they said that because hepatitis was endemic at Willowbrook, newly admitted children would be exposed to the disease anyway. By participating in the experiment, child subjects would gain immunity to an illness they would otherwise surely contract.

Beecher returned to the Willowbrook studies in a 1970 book, *Research and the Individual*; in it he devoted six pages to the hepatitis experiments, now identifying the study by name. He raised questions about coercion and the legitimacy of parental consent. He noted that the NYU researchers had nowhere discussed possible long-term liver damage from hepatitis. Beecher went on to question evidence bearing on the assertion that children housed in the general wards at Willowbrook would inevitably have a bout of hepatitis.

Another Ivy League academic also took aim at the Willowbrook experiments. Paul Ramsey, Princeton theologian and an early contributor to the field of bioethics, included a twelve-page analysis of the studies in his 1970 volume, *The Patient as Person*. He took issue with the withholding of gamma globulin from some subjects and the use of what he called a "captive population" of minors for purely experimental purposes. Ramsey argued that the researchers should have conducted the experiments on adults rather than children. He also declared that, faced with endemic hepatitis at Willowbrook, the NYU team should have focused their efforts on cleaning up conditions that allowed the disease to fester.

What happened next signaled just how acrimonious the divide in professional opinion had become. Between April and July 1971, the British journal *Lancet* carried a series of warring editorial letters about the ethics of experiments at Willowbrook. The first to appear was an essay by Stephen Goldby, a clinician in Oxford. Goldby argued that experiments on children with no benefits for them were unjustified, no matter the researchers' aims. He rebuked *Lancet* for failing to condemn the studies on ethical grounds. Eight letters followed Goldby's salvo, including communications from Krugman, Giles, Pappworth, Beecher, and Edsall. The claims and counterclaims were not new; by this time, major arguments concerning the hepatitis studies at Willowbrook were well-traveled terrain.

What was new was the vitriolic and very visible split within the top stratum of the medical community. In response to Goldby's letter, the *Lancet* editor wrote that although he had held out the hope that experiments at Willowbrook would yield tools for preventing hepatitis, this "could not justify the giving of infected material to children who would not directly benefit." Three months later, *JAMA* published a paper from Krugman's team announcing success in immunizing against hepatitis B using heat-treated serum.

JAMA had been printing celebratory editorials about the NYU team's accomplishment in issues containing the group's scientific reports; this time was no exception. In its accompanying commentary, *JAMA* applauded the group's contribution to preventing hepatitis B, declaring, "Mission accomplished!" The editor then rebuked *Lancet* for adopting a "pious tone" and a misguided stance on the ethics of the Willowbrook studies. *JAMA*'s remarks ended with a final swipe: *"Lancet*'s editor would have been well advised to keep his pen away from paper." Two major medical journals were very openly at loggerheads.

Medical press outlets were now filled with reports of conflicting positions on the Willowbrook experiments, with the coverage slanting toward criticism. A 1971 article in *Medical World News* echoed Ramsey's critique, taking issue with the NYU team for withholding gamma globulin from some of its subjects. The *News* also flatly rejected the claim that children at Willowbrook were destined to get infectious hepatitis. "This is not true," the authors stated bluntly, because the investigators could have administered gamma globulin to all. The display of contentious arguments among experts undermined the legitimacy not only of experiments at Willowbrook but of biomedical research in general.

While disputes within the medical profession over hepatitis experiments were simmering, the mounting outcry over deplorable patient care at Willowbrook was having consequences for Krugman's research program. In the mid-1960s, Willowbrook had become ground zero for a movement insisting on the humane treatment of persons with intellectual impairments. At that time, Willowbrook had the unwelcome distinction of being the country's largest "training school"—a widely used euphemism—and conditions there were appalling. Initial efforts at amelioration focused on securing adequate state funding. In 1965, Robert F. Kennedy, then a U.S. senator from New York, visited Willowbrook and delivered a report to the state legislative committee on mental retardation. In remarks reported by New York City papers, Kennedy called the facility a "snake pit," with inmates "living in filth and dirt, their clothes in rags, in rooms less comfortable and cheerful than the cages in which we put animals in a zoo." He considered the abysmal conditions violations of patients' civil liberties and civil rights. Activists at Willowbrook would later escalate such complaints and, while the protests were not directed at the hepatitis studies, they would nonetheless confound the NYU research team.

In the years following Kennedy's visit, the situation for the facility's residents deteriorated still further. During the early 1970s, New York State faced budget impasses and slashed funding for its Department of Mental Health. Public hospitals imposed hiring freezes, and staffing levels at Willowbrook dropped. In August 1971, the *Staten Island Advance* reported that three hundred positions at Willowbrook were unfilled. The care of residents fell to a new low. In the autumn, a citizens' Board of Visitors sent a letter to the governor saying it was "shocked and appalled by conditions" there. In some wards, patients were unfed, naked, and covered with excrement.

The long-cautious Willowbrook Benevolent Society implored state officials to address the crisis. When the usual routes of complaint failed to bring relief, efforts to secure improvements became confrontational. Willowbrook had several young activists on its professional staff, including doctors William Bronston and Michael Wilkins and social worker Elizabeth Lee. They began meeting with a number of aggrieved parents and, in the fall and winter of 1971–72, the group mobilized demonstrations with placards and picket lines outside Willowbrook's administration building. The *Staten Island Advance* covered these protests.

In January 1972, Willowbrook's director Jack Hammond fired Wilkins and Lee for meeting with parents. Wilkins still had his keys to the buildings, and very early on the day after his dismissal, he brought his friend, TV news reporter Geraldo Rivera, and a camera crew into some of Willowbrook's wards. The crew filmed conditions that day and returned on later days for additional footage. On January 6, 1972, Rivera began airing images from Willowbrook on ABC's local evening news. On February 2, the channel ran a half-hour documentary Rivera's team had assembled called *Willowbrook: The Last Great Disgrace*. Televised images of conditions at Willowbrook stunned viewers and gripped the public's attention. A *New York Times* article reporting Rivera's coverage ran with the headline "Willowbrook State School, 'the Big Town's Leper Colony.'"

Demonstrations targeting Krugman and the hepatitis experiments began during the months immediately following Rivera's TV exposé. Protesters were demanding that NYU scientists end hepatitis experiments and improve the care of Willowbrook residents. When members of

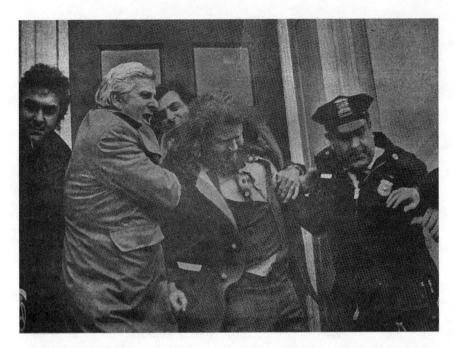

Malachy McCourt, Diana McCourt's husband, meets resistance during a protest from a security guard at the door of the Willowbrook administration building. (Photo by Eric Aerts. 1972 *Staten Island Advance*. All rights reserved. Reprinted with permission.)

the MCHR made this argument, a researcher at the University of Pennsylvania wrote a letter to the organization in exasperation: "I do not doubt that Dr. Krugman deplores conditions at Willowbrook as much as anyone else but I fail to see why the conditions should be laid at his door."

On the ground at Willowbrook, activists launched a new strategy for addressing the plight of the facility's residents. In March 1972, the New York Civil Liberties Union and Legal Aid Society filed a class action suit on behalf of Willowbrook parents. The suit charged that conditions at the facility violated the constitutional rights of patients. The case would yield a consent decree issued in 1975 that required the state to create community placements for the facility's residents. The court order would lead to the deinstitutionalization of many Willowbrook residents, and to the facility's eventual closure in the 1980s.

The movement of patients out of Willowbrook was under way even before the lawsuit's outcome was determined. Early in 1972, Willowbrook

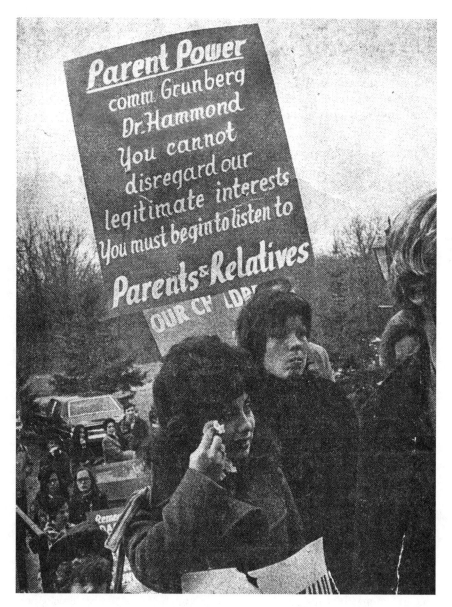

Parents and relatives at Willowbrook, some in tears, protest funding cuts and staff firings implemented by Deputy State Commissioner Frederic Grunberg and Willowbrook director Jack Hammond. (Photo by Eric Aerts. 1972 *Staten Island Advance*. All rights reserved. Reprinted with permission.)

administrators began reducing the facility's population by terminating new admissions and transferring patients to other facilities. Because all participants in hepatitis infection studies had to be new to the institution, the curtailment of admissions meant no possibility of additional research subjects. Action taken at Willowbrook to alleviate overcrowding was the immediate reason for the closure of the NYU research unit.

In May 1972, Krugman informed the Armed Forces Epidemiology Board that the research unit would shut down on August 1 of that year. In December, he reported at a board meeting that he had terminated all hepatitis transmission procedures but planned in the future to conduct retrospective studies using stored serum samples already collected. His tone at this meeting was somber. A close colleague reported later that Krugman had been deeply wounded by the repudiation of his hepatitis research. But the biomedical elite continued to revere him for his scientific contributions; in the years that followed, the research community would bestow on him some two dozen additional awards and honors.

Even as the Willowbrook research unit was closing, disputes over hepatitis studies with children continued. And while Krugman was not launching new interventions, he continued to defend his project. The student council of the NYU School of Medicine held a symposium on the ethics of experiments at Willowbrook in May 1972. Krugman gave a presentation in which he refuted claims that parental consent was coerced, pointed to support from the Willowbrook Benevolent Society, and emphasized the project's achievements in preventing hepatitis. Krugman was asserting a position many within America's biomedical elite still held: that progress in disease prevention required that investigators have leeway to enroll children in experiments not directly related to their medical treatment.

Even as embers from the controversy over the hepatitis studies with disabled children were still burning, additional research scandals unfolded. One of these was immediately explosive. In July 1972, reports of the Tuskegee Syphilis Study burst onto the front pages of newspapers across the country. Jean Heller, an Associated Press journalist, reported that for forty years, Public Health Service investigators had been conducting a study on more than four hundred poor African American men with latent syphilis in which researchers misrepresented the study to subjects and withheld medical treatment. In the weeks after Heller's piece appeared, expressions of outrage flooded newspapers nationwide.

Articles and editorials about the Tuskegee study appearing in the American press during July and August bore damning headlines: "A Nightmare Experiment" (Raleigh *News and Observer*); "A Violation of Human Dignity" (*Houston Chronicle*); "An Immoral Study" (*St. Louis Post-Dispatch*); "Inhuman Experiment" (*Oregonian*); "Horror Story" (*Providence Sunday Journal*); "Blot of Inhumanity" (*Chattanooga Times*); "A Shocking Medical Experiment" (*New Haven Register*); and "Official Inhumanity" (*Los Angeles Times*). One historian commented that the ultimate lesson many Americans learned from the Tuskegee study "was the need to protect society from scientific pursuits that ignored human values." Others emphasized that the Tuskegee study raised issues not only about consent, deception, and exploitation but also about racial injustice.

Six months later, another elaboration of research abuses received media attention. In January 1973, journalist Jessica Mitford published an article in the *Atlantic Monthly* denouncing medical experimentation with prisoners. Among the issues addressed was whether inmates, denied civil liberties, were able to exercise freedom of choice. Mitford declared that there was no such thing as informed consent in prisons.

Objections to enrolling prisoners in medical experiments came relatively late in the course of human research controversies—this despite the tremendous growth in medical studies with prisoners during the postwar years, fueled in large measure by drug companies testing new products. Scandals had surfaced during the late 1960s; critics had pointed to moneymaking schemes for conducting pharmaceutical clinical trials in prisons that involved coercion and exploitation of inmates. But professional associations had assessed the problems to be rectifiable through reform; they had not suggested that the use of prisoners in medical research was inherently flawed. Now, with Mitford's widely cited critique, the practice of enrolling prison inmates in medical experiments was under attack.

By the early 1970s, the American press had been publishing reports of ethically problematic medical research for a decade; this included coverage of studies at JCDH, Willowbrook, and Tuskegee as well as the allegations of Beecher and Mitford. These accounts fundamentally changed public perception and sentiments about human experimentation. Portrayals of unfeeling scientists abusing defenseless subjects replaced the once-dominant depictions of heroic researchers and willing subjects contributing to disease control for the greater good. The transformation empowered critics, who called for new rules for human research and formal constraints on its conduct.

Preliminary regulatory measures had in fact emerged in the wake of discord over studies at JCDH. The NIH had funded Southam's experiments and, during the controversy, its leaders realized that the agency needed guidelines for human research conducted by extramural grant recipients. In 1966, the PHS surgeon general issued a policy directive that required local peer review of experimental protocols receiving agency funding and involving human subjects. The purview of these review committees—later called institutional review boards (IRBs)—was to ensure that prospective experiments entailed an appropriate balance of risks and benefits, and that investigators secured the subjects' informed consent. The initial regulations included no stipulations regarding recruitment from groups now being called vulnerable populations.

In formulating this policy, the NIH was acting as both a federal sponsor of research and an influential branch of America's biomedical elite. The surgeon general's National Advisory Health Council—whose members included medical school deans and university presidents—approved the directive. In the view of biomedical leaders, placing research oversight with local review boards had two advantages: it allowed the NIH to avoid becoming a political target when a grantee's conduct generated condemnation, and it protected the broader scientific community from centralized external control.

Scientists had good reason to be concerned about external regulation of this type. Media coverage of the Tuskegee experiments had created intense pressure for additional action at the federal level. In 1973, members of the Senate introduced several bills pertaining to human experimentation, one of them proposing a permanent, independent research ethics commission. Between February and July 1973, Edward Kennedy, U.S. senator from Massachusetts, oversaw Senate subcommittee hearings on issues in human experimentation. He devoted two days of the hearings to the Tuskegee study. Mitford testified at the hearings, which included a full day on medical experimentation in prisons.

Behind the scenes, a struggle took place over the design of federal policy. The biomedical community lobbied to prevent centralized oversight and a permanently constituted ethics commission. But research ethics had become a matter of public morality, and scientific leaders understood that continuing acrimony and open conflict about investigatory conduct was undermining biomedicine's legitimacy. While not eager to see new rules, particularly rules that restricted their use of some subject pools, the research elite was prepared to compromise so that the turmoil would stop.

In an opinion piece appearing in the *New England Journal of Medicine* during the Kennedy hearings, the *Journal*'s editor Franz Ingelfinger signaled reluctant acceptance of some constraints on experiments with minors. He had previously voiced both support for the Willowbrook studies and strong opposition to prohibiting experiments on children done without therapeutic or preventive intent; such a prohibition was, in his view, "neither observed nor practical." But now he wrote, "Perhaps as a result of the hearings being conducted by Senator Kennedy on human experimentation, or the two bills introduced by Senators Javits and Humphrey, some broadly based system can be set up to determine under what circumstances children or mentally incompetent persons can be used for experimentation not primarily designed for their benefit. This is the only reasonable way."

PHS leaders reached an informal agreement with influential members of Congress about the direction human subjects oversight would take. In 1974, the Department of Health, Education and Welfare (DHEW), the PHS's parent agency, issued the 1966 policy directive as federal regulatory code. In subsequent decades, a full range of federal agencies would adopt versions of the regulations, and its core features would become known as the Common Rule. With governmental guidelines requiring all institutions receiving federal research funds to follow these codes, what emerged over time was a nationwide system of human subjects oversight implemented through local IRBs. The resulting regulatory system placed responsibility for avoiding violations not on the federal agencies that supported—indeed, sought—human experiments, but rather on individual investigators conducting the research and the institutions employing them.

Also in 1974, Congress passed the National Research Act, which created a temporary ethics commission: the National Commission for Protection of Human Subjects of Biomedical and Behavioral Research—widely known as simply the National Commission. Its members would be recognized as among the founders of the field of bioethics. Its mandate was to further delineate guidelines that IRBs would use when evaluating research protocols. This included creating special provisions for experiments with vulnerable groups. DHEW agreed to revise and augment the regulatory code based on the National Commission's recommendations. Among the commission publications were proposed protections for children (released in 1977) and for prisoners (released in 1978). Enhanced DHEW regulations followed: provisions pertaining to prisoners (subpart C of the federal code) in 1978 and for children (subpart D) in 1983.

These new rules codified changes in public sentiment about medical experiments with captive and vulnerable groups—and about research practices more broadly—that had already taken place. After Mitford's article and the Kennedy hearings, efforts to restrict research in prisons had gained momentum. In 1974, the incoming director of the Department of Corrections in Illinois—where malaria infection experiments were still ongoing—announced the termination of medical studies in the state's prisons. Experiments with inmates were, in his view, "immoral and unethical." The *Chicago Tribune* quoted the new director as saying, "Our stand is based on the question of whether an inmate can truly volunteer his services, and we do not believe he can." Ironically, prisoners themselves protested the close of malaria research; the rehabilitative ethos was still alive among Stateville's inmates. The prisoners mobilized a letter-writing campaign urging state officials to allow the research program to continue. It was, they insisted, "a vital force in our rehabilitation" and "the only program here in which we can make a contribution to society." The head of corrections was unswayed.

Action also took place outside DHEW at the federal level. In 1974, a U.S. congressman from Maryland introduced a bill aimed at prohibiting medical experiments in both federal and state prisons. Representative Robert Kastenmeier convened House subcommittee hearings on the proposed legislation. But the Federal Bureau of Prisons preempted congressional action; in 1976, the bureau's head announced he was ending human experiments in federal penitentiaries through administrative edict.

Subpart C of human subjects regulations on prison research curbed the use of incentives for inducing inmates' participation and allowed only experiments that directly addressed the situation of incarcerated persons or medical conditions prevalent among inmates. Subpart D relating to children distinguished studies on the basis of hazards posed to subjects and benefits expected. It imposed the most severe constraints on experiments involving more than minimal risk and those without expected gain for subjects or for children with similar conditions. In all cases, the code required investigators to obtain both consent from parents and assent—meaning active agreement to participate in the research—from minors. The new rules created restrictions but also left many matters of interpretation to the discretion of local IRBs.

With Krugman's project ended and new regulations in place, publicly visible outcries over research with children receded. But disagreements within the medical community over the Willowbrook studies were never resolved. Decades after the experiments were over, debate about their appropriateness was still alive. The authors of a chapter in a 2008 volume on clinical research ethics challenge what they describe as the widespread disparagement of Krugman's hepatitis studies. These Willowbrook defenders were part of a growing movement among researchers and even bioethicists during the 2000s that voiced objections to overly restrictive limitations on medical experiments, particularly studies with children and prisoners. They contend—as did Krugman—that the NYU team conducted the experiments for the benefit of subjects and with the purpose of conferring lasting immunity. They lament misinformed accounts that cast doubt on the ethics of research that, they suggest, would ultimately benefit children. In their view, to characterize "Willowbrook in such a manner dangerously discourages research as a means to ameliorate health conditions for vulnerable populations of children."

But more typical accounts of the studies at Willowbrook castigate Krugman and his team for placing overwhelmed parents in a situation where they felt pressured to provide consent. Investigatory abuse more generally remains a recurrent theme in public depictions of medical research. These narratives underscore the potential for misuse of professional authority and the dangers of science that overreaches by placing the aim of new knowledge above individuals' well-being. They are cautionary tales illustrating the need for researchers to honor the self-determination of research subjects and protect their safety. The emphasis on the investigator's personal accountability is compatible with the core social value of individualism and its dominant place in the professional ethos of bioethics and public health between the 1970s and the early 2000s.

Research abuse narratives are embedded in our collective memory of late twentieth-century biomedical research; they serve to affirm the moral priorities we proudly hold. But the accounts have serious shortcomings as reflections of the past. By focusing exclusively on the individual scientist as the responsible party, they obscure the web of institutional and cultural supports that gave momentum to the now-condemned research. Missing from the picture are the federal sponsorship of virtually all of the repudiated studies; the central role of a military-biomedical elite with its links to defense agencies; the widespread legitimacy of scientists' justificatory claims; the deference of the press; the buy-in from managers of multiple institutions providing access to subjects; and the lived experience of some participants, particularly the conscientious objectors, who actually did willingly sign on to dangerous experiments in hopes of advancing science for the common good.

CHAPTER NINE

An Ending without Closure

WHILE THE HEPATITIS INFECTION program was ongoing, scientists did not understand the delayed harms their experiments were unleashing. Evidence had yet to materialize that a portion of subjects who become hepatitis carriers after receiving blood-borne viruses will go on to develop cirrhosis or liver cancer. But there were abundant signs of lasting problems. These included accounts of patients whose symptoms continued for more than six months after initial infection (1946); anomalous liver function tests among people who had contracted the disease one to five years earlier (1948); case reports linking serum hepatitis to cirrhosis of the liver (1950); and a finding of persistent disabilities following hepatitis B infection in 1 or 2 percent of cases (1951).

Midcentury scientists did recognize the existence of hepatitis carriers. They knew that blood and serum from asymptomatic carriers caused jaundice in recipients and made removing hepatitis B from the blood supply one of their major objectives. The infectivity of child carriers became an issue in the 1970s, when youngsters from Willowbrook were placed in public classrooms; parents of elementary school students vigorously opposed mingling highly infective young hepatitis B carriers with their susceptible offspring.

For years, controlling disease transmission was scientists' overriding concern, not distant health outcomes for virus carriers. When considering the risks and benefits of a hepatitis infection experiment, investigators balanced the chance of immediate fatalities against expected gains for science and national security. They viewed the short-term risk to participants as low and had great confidence that their research efforts would advance the greater good. The possibility of delayed harms to human subjects or their close contacts was not part of scientists' calculus; Stokes's stated reluctance to give serum hepatitis to women of childbearing age was an exception.

Knowledge of the long-term dangers carriers face came from multiple directions after the research program had ended and tests for the hepatitis B antigen were available. Epidemiological studies published in the late 1970s and 1980s showed that, in Asian and African populations, hepatitis B carriers were substantially more likely than noncarriers to develop cirrhosis and liver cancer. And waves of increasingly sophisticated assay techniques allowed scientists to identify the components of hepatitis viruses and discern immune system responses to their presence. These tools also yielded insights into what portion of individuals sickened with blood-borne hepatitis retained the viruses for years after infection and even permanently. The findings varied by hepatitis strain and the person's age at the time of initial infection.

By the 1980s, scientists were in agreement that among adults infected with hepatitis B, between 5 and 10 percent would harbor the virus indefinitely. The emerging picture was considerably more discouraging for children. Researchers had been patently wrong in their belief that hepatitis B is more benign in youngsters than in adults. While their initial symptoms are indeed typically mild, children are much more likely than adults to become long-term carriers. Among those between one and five years of age at the time of infection, 30 to 50 percent become carriers, with the youngest most likely to be permanently affected.

More bad news came in the 1990s when newly available assay techniques for the hepatitis C antigen revealed that between 75 and 85 percent of infected adults never clear that virus. Researchers were unaware of hepatitis C during the years the hepatitis experiments were ongoing. But laboratory studies conducted soon after the program's termination showed that government-sponsored investigators had in fact transmitted hepatitis C to human subjects.

Work conducted at the NIH Division of Biologic Standards during the early 1970s revealed the presence of the C strain in serum administered to some study participants. Serological tests for hepatitis A and B markers had become available, and the Division of Biologics Standards still had access to preserved blood samples from the agency's blood sterilization project twenty years earlier. Jay Hoofnagle, then a young postdoc in a division lab, analyzed specimens from six hepatitis carriers whose serum had been used as infective material in the much earlier study, and from seventy-five prisoners injected with these donors' material. Blood from three of the six donors showed no signs of either hepatitis A or B; nonetheless, thirty-five inmate-subjects inoculated with their serum had well-documented cases of hepatitis. Blood from these sickened prisoners was also negative for both hepatitis A and B. Hoofnagle and his colleagues concluded that a third strain then called hepatitis non-A, non-B—later known as hepatitis C—had caused the illnesses.

No specimens from other virus transmission studies were ever analyzed for their hepatitis C content; as a result, the pervasiveness of this strain in specimens transmitted to subjects in hepatitis experiments more generally remains a mystery.

Further ordeals awaited many of the subjects who became hepatitis B or C carriers. The lingering viruses are slow-moving and insidious, often wreaking internal damage with minimal symptoms. Serious medical problems typically develop two or more decades after initial infection and the ultimate outcome can be devastating. The U.S. Centers for Disease Control and Prevention estimates that one-quarter of hepatitis carriers have died prematurely from cirrhosis or liver cancer. Cures for hepatitis C carriers introduced in the 2010s were too late for study participants.

Hepatitis researchers made periodic attempts to address symptoms and disabilities among subjects that persisted after their studies had ended. Stokes secured private funds to provide several months of additional care for conscientious objectors who had not recovered by the time the Philadelphia Civilian Public Service unit was closing. After World War II, he pressed the Office of the Surgeon General–Army for permission to purchase disability or life insurance for subjects in hepatitis experiments. Other program scientists supported his effort.

Participants in one virus transmission study did receive further attention from researchers following the experiments' completion. After the death of three subjects in the blood sterilization project, Roderick Murray continued medical exams and liver function tests for a period of one to three years on some of the remaining inmates who had received blood-borne viruses. This follow-up period was too short to be of assistance to a person developing cirrhosis or liver cancer.

The NIH's role in the blood sterilization project apparently accounts for Murray's continued monitoring. In his recruitment pitch to McNeil Island inmates, Oliphant—initially lead investigator on the study—made a statement of a sort I had not encountered before nor have I since. He told prospective enrollees, "The Public Health Service, while not legally obliged to care for subjects who were permanently affected or affected for any length of time, had not failed in the past to provide for such contingencies resulting from other such programs." I asked one of the several senior or retired NIH scientists I interviewed for background on the hepatitis infection studies whether he knew about arrangements of the kind Oliphant had mentioned. My informant responded that these things were sometimes done on an informal basis.

For its part, the Defense Department was consistently inhospitable to remuneration or continued care for disabled research subjects. Stokes's government sponsor ordered his team to transfer the unrecovered conscientious objectors in his Philadelphia unit to other CPS camps, none of them able to provide care for the men's continuing symptoms. Agency lawyers prohibited researchers from purchasing disability or life insurance for hepatitis subjects. Defense officials instructed scientists to rely instead on waiver provisions in consent documents and on their own liability insurance. As noted earlier, the only exception I found to the no-compensation rule was payment of burial costs for deceased subjects, with funds drawn from the investigators' research accounts.

No researcher ever conducted—nor did a federal agency support—a long-term study of the health status of subjects in America's hepatitis infection program. John Neefe had hoped to do so. After the war, he made chronic hepatitis and hepatitis carriers his scientific foci and planned to follow patients with histories of hepatitis, including conscientious objectors from the Philadelphia CPS camp. But follow-up studies with past subjects were not conducted and, after three hepatitis deaths in 1952, the Army Epidemiology Board decided that Neefe's proposed studies with virus carriers might result in further casualties and curtailed his funding. During the 1970s and 1980s, researchers with support from the U.S. Department of Veterans Affairs published a series of reports on health outcomes among military veterans sickened with blood-borne hepatitis decades earlier, including those affected by the 1942 vaccine-generated outbreak; subjects in hepatitis infection studies were not included. When closing his research unit in 1972, Saul Krugman said he intended to continue monitoring his Willowbrook subjects, but no follow-up studies were later published. And neither hepatitis program sponsors nor scientists considered examining whether subjects who had become carriers had infected close contacts with blood-borne hepatitis.

The magnitude of delayed harm caused by America's hepatitis infection experiments is difficult to tally. From a combination of published and unpublished reports, I estimate that researchers transmitted blood-borne hepatitis to well over 1,000 persons during the thirty-year course of the program, and that more than 150 of these were children. But extrapolating from these figures to a number of resulting carriers would require knowing the prevalence of hepatitis C in specimens used as inoculants with adults—I found no evidence suggesting that child subjects received hepatitis C—and also the ages of susceptible children receiving unmodified hepatitis B. This information is not available.

I can offer observations about which groups of subjects would have suffered or avoided the brunt of injuries. Healthy young men like those in CPS camps were likely to fully expel hepatitis B pathogens and experience no lasting harm from their exposure to the virus. But the great bulk of subjects infected with blood-borne hepatitis resided in facilities where conditions would likely undermine robust immunological responses; these settings included Lynchburg Colony, Trenton State Hospital, and an array of state and federal prisons. And no matter what the location, children's immunological systems make them highly vulnerable to retaining hepatitis B viruses and experiencing serious long-term health problems.

The adult subjects most likely to become permanent carriers were those inoculated with specimens containing hepatitis C. This would include the thirty-five prisoners that NIH researchers identified as having received serum with non-A, non-B. Among these men and an unknown number of other subjects exposed to hepatitis C, the vast majority would become permanent carriers.

The situation would be grim for carriers who went on to develop cirrhosis or liver cancer. If they remained in a custodial facility, their condition would be unseen from outside. Still in an institution or not, past subjects with progressive liver disease would receive no acknowledgment of or explanation for the cause of their illnesses. They and their families would be isolated and alone, without financial redress or access to physicians with expertise in liver diseases.

The United States provides no readily available compensation for injuries sustained in government-sponsored medical research. Short of

initiating a legal suit, injured subjects have no means for obtaining recompense. Even the rejection of waiver clauses in the 1970s would be of
little help to research participants in America's hepatitis program. To suc-
ceed in court action, persons suffering harm would need to—among
other legal hurdles—document their participation in experiments for
which detailed records may have disappeared, and argue persuasively
that interventions taking place years if not decades in the past had caused
their injuries. Acting alone, precious few have the resources to pursue
such a course, let alone prevail.

On some occasions, the U.S. government has provided compensation for subjects harmed in federally sponsored human experiments. Officials established a program for the Tuskegee Syphilis Study subjects and
their families in the face of a 1974 class action lawsuit. More recently,
other groups of subjects with long-term health problems from midcentury experiments have won remuneration or medical assistance; this includes soldiers exposed to chemical warfare materials or radiation while
on military duty—the latter called "atomic veterans"—and some who, as
civilians, were deliberately exposed to ionizing radiation. But the provisions typically restrict what categories of subjects and illnesses are covered and fall far short of satisfying a full range of complainants. Redress
for injured human subjects has been spotty at best; to the extent it occurs, it has followed some combination of group mobilization, collective
legal action, journalistic exposé, and political pressure. A 1993 National
Academy of Sciences report on veterans who developed medical problems related to experiments with mustard gas and Lewisite—another
gaseous chemical weapon—underscored that the absence of follow-up
studies on long-term health consequences of the interventions greatly
hindered plans for compensation.

Since the 1970s, some within bioethics and policy circles have champi-
oned the introduction of a system of no-fault compensation for medical
research injuries. Such a program might provide for continuing care, disability income, and death benefits for injured research subjects and, in some
circumstances, family members. Advocates place priority on addressing
harm suffered by those who participated in nontherapeutic experiments
conducted for the purpose of increasing medical knowledge. Proponents
point out that many other countries offer no-fault compensation for injured
research subjects.

Still, in the United States, there has been little momentum for
provisions of this kind. A 2011 President's Commission for the Study of

Bioethical Issues looked favorably on compensation for subjects injured in federally sponsored experiments, but its recommendations did not go beyond advocating further study. This is virtually the same position that a previous presidential commission adopted in 1982. After more than thirty years of deliberations, progress on the matter remains at a standstill.

Two well-traversed story lines have dominated depictions of the hepatitis infection studies. One tells of heroic efforts to vanquish a serious disease. The other condemns violations of consent and misuse of vulnerable subjects. Documenting the relative sway of these accounts and the cultural currents supporting them goes far toward explaining how the hepatitis program arose, continued, and eventually came to a close. Yet neither narrative elucidates complex questions about research hazards that lie at the heart of experiments that place human participants in serious danger.

Are there limits to the risks to which healthy subjects should be exposed, even with adequate consent? Whose harms matter and who should be asked—indeed, allowed—to sacrifice their well-being for an expected greater good? How reliable are scientists' assessments of risks when so much of their research borders the limits of medical knowledge? Should risky studies with healthy participants proceed when the science underlying them is rudimentary at best, or has long been stalled? When the government directs researchers to pursue risk-laden human experiments to advance the nation's interest, does it not incur a moral responsibility to care for and compensate resulting injuries, whether immediate or delayed?

During World War II and the Cold War years, U.S. agencies established a system for supporting biomedical studies that included dangerous human experiments. Originally, most clinical investigators were government scientists or university investigators with federal contracts. In recent decades, this regime has undergone significant change. Pharmaceutical firms have sponsored an expanding segment of clinical research, with many relying on for-profit companies to recruit subjects and oversee experiments. A good portion of the research has been exported to developing countries where costs are low and health professionals welcome studies on diseases more common on their soil than in the West. For research taking place in the United States, the economically marginal, including minority populations, have become major sources of healthy subjects for nontherapeutic studies, to a large degree replacing groups whose members are incarcerated, underage, or impaired. By the 2000s, enrollment in clinical trials was, for repeat participants, an informal labor market for people without income security.

Renewed emphasis on science for the common good has accompanied these developments. In the early 2000s, a shift away from a dominant emphasis on subjects' rights gained momentum. Advisory committees convened by the National Academy of Sciences favored loosening restrictions on experiments with children and prisoners, arguing that the constraints impeded potentially beneficial research. And public health bioethicists—members of an emerging and increasingly vocal professional segment—have endorsed rigorous informed consent requirements while also maintaining that human subjects protections have placed inadequate weight on the expected social value of hazardous human experiments.

This reformulated greater-good framework bolsters justifications for responding to public health crises by proceeding with studies that pose very significant dangers to human subjects. The perspective has gained traction and adherents as researchers deliberate risk-laden interventions aimed at understanding and controlling emerging infectious diseases. The language of its proponents is reminiscent of narratives about the nobility of sacrifices for the broader community that prevailed during World War II and the early Cold War. The arrival of COVID-19 triggered a surge of advocacy for disease-inducing experiments with SARS-CoV-2 conducted for science and humanity, even as the long-term health consequences that participants would face remained unknown.

Meanwhile, little change has occurred in how sponsors handle injuries to human subjects. At no point have policy makers introduced a mechanism apart from lawsuits for redressing adverse outcomes from clinical research. Researchers and their patrons have been able to look the other way, particularly when adverse events are delayed. Neither scientists nor their sponsors have envisioned recompense for long-term harms as a collective responsibility. These injuries remain uncounted and unexamined; they are the largely invisible underbelly of America's experiments with human subjects.

Epilogue
Misgivings of Hindsight

ONE OF THE PROMINENT physicians entangled in America's hepatitis infection program was C. Everett Koop, surgeon general of the U.S. Public Health Service between 1982 and 1989 during Ronald Reagan's presidency. On Koop's death in 2013, the *New York Times* noted that he was "widely regarded as the most influential surgeon general in American history." He trained as a pediatric surgeon at the University of Pennsylvania Medical School. At the age of twenty-nine, while a chief resident at Penn, he performed surgical liver biopsies on conscientious objectors who were subjects in hepatitis infection experiments. One of his biopsy patients was Neil Hartman who, like Warren Sawyer, was a draft objector stationed at the Byberry Hospital alternative service camp and a participant in Joseph Stokes Jr.'s hepatitis experiments.

Koop published an autobiography in 1999. Hartman read the memoir and found it striking that Koop barely mentioned his role in the hepatitis project. "I wrote him a fan letter and said he's given me a scar. He answered right away and said . . . something that rather surprised me. He said the reason he didn't talk about that in the book is that it's one thing he was not proud of."

Hartman and Koop discussed their exchange of letters and involvement in hepatitis research in the documentary film *The Good War and Those Who Refused to Fight It*, released in 2000. Koop had this to say about his participation: "I was introduced to this whole program when I, as a young surgeon, was asked to do serial biopsies on [conscientious objectors'] livers to see what the effect of the virus was in the production of the changes in the liver. And in that way, I got to know that a lot of these young men had no idea that the risks they were taking also included death. And some of these youngsters did die and it was a very difficult thing for me to be part of, because you know, you're powerless, when you're part of a big team." Koop went on to say that experiments of this sort could no longer be performed. IRBs would not permit scientists to transmit live virus unless they understood a great deal more about the likely outcome; even then, he doubted that an IRB would approve a study of this type.

Hartman and Sawyer became friends at the Byberry CPS camp, and their camaraderie continued for decades. They both had the good fortune to recover completely and permanently from bouts in their youth with experimentally induced hepatitis. They had survived the deaths of spouses and now lived in the same Quaker retirement community. I interviewed each of them on a clear-skied warm day in June 2014—an account of my conversation with Sawyer appears in the introduction.

I had arranged to meet Hartman, ninety-four, at the sprawling complex's main building. While waiting near the reception desk, I saw a beater car drive into the parking lot. A man got out and walked toward the building with a determined gait, though with the help of a cane. It was Hartman. He was wearing khaki shorts, tennis shoes with crew socks, and a T-shirt with the name of his Friends meetinghouse emblazoned in large red letters. If his frame was slightly bowed with age, it would quickly become apparent that his mind was keen. He had expressive blue eyes and unruly white hair.

When we had settled into a place to talk, I asked Hartman how he became a conscientious objector and a subject in hepatitis infection experiments. He told me that, though raised as a Methodist, he spent summers at Quaker work camps during his youth, and when it was time to register with Selective Service, he applied for conscientious objector status. He received the classification on appeal, and entered the CPS system during the summer of 1942, when he was twenty-one. One of his first assignments was at a land-reclamation camp in Trenton, North Dakota, where the men built an irrigation system and had the option of making spare money by picking potatoes. Hartman's jobs included driving a huge tractor.

He applied to the Byberry camp for his next posting. Before leaving North Dakota, he received a letter asking whether he was willing to be a subject in hepatitis infection research. The project was just starting. Hartman told me he had two reasons for agreeing to participate. Conscientious objectors were being called yellowbellies, and he wanted to show that he was not a coward. And he was drawn to the idea of eradicating illness: "We were helping discover how to cure a disease and that's what we liked doing."

Hartman was a subject in the Philadelphia project's earliest hepatitis experiments. He was one of nine men who received injections of specimens containing hepatitis B virus. All of the men became ill and their laboratory tests showed hepatic disturbance. Stokes's team then proceeded with cross-immunity studies that involved monitoring subjects for the better part of a year. Hartman and five other men in the initial study received two additional exposures to hepatitis virus, one with serum materials used earlier and the other with specimens containing hepatitis A. The scientists reported that the second inoculation with hepatitis B generated no more than transient symptoms, while five of the six subjects receiving hepatitis A became acutely ill. Hartman was among them.

"The serum one, I didn't know I had it till a week afterwards. They looked at my chart and said, 'You were sick.' It was very mild. But the infectious," he said, referring to hepatitis A, "the infectious was really bad." He spent several weeks as an inpatient at the University of Pennsylvania Hospital.

The surgical procedures came later. "They asked five of us if they could do a biopsy 'to prove that the cells returned to normal.'" Hartman's liver biopsy did not go entirely smoothly. "I came open and got infected." He was on an extended furlough during his convalescence. When he finally recovered, Hartman transferred out of the unit. He had spent the better part of two years living at Byberry and serving as a research subject at Penn. "I left the unit because I was no longer of value to them," referring to the Penn research team. "I mean they more or less kicked me out."

Hartman showed me a journal reprint from the Penn hepatitis project, turning to a figure depicting a subject's laboratory tests labeled "N.H.H." "Here," he said, "that's Neil Hartman."

Hartman was proud of his participation in the experiments. He wanted to believe that his service mattered, that he had contributed to the prevention of a serious illness. But he was left unsettled by what Koop had said about the men not being aware of the hazards. His discomfort was evident when I asked him questions about the matter of consent.

"Is it fair to say that you felt your participation was voluntary; you weren't coerced at all?"

He responded, "Oh, yes, it was voluntary. There was no coercion."

"Did you feel you were induced in any way?"

"No, not at all," he said. "I got this letter when I was at Trenton. I volunteered from Trenton. And, as I said, I was happy to volunteer, because I was called a yellowbelly and that sort of thing."

"Do you think they accurately informed you about the risks?"

At this point, Hartman looked away. Speaking softly, he said, "No," and after a pause, "No" again.

"Do you think they informed you to the extent that they knew what the story was, or do you think they were minimizing the risks?"

"I don't think they were hiding anything. But they didn't really sit us down and tell us the risks—they didn't with me."

I asked Hartman what Koop had said in his letter about the risks.

"He said a person died. . . . He said it was too dangerous and he wouldn't do it again. . . . I thought, I wish you'd told me that before—that it was too dangerous."

When the war was over but Hartman was still in CPS, he volunteered for overseas duties in projects run by the United Nations Relief and Rehabilitation Administration. Following his discharge from CPS, he taught at a Quaker boarding school for a time. He married and moved with his wife to Japan, where they ran a community center for the American Friends Service Committee. He had taught in a public school before entering CPS, and when he and his family returned to the United States, Hartman took a position at a Friends day school, where he taught math and science for thirty-three years. He maintained ties with the CPS community and particularly with conscientious objectors he had met at Byberry, who remained among his close friends.

In 1996, the Friends Service Committee held a conference for World War II CPS men. The organizers set up a panel for those who had served as subjects in a variety of medical experiments; the session was called "Ethics and the Guinea Pig Experiments." Hartman presided. The attendees spoke about their experiences in a range of wartime medical studies: semi-starvation experiments, research on tolerance for high-altitude conditions, and studies with anti-malaria drugs. Their topics included whether research enrollees had been informed about research hazards, and whether they had been vulnerable to inducements like the attraction of an urban setting. The men were aware that in the half century since their service as research subjects, marked shifts had occurred in notions about acceptable human experiments. Participating in studies that might advance medical knowledge had once seemed unambiguously good. Now it appeared that the whole endeavor was fraught with ethical pitfalls.

Reigning moral frameworks are ineffable; we experience them as the natural order of things. After they have undergone fundamental change, it is difficult for us to imagine how things could have looked so different in the past.

At the conference session, Hartman puzzled over the chasm between sensibilities about human subjects research that prevailed in the 1990s and the moral perspectives of his youth. CPS men had carried on long discussions about matters of conscience related to the war. At the North Dakota camp, these included lively debates about whether picking potatoes for spare money was consistent with pacifist convictions. Hartman observed, "We had much more ethical discussion on picking potatoes"—which might feed soldiers and thus prolong the war—"than we ever did on whether we should be guinea pigs in the hepatitis unit. And I don't—" Hartman broke off. "That's something to ponder. I don't understand that myself."

Glossary

Albumin: A serum protein that is the main component of blood plasma. Derived from the process of fractionation, human albumin was used as a substitute for whole blood.

Animal model: An animal susceptible to a disease that afflicts humans. Scientists use animal hosts to conduct basic research on infectious diseases and to develop and test experimental immunizing agents.

Antibodies: Proteins the immune system produces in an effort to disarm substances it identifies as foreign, including disease-causing bacteria and viruses. Antibodies target specific antigens.

Antigens: Proteins—notably components of bacteria and viruses—the immune system identifies as foreign and that trigger the production of protective antibodies. Identification of the hepatitis B surface antigen in the late 1960s was a boon to the development of effective measures to control the disease.

Assay techniques: Laboratory tests that identify the presence and measure the quantity of a targeted substance—in this case, antigens and antibodies. Progressively more sophisticated assay techniques allowed researchers to identify hepatitis carriers and understand the immune system's responses to the presence of hepatitis viruses.

Challenge procedure: An intervention that deliberately exposes individuals to a disease pathogen. Originally, scientists restricted use of the term to procedures aimed at determining immunity to infection. Early vaccine investigators employed challenge procedures to demonstrate the effectiveness of a previously administered immunizing agent. With increasing frequency beginning in the early 1940s and for the purpose of gathering systematic evidence on vaccine efficacy, researchers administered challenge inoculations to both individuals who had been vaccinated (an experimental group) and those who had not (a control group).

Cirrhosis: A disease characterized by inflammation and scarring of liver tissue and progressive erosion of organ function. Typically the result of either alcoholism or chronic hepatitis infection, cirrhosis has a high mortality rate.

Fulminant hepatitis B: An overwhelming infection in which the immune system, in an effort to eliminate hepatitis B viruses, attacks and destroys massive numbers of liver cells. Now often referred to as "acute liver failure." While rare, the ailment is almost always fatal.

Gamma globulin: A blood product made from pooled donations—produced through a process called fractionation—and containing high concentrations of antibodies. Physicians have used it to provide short-term, passive immunity to a variety of disease pathogens.

Hepatitis: A condition characterized by inflammation of the liver in which the patient may experience jaundice, fever, loss of appetite, abdominal pain, nausea and vomiting, diarrhea, muscle and joint aches, and exhaustion. While the trigger can be noninfectious, viruses generate the great majority of cases. The acute phase of pathogen-triggered disease can last six to eight weeks. *Hepatitis* is also shorthand for the viruses that cause liver inflammation.

Hepatitis A: An illness caused by a strain of virus with a fecal-oral route of infection and a typical incubation period of two to six weeks. The usual source of infection is contaminated food or water. The Food and Drug Administration licensed the first hepatitis A vaccine in 1995.

Hepatitis B: An illness caused by a strain of virus transmitted through bodily fluids, including blood and blood products, with an incubation period of two weeks to six months. Between 5 and 10 percent of adults who contract this strain retain the virus indefinitely. The prevalence of carriers is much higher among those who contract the disease as children, with the youngest the mostly likely to continue harboring the pathogen. Researchers developed an initial vaccine for hepatitis B during the early 1980s and other immunizing agents followed. But as of 2021 there was no antiviral cure for hepatitis B carriers.

Hepatitis C: An illness caused by a strain of virus transmitted through bodily fluids, including blood and blood products, with an incubation period that ranges from two weeks to six months. Infection with hepatitis C often triggers few early symptoms but generates a very high rate of carriers. Among infected adults, between 75 and 85 percent carry the virus permanently. In 2011, the first direct-acting antiviral drug for hepatitis C carriers became widely available; but as of 2021 there was no vaccine for hepatitis C.

Hepatitis carrier: A person whose immune system has failed to clear hepatitis B or C viruses after the initial phase of infection. Carriers may be symptom-free but are nonetheless at heightened risk for progressive liver disease—cirrhosis and liver cancer—two to four decades after contracting the infection. Researchers estimate that between 850,000 and 2.2 million Americans are hepatitis B carriers and that 3.5 million have been carriers of hepatitis C.

Hepatitis non-A, non-B: An early name for the hepatitis C virus strain.

Immune globulin: Sometimes used interchangeably with *gamma globulin.* In other contexts, the term refers to a fractionated blood product made from pooled donations of individuals believed to have antibodies against a specific disease-causing pathogen. The product is used to provide short-term, passive immunity to that disease agent.

Incubation period: The time between exposure to a disease pathogen and the appearance of symptoms.

Infectious (epidemic) hepatitis: An early name for hepatitis A.

Jaundice: Yellowing of the skin and eyes that can accompany liver inflammation. One of the liver's functions is to assist in recycling red blood cells. The yellow coloration in jaundice is from bilirubin, a byproduct from the breakdown of hemoglobin contained in red blood cells.

Liver cancer: The technical term is hepatocellular carcinoma. Through the carriers they generate, hepatitis B and C are responsible for the vast majority of primary liver cancers worldwide.

Liver function tests: Blood tests measuring liver proteins and enzymes that provide information on degrees of cellular integrity and liver injury. Early researchers used these tests with hepatitis-sickened subjects to learn about the course of the illness.

Passive immunity: Temporary immunity generated by the injection of an antibody-rich blood product. It is distinct from active immunity, which develops when the body's immune system produces antibodies in response to the presence of an antigen from either natural exposure or vaccination.

Plasma: The liquid portion of blood with cells removed but clotting factors retained and anticoagulant added. Commercial laboratories combined large batches of donated blood when processing plasma and medical providers used the resulting product as a blood substitute.

Sequelae: Conditions that are the consequence of a previous infection.

Serial passage: The transfer of a pathogen repeatedly through an animal host or cell line. This process can decrease the microbe's virulence.

Serum: The liquid portion of blood with both cells and clotting factors removed. Researchers used serum from patients with known or suspected cases of hepatitis B when transferring the disease to human subjects.

Serum hepatitis: An early name for hepatitis B.

Specimens: Samples of bodily tissues (blood included) or waste products. Investigators used hepatitis-containing specimens from infected patients to induce the disease in research participants.

Tissue culture: A growth medium derived from living tissue used for cultivating viruses.

Unmodified pathogens: Fully virulent disease microbes, in contrast to attenuated or killed pathogens that have been the active ingredients in many vaccines.

Record Group Abbreviations

AFSC CPS   Civilian Public Service Records, American Friends Service Committee Archives, Philadelphia

APS Stokes   Joseph Stokes Jr. Papers, American Philosophical Society Archives, Philadelphia

Bancroft Meyer   Karl F. Meyer Papers, Bancroft Library, University of California, Berkeley

Bentley Francis   Thomas Francis Jr. Papers, Bentley Historical Library, University of Michigan, Ann Arbor

Countway Beecher   Henry K. Beecher Papers, Center for the History of Medicine, Countway Library of Medicine, Harvard University, Cambridge

CSI Clippings   Willowbrook State School News Clippings Collection, Archives and Special Collections, College of Staten Island, City University of New York

CSI McCourt   Diana McCourt Collection, Archives and Special Collections, College of Staten Island, City University of New York

Harvard Nuremberg Digital   Nuremberg Trial Project, Digital Document Collection, Historical and Special Collections, Harvard Law School Library, Cambridge

LVA Hospital Board   Accession 42741 (State Mental Health, Mental Retardation, and Substance Abuse Service Board), State Government Records Collection, Archives and Manuscripts, Library of Virginia, Richmond

NARA AEB Boards	RG 112 (Office of the Surgeon General–Army), Entry 31 (World War II), Zone I (Interior), Decimal 334 (Boards), National Archives and Records Administration, College Park, MD
NARA AEB Histories	RG 112 (Office of the Surgeon General–Army), Entry 31 (World War II), Zone I (Interior), Decimal 314.7 (Unpublished Histories), National Archives and Records Administration, College Park, MD
NARA AFEB	RG 334 (Interservice Agencies), Entry 14 (Armed Forces Epidemiology Board—Commissions, 1947–63), National Archives and Records Administration, College Park, MD
NARA AFEB Accession	RG 334 (Interservice Agencies), Unprocessed Accession, National Archives and Records Administration, College Park, MD
NARA AFEB Meetings	RG 334 (Interservice Agencies), Entry 13A (Armed Forces Epidemiology Board—Board Meetings, 1948–63), National Archives and Records Administration, College Park, MD
NARA NIH Director	RG 443 (National Institutes of Health), Office of the Director, Central Files, 1960–82, National Archives and Records Administration, College Park, MD
NARA NIH Org Files	RG 443 (National Institutes of Health), Individual Institutes (Organizational Files), National Archives and Records Administration, College Park, MD
NARA NIH Planning	RG 443 (National Institutes of Health), Office of the Director, Office of Research and Planning, Subject Files, 1948–56, National Archives and Records Administration, College Park, MD
NARA OSRD CMR	RG 227 (Office of Scientific Research and Development), Entry 165 (Committee on Medical Research General Records, 1942–46), National Archives and Records Administration, College Park, MD

NARA OTSG Diseases   RG 112 (Office of the Surgeon General–Army), Entry 31 (World War II), Zone I (Interior), Decimal 710 (Diseases), National Archives and Records Administration, College Park, MD

NARA OTSG R & D   RG 112 (Office of the Army Surgeon General), Entry 389 (U.S. Army Research & Development Command), National Archives and Records Administration, College Park, MD

NARA SOD   RG 330 (Secretary of Defense), National Archives and Records Administration, College Park, MD

NARA SSS   RG 147 (Selective Service System), Entry 23 (Conscientious Objectors, General Files 1941–47), Decimal 450 (Camp Operations), National Archives and Records Administration, College Park, MD

NAS Blood Related   Committee on Blood and Related Problems, Division of Medical Sciences, 1946–1973, National Research Council, National Academy of Sciences Archives, Washington, DC

NAS Liver   Subcommittee on Liver Disease, Division of Medical Sciences, 1946–1973, National Research Council, National Academy of Sciences Archives, Washington, DC

NAS Plasma   Committee on Plasma and Plasma Substitutes, Division of Medical Sciences, 1946–1973, National Research Council, National Academy of Sciences Archives, Washington, DC

NAS Sterilization   Subcommittee on Sterilization of Blood and Plasma, Division of Medical Sciences, 1946–1973, National Research Council, National Academy of Sciences Archives, Washington, DC

NAS Tropical Meetings   Subcommittee on Tropical Diseases Meeting Minutes (microfiche), Committee on Medicine, Division of Medical Sciences, 1940–1945, National Research Council, National Academy of Sciences Archives, Washington, DC

NAS Tropical Misc   Subcommittee on Tropical Diseases, 1942,
                                   Committee on Medicine, Division of Medical
                                   Sciences, 1940–1945, National Academy of
                                   Sciences Archives, Washington, DC

NAS WBC   Committee on Biological Warfare, War Bureau of
                                   Consultants, National Research Council,
                                   National Academy of Sciences Archives,
                                   Washington, DC

NJSA Board Minutes   SZCTR001 (Minutes of the State Board of Control),
                                   New Jersey State Archives, Trenton

NJSA Clinton   SINCL004 (New Jersey State Reformatory for
                                   Women at Clinton, Annual Reports), New Jersey
                                   State Archives, Trenton

NJSA Commissioner   SINCO001 (Department of Institutions and
                                   Agencies, Commissioner's Office), New Jersey
                                   State Archives, Trenton

NJSA Trenton Reports   SHUTP003 (Monthly Reports of New Jersey State
                                   Hospital at Trenton, 1939–52), New Jersey State
                                   Archives, Trenton

NLM Bayne-Jones   MSC 155 (Stanhope Bayne-Jones Papers), National
                                   Library of Medicine, Bethesda, MD

NLM Henle   MSC 460 ("Growing Up with Virology: An
                                   Annotated Bibliography of Werner and Gertrude
                                   Henle," 1986 typescript), National Library of
                                   Medicine, Bethesda, MD

NLM NIH Director   MSC 536 (NIH Director's Files), National Library
                                   of Medicine, Bethesda, MD

NYU Krugman   Saul Krugman Papers, 1949–2002, Lillian &
                                   Clarence de La Chapelle Medical Archives, New
                                   York University Health Sciences Library, New
                                   York City

Penn MCHR   MS 641 (Medical Committee on Human Rights),
                                   Special Collections, University of Pennsylvania
                                   Library, Philadelphia

RAC Bauer Diary   Rockefeller Foundation, RG 12 (Officer's Diaries),
                                   Box 16, Folder: Johannes Bauer, 1940–44,
                                   Rockefeller Archive Center, Sleepy Hollow, NY

RAC IHD Admin   Rockefeller Foundation, RG 3.1 (Administration,
                         Program and Policy), Series 908 (IHD),
                         Rockefeller Archive Center, Sleepy Hollow, NY
RAC RF International   Rockefeller Foundation, RG 1 (Projects), Series 100
                         (International), Rockefeller Archive Center,
                         Sleepy Hollow, NY
RAC Virus Lab   Rockefeller Foundation, RG 5 (International Health
                         Board and Division), Series 4 (Virus Laboratory),
                         Rockefeller Archive Center, Sleepy Hollow, NY
SCPC AFSC CPS   DG 02 (American Friends Service Committee,
                         Civilian Public Service), Swarthmore College
                         Peace Collection, Swarthmore, PA
TMC Melnick   Joseph Melnick Papers, McGovern Historical
                         Center, Texas Medical Center Library, Houston
Winkler Sabin   Albert B. Sabin Papers, Henry R. Winkler Center
                         for the History of Health Professions, Health
                         Sciences Library, University of Cincinnati
WRAIR AEB   Army Epidemiology Board Records, Gorgas
                         Memorial Library, Walter Reed Army Institute of
                         Research, Silver Spring, MD
Yale Enders   John Enders Papers, Manuscripts and Archives, Yale
                         University Library, New Haven, CT

Notes

Preface

Waiver and release forms for hepatitis experiments among Stokes's papers ("WAIVER AND RELEASE"; *"for the purpose of experiments"*): APS Stokes (unprocessed), Folder: Measles Volunteers #1. (Currently reorganized into Series VI, Folders: Measles #39 through Measles #42.) Italics added.

Introduction

Estimates of the numbers and characteristics of hepatitis infection subjects: Thirty-seven hundred is a cumulative estimate based on the combination of scientific publications, unpublished research reports, and researchers' statements in correspondence or professional meetings. Not all of these subjects developed an identified case of hepatitis. Some were apparently unaffected; others contracted what researchers described as mild illness, while many had full-blown bouts with hepatitis. Research reports sometimes note the age and sex of subjects but rarely their race or ethnicity. Documents that include designations of race are classified as patient records and are excluded from repository collections or are otherwise inaccessible. My information on participants' race comes from sources on the institutions housing subjects—one nonprison facility where hepatitis experiments took place admitted whites only—and from sparse documents with information on race that I occasionally found among archived materials.

Researchers used waiver and release clauses before the 1940s: Sydney A. Halpern, *Lesser Harms: The Morality of Risk in Medical Research* (Chicago: University of Chicago Press, 2004), 100–102, 104.

With World War II, medical research became an organized program: On the transformation in medical research with the advent of World War II, David J. Rothman wrote, "A cottage industry turned into a national program";

found in *Strangers at the Bedside* (New York: Basic Books, 1991), 30. Rothman also noted that a wartime utilitarian ethos enabled hazardous experiments; see *Strangers at the Bedside*, 49–50; and David J. Rothman, "Ethics and Human Experimentation: Henry Beecher Revisited," *New England Journal of Medicine* 317, no. 19 (November 5, 1987): 1198.

Precedents for the notion of a military-biomedical elite: Similar concepts are found in literature on physical sciences and the state. Paul Hoch uses the term *boundary elite* in "The Crystallization of a Strategic Alliance: The American Physics Elite and the Military in the 1940s," in *Science, Technology and the Military*, vol. 12, ed. Everett Mendelsohn, Merritt R. Smith, and Peter Weingart (Dordrecht, Netherlands: Kluwer Academic, 1988), 87–116. Daniel L. Kleinman develops the notion further in *Politics on the Endless Frontier: Postwar Research Policy in the United States* (Durham, NC: Duke University Press, 1995). Concerning the biomedical arena, Kayte Spector-Bagdady and Paul A. Lombardo allude to the existence of a research elite in their discussion of early postwar STD experiments in Guatemala. They note that multiple government-sponsored scientific panels composed of prestigious and well-connected investigators approved those studies' conduct. "'Something of an Adventure': Postwar NIH Research Ethos and the Guatemala STD Experiments," *Journal of Law, Medicine and Ethics* 41, no. 3 (Fall 2013): 697–710.

Wartime researchers used challenge procedures for testing vaccines: Jonas Salk and Thomas Francis Jr. administered challenge procedures of unmodified influenza to vaccinated and unvaccinated subjects at Ypsilanti State Hospital, a mental institution in Michigan. One report of this work is Jonas E. Salk et al., "Protective Effect of Vaccination against Induced Influenza B," *Journal of Clinical Investigation* 24, no. 4 (July 1945): 547–53. Francis describes the broader AEB-sponsored program in "History of the Commission on Influenza, February 1942–December 1945," Bentley Francis, Box 32, Folder: History of Influenza Commission. Papers on challenge procedures testing measles vaccines include Elizabeth P. Maris et al., "Studies in Measles: V. The Results of Chance and Planned Exposure to Unmodified Measles Virus in Children Previously Inoculated with Egg-Passage Measles Virus," *Journal of Pediatrics* 22, no. 1 (January 1943): 17–29. Other challenge studies from Stokes's team include Werner Henle, Gertrude Henle, and Joseph Stokes Jr., "Demonstration of the Efficacy of Vaccination against Influenza Type A by Experimental Infection of Human Beings," *Journal of Immunology* 46, no. 3 (March 1943): 163–75; and Werner Henle et al., "Experimental Exposure of Human Subjects to Viruses of Influenza," *Journal of Immunology* 52, no. 2 (February 1946): 145–65. The Stokes group's subjects were institutionalized children in Pennsylvania and New Jersey. Howard J. Shaughnessy et al. report challenge procedures in "Experimental Human Bacillary Dysentery," *JAMA* 132, no. 7 (December 19, 1946): 362–68; their subjects were inmates at the Illinois State Penitentiary at Joliet, also called Joliet Penitentiary.

Wartime scientists transmitted unmodified pathogens for purposes other than vaccine testing: John R. Paul reports human infection experiments with sand-fly fever and dengue in "History of the Commission on Neurotropic Virus Diseases, 1941–45," Army Epidemiology Board, NARA AEB Histories, Box 226, Folder: Army Epidemiology Board, Neurotropic Virus Diseases, History of the Commission. Albert Sabin elaborates on the AEB's research program with dengue and sand-fly fever in "Research on Dengue during World War II," *American Journal of Tropical Medicine and Hygiene* 1, no. 1 (January 1952): 30–50. Among the journal publications on experiments with atypical pneumonia is Commission on Acute Respiratory Diseases, "Transmission of Primary Atypical Pneumonia to Human Volunteers," *JAMA* 127, no. 3 (January 20, 1945): 146–49. Literature on the U.S. malaria infection program includes Karen M. Masterson, *The Malaria Project: The U.S. Government's Secret Mission to Find a Miracle Cure* (New York: Penguin, 2014); Bernard E. Harcourt, "Making Willing Bodies: The University of Chicago Human Experiments at Stateville Penitentiary," *Social Research* 78, no. 2 (Summer 2011): 443–78; and Nathaniel Comfort, "The Prisoner as a Model Organism: Malaria Research at Stateville Penitentiary," *Studies in the History and Philosophy of Science, Part C: Studies in History and Philosophy of Biological and Biomedical Sciences* 40, no. 3 (September 2009): 190–203. Researchers recruited conscientious objectors as subjects in transmission experiments with atypical pneumonia. Most of the participants in human infection studies with sand-fly fever, dengue, and malaria were prison inmates.

What the Tuskegee Syphilis Study did and did not involve: Sources on the Tuskegee Syphilis Study include Allan Brandt, "Racism and Research: The Case of the Tuskegee Syphilis Study," *Hastings Center Report* 8, no. 6 (December 1978): 21–29; James H. Jones, *Bad Blood: The Tuskegee Syphilis Study* (New York: Free Press, 1981); Susan M. Reverby, ed., *Tuskegee's Truths: Rethinking the Tuskegee Syphilis Study* (Chapel Hill: University of North Carolina Press, 2000); and Susan M. Reverby, *Examining Tuskegee: The Infamous Syphilis Study and Its Legacy* (Chapel Hill: University of North Carolina Press, 2009).

The PHS conducted STD infection experiments in Guatemala: Susan M. Reverby, "'Normal Exposure' and Inoculation Syphilis: A PHS 'Tuskegee' Doctor in Guatemala, 1946–48," *Journal of Policy History* 23, no. 1 (January 2011): 6–28; and Susan M. Reverby, "Ethical Failures and History Lessons: The U.S. Public Health Service Research Studies in Tuskegee and Guatemala," *Public Health Reviews* 34, no. 1 (June 2012): 1–18. PHS researchers issued no publications from this research, and it remained hidden for sixty years.

Records bearing on the race of prisoners in hepatitis experiments: Participation of people of color was apparently most common in experiments taking place at prisons. A publication from experiments conducted in 1945 at Jackson State Prison in Michigan (near Detroit) reveals that among a subset of eight participants, two (25 percent) were African American. Documents on hepatitis transmission studies from the late 1960s at Joliet Penitentiary (near Chicago) suggest that, in some rounds of experiments, 25 to 44 percent of subjects were African American. Among hepatitis infection subjects overall, approximately 45 percent were prison inmates.

Literature on the rise and fall of dominant systems of beliefs: The question of how a system of beliefs takes hold has been the subject of scholarly debate. French sociologist Pierre Bourdieu highlights the role of cultural capital in establishing belief systems within a social field and the importance of personally embodied understandings of the social world in generating system stability. Focusing on the possibilities of disruption and system change, American field theorists Neil Fligstein and Doug McAdam emphasize the importance of state actors and interplay among disparate social fields. See Pierre Bourdieu and Loïc J. D. Wacquant, *An Invitation to Reflexive Sociology* (Chicago: University of Chicago Press, 1992); and Neil Fligstein and Doug McAdam, *A Theory of Fields* (New York: Oxford University Press, 2012). My analysis details processes of change highlighting the impact of both the historical context and actors who leverage powerful cultural imagery; this perspective draws on Ann Swidler, "Culture in Action: Symbols and Strategies," *American Sociological Review* 51 no. 2 (April 1986): 273–86.

Stokes states he enrolled fourteen hundred subjects in hepatitis studies: Discussion following "Infectious Hepatitis," *Transactions of the Conference on Liver Injury* 11 (April 30–May 1, 1952): 24; and Joseph Stokes Jr., "Gordon Wilson Lecture: Viral Hepatitis," *Transactions of the American Clinical and Climatological Association* 64 (1953): 117. Elsewhere Stokes stated he had enrolled more than fifteen hundred subjects in hepatitis transmission studies.

Stokes says proudly he had no deaths from hepatitis experiments: Stokes, "Gordon Wilson Lecture," 117.

Stokes shows that gamma globulin slowed the spread of hepatitis A during epidemics: Stokes's group first tested gamma globulin for hepatitis A abatement during an outbreak at a summer camp for children in the Pocono Mountains during August 1944. Joseph Stokes Jr. and John R. Neefe, "The Prevention and Attenuation of Infectious Hepatitis by Gamma Globulin," *JAMA* 127, no. 3 (January 20, 1945): 144–45. Then, with the approval of the army surgeon general, members of his team together with army medical officers conducted field trials of gamma globulin during hepatitis A outbreaks among military personnel in the Mediterranean region. The trials, which took place during the fall of 1944 and winter of 1944–45, showed that gamma globulin had a protective effect. Sydney S. Gellis et al., "The Use of Human Immune Serum Globulin (Gamma Globulin) in Infectious (Epidemic) Hepatitis in the Mediterranean Theater of Operations," *JAMA* 128, no. 15 (August 11, 1945): 1062–63.

Written accounts of the smallpox challenge procedure of Stokes's forebear: The story was passed down as oral tradition before entering the written record. According to local historian George Decou, John Hinchman Stokes, who began practicing medicine in Moorestown, New Jersey, in 1786, "was the first physician in Burlington County to accept Jenner's theory of vaccination and was so confident of its efficacy that he inoculated his little daughter Hannah and laid her on the bed with one of his smallpox patients in order to convince his skeptical friends and patients." *Moorestown and Her Neighbors, Historical Sketches*

(Philadelphia: Harris & Partridge, 1929), 44. In his acknowledgments, Decou lists Dr. Joseph Stokes—likely Stokes Sr., Szanton's grandfather. A briefer version of the story is found in Evens M. Woodward and John F. Hageman, *History of Burlington and Mercer Counties, New Jersey* (Philadelphia: Everts & Peck, 1993), 78.

Jenner's challenge procedures demonstrating the efficacy of cowpox vaccination: Halpern, *Lesser Harms*, 13, 25–28. Before widespread acceptance of vaccination against smallpox using cowpox specimens, inoculation with human smallpox specimens was common. When successfully administered, this intervention generated a case of smallpox that conferred immunity to future infection. While the procedure carried very real risks, rates of fatalities from inoculated smallpox were substantially lower than death rates from the naturally contracted disease. When Jenner challenged his eight-year-old subject with human smallpox, he was employing a medical procedure in wide use at that time.

Thomas Jefferson adopted Jenner's method and arranged for a challenge demonstration: Todd L. Savitt, *Medicine and Slavery: The Disease and Health Care of Blacks in Antebellum Virginia* (Champaign: University of Illinois Press, 1978), 294–97. Relevant primary documents are reprinted in Robert H. Halsey, *How the President, Thomas Jefferson, and Dr. Benjamin Waterhouse Established Vaccination as a Public Health Procedure* (New York: New York Academy of Medicine, 1936). Savitt notes that Jefferson had family members inoculated with human smallpox before he arranged for the cowpox vaccinations and the subsequent challenge procedure.

Chapter One. In the National Interest

Paul describes the 1942 hepatitis outbreak ("the great epidemic"; "fell upon the troops"): John R. Paul and Horace T. Gardner, "Viral Hepatitis," in *Preventive Medicine in World War II*, vol. 5 (Washington, DC: Office of the Surgeon General, U.S. Army, 1960), 411.

On the numbers of personnel infected in the 1942 hepatitis epidemic: Stimson released the 28,500 figure in "Jaundice Danger in Army from Yellow Fever Vaccine Now Over," issued by the War Department Bureau of Public Relations, July 28, 1942, NARA OTSG Diseases, Box 1125, Folder: Virus Disease, Jaundice—Publicity on the Effect of Yellow Fever Vaccine. Walter Paul Havens Jr. cites the figure of 50,000 hospitalizations in "Viral Hepatitis," in *Internal Medicine in World War II*, vol. 3: *Infectious Diseases and General Medicine* (Washington, DC: Office of the Surgeon General, U.S. Army, 1968), 332. Many sickened soldiers, having not received inpatient care, went uncounted. Leonard B. Seeff et al. put the number of infected personnel at 330,000 in "Serologic Follow-up of the 1942 Epidemic of Post-vaccination Hepatitis in the United States Army," *New England Journal of Medicine* 316, no. 16 (April 16, 1987): 965.

War Department withheld information on total hepatitis fatalities: Johannes Bauer, head of the Rockefeller Foundation's Virus Laboratory, wrote of the army's refusal to share figures on post-vaccination hepatitis deaths: "It is considered confidential and cannot be made available, even to us." RAC Bauer Diary, April 13, 1943.

Bayne-Jones reports the commander's reaction to the epidemic ("It was more shocking"; "was won by pilots"): Stanhope Bayne-Jones, "An Oral History Interview," conducted in 1966 by Harlan B. Phillips, 691, 547. Transcript available at the National Library of Medicine, Bethesda, MD.

The 1918 flu pandemic sickened a large portion of American military personnel: Carol R. Byerly, "The U.S. Military and the Influenza Pandemic of 1918–1919," *Public Health Reports* 125, Suppl. 3 (2010): 82–91.

On the army's World War II vaccine program: Arthur P. Long, "The Army Immunization Program," in *Preventive Medicine in World War II*, vol. 3: *Personal Health Measures and Immunizations* (Office of the Surgeon General, U.S. Army, 1955), 271–341.

Bayne-Jones's description of Simmons ("a preventive medicine evangelist"): Albert E. Cowdrey, *War and Healing: Stanhope Bayne-Jones and the Maturing of American Medicine* (Baton Rouge: Louisiana State University Press, 1992), 147.

IHD scientists developed the yellow fever vaccine: John Farley, "Yellow Fever Vaccines: A Slap in the Face," in *To Cast out Disease: A History of the International Health Division of the Rockefeller Foundation, 1913–1951* (New York: Oxford University Press, 2004), 167–82. Farley's chapter also provides an account of events surrounding the 1942 hepatitis epidemic. Other sources on the early development of yellow fever vaccine include Nancy Leys Stepan, *Eradication: Ridding the World of Disease Forever?* (Ithaca, NY: Cornell University Press, 2011); Greer Williams, *Plague Killers* (New York: Scribner's, 1969); Hugh H. Smith, "Controlling Yellow Fever," in *Yellow Fever*, ed. George K. Strode (New York: McGraw-Hill, 1951), 539–628. Max Theiler performed the laboratory work for development of the IHD's yellow fever vaccine and received the 1951 Nobel Prize in medicine for his accomplishment.

The NRC recommends limited use of the IHD yellow fever vaccine: NAS Tropical Meetings, Minutes of June 19, 1940. The initial number of doses requested is from L. R. Thompson, NIH director to the PHS surgeon general, August 16, 1940, NARA NIH Org Files (1930–48), Box 140 (Microbiology 1930–48), Folder: Yellow Fever Vaccine.

The War Department expands its mandate for yellow fever vaccination: "Stimson Orders All in Army Vaccinated against Yellow Fever," *New York Times*, February 13, 1942, 1. Farley notes the number of doses that were eventually distributed in "Yellow Fever Vaccines," 173.

Japanese researchers tried to obtain yellow fever virus: The scientists were Ryōichi Naitō and Yonetsugi Miyagawa. Peter Williams and David Wallace, *Unit 731: The Japanese Army's Secret of Secrets* (London: Hodder & Stoughton, 1989), 92–93, 152–53.

The War Bureau of Consultants recommends vaccination ("one of those most to be feared"; "the method of choice"): NAS WBC, Box 2, Report of February 19, 1942, 8.

Fear of germ warfare spurred yellow fever vaccine policy ("used this scare"): Bayne-Jones, "Oral History," 516. The quotation ("could be traced to") is from Cowdrey, *War and Healing*, 145. Cowdrey discusses Simmons's convictions about yellow fever and biological warfare in *War and Healing*, 141–45; the author also notes that the administration spent $40 million on building and equipment costs for its World War II germ warfare program. The United States also began research with chemical warfare agents; Susan L. Smith examines the program of human experiments with mustard gas in *Toxic Exposures* (New Brunswick, NJ: Rutgers University Press, 2017).

Bayne-Jones's character and professional biography ("to master the detail"): Cowdrey describes Bayne-Jones's temperament in *War and Healing*, 85, 147–49. On his first six months at the OTSG, see Bayne-Jones, "Oral History," 689.

Consultants investigate hepatitis at West Coast military installations: Karl F. Meyer, *Medical Research and Public Health*, an interview by Edna T. Daniel in 1961 and 1962 (Berkeley, CA: Bancroft Library, 1976), 227–30. The consultants later issued a full account of the investigation in two consecutive journal issues: Wilbur A. Sawyer et al., "Jaundice in Army Personnel in the Western Regions of the United States and Its Relation to Vaccination against Yellow Fever," *American Journal of Hygiene* 39 (January–May 1944): 337–430, and 40 (July–November 1944): 35–107.

Publications report hepatitis following yellow fever vaccination: These included G. M. Findlay and F. O. MacCallum, "Note on Acute Hepatitis and Yellow Fever Immunization," *Transactions of the Royal Society of Tropical Medicine and Hygiene* 31, no. 3 (November 1937): 297–308; G. M. Findlay and F. O. MacCallum, "Hepatitis and Jaundice Associated with Immunization against Certain Virus Diseases," *Proceedings of the Royal Society of Medicine* 31 (1938): 799–806; and R. L. Soper and H. H. Smith, "Yellow Fever Vaccination with Cultivated Virus and Immune and Hyperimmune Serum," *American Journal of Tropical Medicine* 18 (March 1938): 111–34.

Simmons resists ending yellow fever vaccinations ("Col. Simmons was particularly emphatic"): Bauer to Sawyer, April 11, 1942, RAC RF International, Box 16, Folder 131: Jaundice, April 1942.

Bayne-Jones never believed the heat method would kill hepatitis: RAC Bauer Diary, April 10, 1942.

IHD researchers examine blood donor records: Bauer describes the review of donor records in RAC Bauer Diary, May 18, 1942.

Simmons reacts to news that the vaccine caused hepatitis ("Can't be"): Meyer, *Medical Research*, 228.

The 1942 hepatitis outbreak was humiliating for the IHD ("The most embarrassing episode"): Farley, "Yellow Fever Vaccines," 169.

As outbreak's source becomes clear, critics take aim at Sawyer: Meyer's complaints about Sawyer are found in *Medical Research*, 230–32. IHD scientist Lewis W. Hackett's unfinished history of the IHD describes the judgments of Sawyer's colleagues. These materials include a six-page typescript, "Sawyer and the Army Hepatitis Outbreak." RAC IHD Admin, Box 4, Folder 27: History— Lewis Hackett Notes—Yellow Fever. Also informative is a summary of interviews titled "Sawyer," at RAC IHD Admin, Box 7H, Folder: 86.098.

News coverage of the outbreak is a nightmare for the War Department ("A Grievous Error"; "How did it happen"; "In the war thus far"): *Chicago Tribune*, July 27, 1942. Another call for an investigation is reported in "Rep Thomas Demands Congress Inquiry into Widespread Jaundice Epidemic in Army," *Washington Times-Herald*, July 30, 1942. *JAMA* entered into the fray, calling the *Tribune*'s editorial "unwarranted" and "a disservice to American medicine" in "Jaundice following Yellow Fever Vaccination" *JAMA* 119, no. 14 (August 1, 1942): 1110. (*JAMA* made this commentary available prior to the publication date.) The *Chicago Tribune* covered the *JAMA*'s objections in "Medical Journal Hits *Tribune* Editorial on Jaundice in Army" (July 28, 1942). Press coverage of Stimson's effort at damage control includes "Jaundice Cases Reach 28,585 in Army; 62 Die," *Chicago Tribune*, July 25, 1942; and "Army Jaundice Epidemic over, Stimson Finds," *Chicago Tribune*, August 28, 1942.

Scientists meet on June 13 and 17 in response to the vaccine problem: An account of the June 13 meeting is at RAC RF International, Box 16, Folder: 130, Jaundice, January–March 1942. Summaries of the June 17 meeting are found in Francis Blake to Sawyer, June 20, 1942, RAC RF International, Box 16, Folder 134: Jaundice, June 15–30, 1942; and Blake to surgeon general of the navy, same date, NAS Tropical Misc, 1942. IHD scientific directors attending the June 17 meeting were Thomas Parran (PHS surgeon general), Kenneth F. Maxcy, Ernest W. Goodpasture, and Thomas M. Rivers.

Fateful meeting takes place on July 8 at the National Academy of Science ("The consensus"): NAS Tropical Meetings, Minutes for July 8, 1942. Another account is at RAC RF International, Box 16, Folder 130: Jaundice, January–March 1942.

Some matters are excluded from the July 8 meeting minutes: On July 18, 1942, Robert B. Watson wrote Sanford V. Larkey at the NRC Division of Medical Sciences saying, "Doubtless you have already written [Sawyer] concerning the secret nature of some of the information received by the Subcommittee." NAS Tropical Misc, 1942.

Scientists had made attempts at animal transmission of hepatitis: The IHD researcher conducting animal research was Eaton Monroe. From correspondence in Bancroft Meyer, Box 28, Folder: I Misc.

Precedents for transmitting unmodified pathogens to human subjects: Sources on Walter Reed's yellow fever experiments include Susan E. Lederer, *Subjected to Science: Human Experimentation in America before the Second World War* (Baltimore, MD: Johns Hopkins University Press, 1995); Susan E. Lederer,

"Walter Reed and the Yellow Fever Experiments, in *Oxford Textbook of Clinical Research Ethics*, ed. Ezekiel Emanuel et al. (New York: Oxford University Press, 2008), 9–17; and Enrique Chavez-Carballo, "Clara Mass, Yellow Fever and Human Experimentation," *Military Medicine* 178 (May 2013): 557–62. Publications from the influenza transmission studies following the 1918 pandemic include Milton J. Rosenau, "Experiments to Determine Mode of Spread of Influenza," *JAMA* 73, no. 5 (August 2, 1919): 311–13; and H. R. Wahl, George B. White, and H. W. Lyall, "Some Experiments on the Transmission of Influenza," *Journal of Infectious Diseases* 25, no. 5 (November 1919): 419–26. British scientists began human transmission experiments with hepatitis around the same time as American researchers, although it is unclear whether Bayne-Jones and AEB researchers were aware of this during the spring or summer of 1942. Sources on the British hepatitis infection studies include F. O. MacCallum, "Discussion on Infective Hepatitis, Homologous Serum Hepatitis and Arsenotherapy Jaundice," *Proceedings of the Royal Society of Medicine* 37, no. 8 (June 1944): 449–60; Wilbur Sawyer et al., "Jaundice in Army Personnel" (July–November, 1944): 71–72; and Jenny Stanton, "'I Have Been on Tenterhooks': Wartime Medical Research Council Jaundice Committee Experiments," in *Useful Bodies: Humans in the Service of Medical Science in the Twentieth Century*, ed. Jordon Goodman et al. (Baltimore, MD: Johns Hopkins University Press, 2003), 109–32.

Bauer reports that serum used in vaccine production contained hepatitis ("One thing is quite definite"): Bauer to M. V. Hargett at the PHS Rocky Mountain Laboratory, with a copy to Bayne-Jones, May 21, 1941, RAC Virus Lab, Box 31, Folder 347 (USPHS).

Bayne-Jones promotes transmission experiments with the infective vaccine ("It would be a great achievement"): Bayne-Jones to Bauer, May 25, 1942, RAC RF International, Box 16, Folder 132: Jaundice, May 1942. What Bayne-Jones meant by "designed and controlled experiment" was a replicable laboratory study in which an experienced investigator anticipated and took into account conditions that might bias results. On evolving notions of controlled trials, see Harry M. Marks, *Progress of Experiment* (New York: Cambridge University Press, 1997), 28–32.

The AEB endorses human experiments with hepatitis-containing vaccine ("After thorough discussion"): NARA AEB Boards, Box 615, Folder: Board Meeting, May 12–13, 1942. Emphasis added.

Meyer points to risks of deliberate human transmission of hepatitis ("Experiments in human volunteers"): Meyer to Sawyer, July 1, 1942, Bancroft Meyer, Box 28, Folder: I Misc.

Bauer sends Dyer vaccine from hepatitis-containing lot 331: Bauer to Dyer, July 10, 1942, RAC Virus Lab, Box 31, Folder 347 (USPHS, 1941–44, 1946).

NIH asks for an additional supply of infective vaccine ("since our work is"): M. V. Veldee to Bauer, July 31, 1942, RAC Virus Lab, Box 31, Folder 347 (USPHS, 1941–44, 1946).

PHS researchers investigated hepatitis in the Virgin Islands: The PHS group included Oliphant, Alexander G. Gilliam, and Carl L. Larson. Soon after the hepatitis infection studies began, Larson, the senior officer in the group, became director of the PHS Rocky Mountain Laboratory; Gilliam also moved on to other work.

Bayne-Jones meets with NIH researchers before human studies commence: Memo from Bayne-Jones, August 3, 1942: "Conference held in the office of Colonel Simmons today. Present: Dr. Dyer, Dr. Veldee, Dr. Oliphant, Captain Stephenson and myself." NARA OTSG Diseases, Box 1119, Folder: Virus Disease—Jaundice, Infectious Hepatitis, Incidences in the Caribbean: Virgin Islands.

Oliphant submits a memo on the soon-to-begin transmission studies ("A safe and reliable"; "Prompt solution"; "it is deemed by us"; "Approved by R. E. Dyer"): NARA NIH Org Files (1939–51), Box 139, Folder: 1973.

Documents reveal Oliphant's background: Performance evaluations of Oliphant are from Department of Health and Human Services FOIA #15-0347. Oliphant voiced an affinity for clinical and field investigations and a willingness to serve agency needs in a memo to Dyer dated July 1, 1948. NARA NIH Director, Box 159, Folder: National Institute of Allergy and Infectious Diseases, Rocky Mountain Lab, 1947–1979.

Sterilizations and hepatitis experiments take place at Lynchburg State Colony: Lynchburg Colony was also the site of the famous *Buck v. Bell* Supreme Court case in 1927 that resulted in the compulsory sterilization of Carrie Buck. Paul A. Lombardo, *Three Generations, No Imbeciles: Eugenics, the Supreme Court and* Buck v. Bell (Baltimore, MD: Johns Hopkins University Press, 2008). Lombardo provides an account of Lynchburg virus transmission experiments in "'Of Utmost National Urgency': The Lynchburg Colony Hepatitis Study, 1942," in *In the Wake of Terror: Medicine and Morality in a Time of Crisis*, ed. Jonathan D. Moreno (Cambridge, MA: MIT Press, 2004), 3–15.

PHS researchers' papers on hepatitis experiments at Lynchburg: John W. Oliphant, Alexander G. Gilliam, and Carl L. Larson, "Jaundice following Administration of Human Serum," *Public Health Reports* 48, no. 33 (August 13, 1943): 1233–43; John W. Oliphant, "Jaundice following the Administration of Human Serum," *Bulletin of the Academy of Medicine* 20, no. 429 (August 1944): 254–72; John W. Oliphant, "Infectious Hepatitis: Experimental Study of Immunity," *Public Health Reports* 59, no. 50 (December 15, 1944): 1614–16. A fourth publication reported ultraviolet-inactivation studies: John W. Oliphant and Alexander Hollaender, "Homologous Serum Jaundice: Experimental Inactivation of Etiological Agent in Serum by Ultraviolet Irradiation," *Public Health Reports* 61, no. 17 (April 26, 1946): 598–602.

Researchers routinely called research subjects volunteers: Susan E. Lederer, "Political Animals: The Shaping of Biomedical Research Literature in Twentieth Century America," *Isis* 83, no. 1 (March 1992): 76; and Halpern, *Lesser Harms*, 111–13.

Lynchburg Colony annual reports mention PHS studies ("the entire year"; "selected the institution"): *Thirty-Fourth Annual Report of the Lynchburg State Colony* (July 1942–June 1943), 14. Additional entries on the studies appear in *Thirty-Fifth Annual Report of the Lynchburg State Colony* (July 1943–June 1944), 14, and *Thirty-Sixth Annual Report of the Lynchburg State Colony* (July 1944–June 1945), 14. All reports are at the Library of Virginia, Richmond.

Virginia Hospital Board discusses PHS studies at Lynchburg Colony ("Several of the hospitals"; "It was the expressed wish"): LVA Hospital Board, Minutes of March 17, 1944. Initial discussion of the PHS study is in LVA Hospital Board, Minutes of Executive Session, February 10, 1944.

Attitudes about the intellectually impaired were inhospitable: James W. Trent Jr., *Inventing the Feeble Mind: A History of Mental Retardation in the United States* (Berkeley: University of California Press, 1994); Steven Noll, *Feeble-Minded in Our Midst: Institutions for the Mentally Retarded in the South, 1900–1940* (Chapel Hill: University of North Carolina Press, 1995); and Allison Carey, *On the Margins of Citizenship: Intellectual Disability and Civil Rights in Twentieth Century America* (Philadelphia: Temple University Press, 2009).

Local journalist wrote about hepatitis studies at Lynchburg ("did as we were told"; "They took their records"): Statements of Bertha Corr from Cynthia T. Pegram, "Training Center Residents Used in World War II Experiment," *Lynchburg News & Advance*, April 25, 1995. Reporter Peter Hardin provides another account of the experiments in "State Patients Once Used as Guinea Pigs," *Richmond Times-Dispatch*, November 25, 2001.

NIH seeks approval from Bayne-Jones for Oliphant's journal article ("anything in this article"): Dyer to Bayne-Jones, August 4, 1943, NARA OTSG Diseases, Box 1135, Folder: Jaundice and Diet (Nutrition).

Oliphant sends Bayne-Jones preliminary findings ("*CONFIDENTIAL*"): Oliphant to Bayne-Jones, July 6, 1943, NARA OTSG Diseases, Box 1135, Folder: Jaundice and Diet (Nutrition). The document bears a declassification stamp dated 1958.

Bayne-Jones congratulates Oliphant on study outcomes ("I am greatly obliged"; "I think this is"): Bayne-Jones to Oliphant, July 9, 1943 and August 29, 1943, both at NARA OTSG Diseases, Box 1122, Folder: Virus Disease, Jaundice, Experiments on Animals and Humans.

Oliphant receives a promotion for his hepatitis research: Memo of March 9, 1945, Department of Health and Human Services FOIA #15-0347.

Bauer summarizes results from hepatitis studies at Lynchburg ("Jaundice following yellow fever vaccination"; "agent can be inactivated"): RAC Bauer Diary, March 2, 1944.

Chapter Two. Logistics on the Medical Battlefront

Hepatitis continues to be a problem for the military ("Hepatitis is the disease"): John R. Paul to Stanhope Bayne-Jones, December 6, 1943, NARA AEB Boards, Box 660, Folder: Commission on Neurotropic Disease—Hepatitis

Infections, Africa; ("The nature of its cause"): Statement by Paul, NARA AEB Boards, Box 655, Folder: Commission on Neurotropic Virus Diseases—Board Meeting, April 6, 1944.

Paul contracts hepatitis B while on assignment in the Mediterranean region: In late November 1943, Paul was hospitalized with hepatitis at a British installation outside Cairo. Two weeks into his illness, he wrote Albert Sabin— who had been on the mission but was already back in the United States—from his hospital bed: "An unkind fate is still holding me down in Ward #30, and I imagine that it still will be a matter of some weeks before I am turned loose." Paul to Albert Sabin, December 15, 1943, WRAIR AEB, Folder: Neurotropic Virus Diseases, Commission on, North Africa (Dr. Paul), February 1943–January 1944.

Bayne-Jones rejects hepatitis experiments with soldiers ("Use of soldiers"; "a *suitable* institution"): Bayne-Jones to Paul, March 31, 1944, NARA AEB Boards, Box 661, Folder: Commission on Neurotropic Disease—Hepatitis Project, Human Subjects and Laboratory Workers. Emphasis added. In 1918–19, government researchers did enroll navy enlistees in experiments attempting to transmit influenza. The subjects were isolated in quarantine hospitals in Boston Harbor. Milton J. Rosenau, "Experiments to Determine Mode of Transmission of Spread of Influenza," *JAMA* 73, no. 5 (August 2, 1919): 311–13.

Bayne-Jones prohibits housing hepatitis subjects on farms ("the possibility of the spread of disease"): Bayne-Jones to Stokes, April 14, 1943, NARA AEB Boards, Box 650, Folder: Commission on Measles and Mumps—Hepatitis Studies in Human Subjects. Bayne-Jones was not the only one worried about contagion. In the spring of 1944, Stokes sought access to Philadelphia General Hospital for care of subjects in hepatitis experiments. The city lawyer depicted the proposal as "involving possible danger of contagion to visitors, inmates, attendants and others," warning that if it was approved by the mayor and city council, the city would need to secure indemnification for damages in the event the disease spread. Letter to Stokes from Rufus Reeves, director, Philadelphia Department of Public Health, May 8, 1944, APS Stokes (unprocessed), Folder: U.S. War Dept #6.

Corruption was a problem at Jackson State Prison: "The Big Playhouse," *Newsweek*, August 6, 1945, NARA AEB Boards, Box 642, Folder: Jaundice, Dr. Thomas Francis. A comprehensive account of the political context at Jackson State Prison is found in "The Downfall of Harry Jackson," in "A History of Jackson Prison, 1920–75" (research paper by Charles Bright and students at University of Michigan, Winter 1979), MS 89-80, Archives of Michigan, Lansing.

Conscientious objectors strike at Danbury prison: Mulford Q. Sibley and Philip E. Jacobs discuss two hunger strikes at Danbury in *Conscription of Conscience: The American State and the Conscientious Objector, 1940–1947* (Ithaca, NY: Cornell University Press, 1952), 374, 377. The *Hartford Courant* reported several more. Paul's team conducted hepatitis infection procedures at the prison during the fall of 1944.

Francis conducts hepatitis experiments at Eloise Hospital: Francis's papers include signed waiver forms dated late January and early February 1945 for six patients at Eloise Hospital. The subjects were men between the ages of twenty-two and forty-two with spinal cord abnormalities. An accompanying document shows that the plan was to see whether materials from mosquitoes that fed on a hepatitis patient would generate the disease in subjects. Bentley Francis, Box 32, Folder: Hepatitis: Experiment at Eloise.

Multiple parties were involved in creating and overseeing CPS: Sources include Sibley and Jacobs, *Conscription of Conscience*; George Q. Flynn, *Lewis B. Hershey: Mr. Selective Service* (Chapel Hill: University of North Carolina Press, 1985); and Mitchell Lee Robinson, "Civilian Public Service during World War II: The Dilemmas of Conscience and Conscription in a Free Society" (PhD diss., Cornell University, 1990). The $7 million figure for peace church expenditures is from Sibley and Jacobs, *Conscription of Conscience*, 326.

Selective Service exerts control over management of CPS camps ("The peace churches"; "are draftees"): Albert N. Keim and Grant M. Stoltzfus quote Korsch's statements in *Politics of Conscience: The Historic Peace Churches and America at War, 1917–1955* (Scottdale, PA: Herald, 1988), 119.

Peace churches initiate use of CPS men in medical research: French to Thomas Parran, PHS surgeon general, and Lewis F. Kosch, June 16, 1942, NARA SSS, Box 196, Folder: Special Projects 1942–45, General.

Religious pacifists believe in testimony through work: Sibley and Jacobs, *Conscription of Conscience*, 309.

Experiments with CPS men as subjects begin in 1942: Alison Bateman-House reports that the first experiment with CPS men as subjects was a study of pesticides for control of lice conducted at a CPS camp in New Hampshire. "Men of Peace and the Search for the Perfect Pesticide: Conscientious Objectors, the Rockefeller Foundation, and Typhus Control Research," *Public Health Reports* 124, no. 4 (July–August 2009): 594–602. She provides an overview of the participation of CPS men in wartime research in Alison S. Bateman-House, "Compelled to Volunteer: American Conscientious Objectors to World War II as Subjects in Medical Research" (PhD diss., Columbia University, 2014).

The enrollment of CPS men in medical experiments expands: The report of eight OSRD projects is from A. S. Imirie, assistant chief of camp operations, to Major Culligan, February 14, 1943, NARA SSS, Box 196, Folder: Special Projects 1942–45, General. Standard sources, including Sibley and Jacobs, *Conscription of Conscience*, 143, give five hundred as the total number of CPS men enrolled in wartime medical studies. DeLisle Crawford compiled a list of forty-eight projects with more than one thousand men participating in "A Civilian Public Service through Medical Research," October 1944, SCPC AFSC CPS, Part 5, Box 15, Folder: Scientific Research Projects: Human Guinea Pigs, 1944. Crawford was head of publications for the AFSC's CPS division. His compilation did not include all studies conducted during the final year of the war. Bayne-Jones chronicled the AEB's use of CPS men in handwritten notes dated

October 1, 1949, NLM Bayne-Jones, Container 71, Folder: AEB—Religious Objectors, 1944–50.

Stokes helps arrange access to conscientious objectors for hepatitis studies: On June 3, 1943, Bayne-Jones sent a memo to the army surgeon general reporting that Stokes had "already laid the ground work by getting the cooperation and consent" of AFSC personnel in charge of human volunteers. NARA AEB Boards, Box 650, Folder: Commission on Measles and Mumps—Hepatitis Studies Including Religious Objectors. On June 10, Bayne-Jones wrote Lewis Kosch requesting use of CPS men for AEB hepatitis research. WRAIR AEB, Folder: Commission on Measles and Mumps—Studies on Epidemic Jaundice, June 1943–December 1944.

Stokes serves as medical advisor to the AFSC's CPS division: Report of CPS Medical Advisory Committee Meeting, March 18, 1942, AFSC CPS, 1942 Medical Committee.

Five CPS camps are sites for hepatitis experiments: Three of the camps were situated at mental hospitals: Byberry, Middletown, and Norwich. The Brethren Service Committee sponsored the unit at Norwich. Kosch later approved two additional AFSC camps in Philadelphia and New Haven.

Connecticut official resists diverting CPS men for uses other than staffing state institutions ("in such a depleted condition"): Paul to Bayne-Jones, March 29, 1944, reporting the state's concern about a severe shortage of workers at Middletown. NARA AEB Boards, Box 661, Folder: Commission on Neurotropic Virus Disease—Hepatitis Project, Human Subjects and Lab Workers. The state official was Glendon Scorboria, personnel director of the Connecticut Department of Finance and Control.

Harrisburg official asks about responsibility for injuries to CPS men who participate in medical experiments: S. M. R. O'Hara to Dr. Charles Zeller (superintendent of Philadelphia State Hospital at Byberry), August 4, 1943, NARA AEB Boards, Box 650, Folder: Commission on Measles and Mumps—Hepatitis Studies Including Religious Objectors.

Bayne-Jones negotiates with state agencies to allow medical studies with CPS men assigned to state facilities ("long, drawn-out negotiation[s]"): Bayne-Jones to Paul, March 31, 1944. Bayne-Jones stated that he had learned from previous negotiations with Pennsylvania officials that conscientious objectors assigned to work in hospitals could not be used as subjects unless replacement workers were provided. NARA AEB Boards, Box 661, Folder: Commission on Neurotropic Virus Disease—Hepatitis Project, Human Subjects and Lab Workers.

The War Department would not compensate for research injuries ("I have been informed"): Bayne-Jones to Stokes, August 10, 1943, NARA AEB, Box 650, Folder: Commission on Measles and Mumps—Hepatitis Studies Including Religious Objectors. However, the agency did allow workmen's compensation coverage for CPS men performing jobs at university-based CPS camps that began operating in 1945. On March 31, 1945, Aims McGuinness at the OTSG wrote John Paul saying that the army would approve the purchase of workmen's compensation insurance for CPS assignees holding work positions at Yale University so long as the policy showed the university as the employer and it excluded coverage of illnesses. WRAIR AEB, Folder: Commission on Neurotropic Viral Diseases—Jaundice, January 1945–June 1945.

Stokes's recruitment announcement describes hazards of hepatitis: "The symptoms last for anywhere from a few days to several months. The disease is seldom fatal, about one death occurring in every thousand cases. . . . Although jaundice is not one of the most serious diseases, there is a degree of danger involved (the mortality rate runs about .001)." From "Infectious Hepatitis— (Catarrhal Jaundice), Philadelphia Project," CPS Personnel News, P-33, October 20, 1944, SCPC AFSC CPS, Part 1, Box 40a, Folder: University of Pennsylvania Yellow Jaundice, Dr. Neefe, 1943–1944 (referred to hereafter as SCPC AFSC CPS, Neefe, 1943–1944).

Men at Big Flat camp raise questions about risks of hepatitis studies ("if he is not given some assurance"; "The Service Committee ought"): Jim Read, assistant camp director at Big Flats (Camp 46), to Lou Schneider, AFSC CPS assistant executive director, November 18, 1944, SCPC AFSC CPS, Neefe, 1943–1944.

Camp Operations rebuffed the AFSC's request for insurance: "Regarding insurance, we have introduced the subject several times but without avail." Houston Westover, head of personnel at AFSC CPS, to Lou Schneider, November 22, 1944, SCPC AFSC CPS, Neefe, 1943–1944.

The AFSC reviews its approach to vetting research risks: Westover to Schneider, November 22, 1944, SCPC AFSC CPS, Neefe, 1943–1944.

Burgess assesses hepatitis risk to be low ("outweighs that of any number"): Alex Burgess to Lou Schneider, November 22, 1944, SCPC AFSC CPS, Neefe, 1943–1944. Stokes and Burgess had served together on the AFSC Medical Committee for CPS since March 1942. From Minutes of CPS Medical Committee Meetings, March 18, March 22, and May 21, 1942, AFSC CPS, 1942, Medical Committee.

AFSC leaders dismiss concerns of Big Flats men ("It is our judgment"): Lou Schneider to Jim Read, November 29, 1944, SCPC AFSC CPS, Neefe, 1943–1944.

Samuel Burgess reports his brother's later regrets ("If he knew then"): Steven J. Taylor, *Acts of Conscience: World War II, Mental Institutions and Religious Objectors* (Syracuse, NY: Syracuse University Press, 2009), 88.

African American inmate dies in hepatitis experiment at Michigan prison: Specimens used in the experiment were from a soldier in Italy who contracted hepatitis and subsequently died after receiving serum from a donor who began to show symptoms of hepatitis forty-eight hours after giving blood. The published paper from the research interventions is Thomas Francis Jr., Arthur W. Frisch, and J. J Quilligan Jr., "Demonstration of Infectious Hepatitis Virus in Presymptomatic Period After Transfer by Transfusion," *Proceedings for the Society* *for Experimental Biology and Medicine* 61 (March 1946): 276–80. Uncharacteristically, this paper identifies the race of eight of the study's subjects; table 1 shows that of these participants, two (25 percent) were "C," a notation meaning "colored" (278). The authors report striking variation in the severity of participants' illnesses and state without further comment that the study resulted in the "fatal termination" of one subject (279). Ford is identified by name in both archived documents and press reports. His death certificate lists his race as Negro. In 1945, 33 percent of inmates admitted to state correctional facilities were black. Patrick A. Landan, "Race of Prisoners Admitted to State and Federal Institutions, 1926–86," from the Bureau of Justice Statistics, U.S. Department of Justice, 1991, available at the Bureau of Justice Statistics website, www.bjs.gov.

Another death in World War II studies preceded the Michigan prison fatality: Jon Harkness recounts events surrounding the death of Norfolk prisoner Arthur St. Germaine in "Research behind Bars: A History of Nontherapeutic Research on American Prisoners" (PhD diss., University of Wisconsin, Madison, 1996), 73–87. Susan E. Lederer discusses research deaths more generally in "Dying for Science: Historical Perspectives on Research Participants' Deaths," *AMA Journal of Ethics* 17, no. 12 (December 2015): 1166–71.

Warden asks whether deceased prisoner's family will receive compensation: Francis, "Memo concerning Hepatitis Studies at Jackson," May 31, 1945, NARA AEB Boards, Box 642, Folder: Jaundice: Dr. Thomas Francis.

Common-law wife of inmate seeks compensation ("I understand my husband"; "told me to write"; "I do not believe"): Helen H. to Francis, June 23, 1945, NARA AEB Boards, Box 642, Folder: Jaundice: Dr. Thomas Francis.

War Department instructs Francis on responding to possible claimant ("try to make a claim"): In response to Francis's request for assistance (in a letter dated July 27, 1945), Bayne-Jones forwards him instructions from the Legal Division on July 31, 1945. Francis then wrote Helen H. on August 2, 1945. All documents at NARA AEB Boards, Box 642, Folder: Jaundice: Dr. Thomas Francis.

Deceased subject had signed a waiver form ("any ill effects"; "permanent disability or death"): Francis's waiver document accompanies his correspondence to Bayne-Jones of July 27, 1945. NARA AEB Boards, Box 642, Folder: Jaundice: Dr. Thomas Francis.

Local newspapers report inmate's death ("a new serum for jaundice"): "Human Guinea Pig Dies," *Detroit Free Press*; and "Death of Prison Inmate under Investigation," *Ann Arbor News*, both June 2, 1945, NARA AEB Boards, Box 642, Folder: Jaundice: Dr. Thomas Francis.

Prison physician pressures Francis to allow press coverage ("wildcat type of publicity"): Francis to Bayne-Jones, September 27, 1945, NARA AEB Boards, Box 642, Folder: Jaundice: Dr. Thomas Francis. Francis reported he had received a call from William Huntley, prison physician, who thought it was time to allow newspaper coverage. Some reporters were calling persistently and Huntley thought a factual account of the research program would prevent the kind of publicity that had occurred earlier. Huntley stated that the desire was not to publicize the death but rather to convey the part inmates had played in helping to find a solution to problems facing the army.

Francis writes an account of the prison studies for release to the press: Three-page typescript stamped October 1, 1945. Bayne-Jones approved the release on October 9, 1945, with the provision that any stories to appear in the press be sent to him for clearance before publication. Both documents at Bentley Francis, Box 32, Folder: Bayne-Jones, Correspondences.

Stokes attends meeting to arrange experiments at Trenton State Hospital ("They showed great interest"): Stokes to Bayne-Jones, March 26, 1944, NARA AEB Boards, Box 650, Folder: Commission on Measles and Mumps—Hepatitis Studies Including Religious Objectors. Officials attending the meeting included William Ellis (New Jersey commissioner of institutions and agencies), Joseph Raycroft (physician and longtime member of the hospital board), and James Spradley (senior physician at Trenton State). Spradley replaced Robert G. Stone as hospital director in May 1944.

Bayne-Jones approves experiments with mental patients ("I hope these plans"): Bayne-Jones to Stokes, March 27, 1944, NARA AEB Boards, Box 650, Folder: Commission on Measles and Mumps—Hepatitis Studies Including Religious Objectors.

The army surgeon general thanks Trenton State director: Major General Norman T. Kirk, surgeon general of the army, to James B. Spradley, Trenton State Hospital director, May 23, 1946. "These studies have been particularly difficult. In spite of difficulties, results have been obtained which are of importance to both civilian and military medicine. I appreciate your part in making these advances possible." NARA AEB Boards, Box 660, Folder: Commission on Neurotropic Disease—Hepatitis Project.

Hospital physicians are to evaluate hepatitis as therapy for psychosis ("that they use"): Stokes to Bayne-Jones, March 26, 1944, NARA AEB Boards, Box 650, Folder: Commission on Measles and Mumps—Hepatitis Studies Including Religious Objectors.

Authors describe early twentieth-century therapies for psychotic disorders: Gerald N. Grob provides an overview of practices in *Mental Illness and American Society, 1875–1940* (Princeton, NJ: Princeton University Press, 1983), 123–26, 291–308. The Austrian physician who received a Nobel Prize for introducing malaria fever therapy for neuro-syphilis was Julius Wagner-Jauregg. Discussions of the use of malaria-induced fever in the United States include Edward M. Brown, "Why Wagner-Jauregg Won the Nobel Prize for Discovering Malaria Therapy for General Paresis of the Insane," *History of Psychiatry* 11 (December 2000): 371–82; Margaret Humphreys, "Whose Body? Which Disease? Studying Malaria while Treating Neurosyphilis," in *Useful Bodies: Humans in the Service of Medical Science in the Twentieth Century*, ed. Jordan Goodman, Anthony McElligott, and Lara Marks (Baltimore, MD: Johns Hopkins University Press, 2003), 53–77; Howard I. Kushner, "Cutting Edge Psychiatry," *Cerebrum* 7, no. 3 (Summer 2005): 71–80; and Matthew Gambino, "Fevered Decisions: Race, Ethics, and Clinical Vulnerability in the Malaria Treatment of Neurosyphilis, 1922–1953," *Hastings Center Report* 45, no. 4 (July–August 2015): 39–50. Gambino reports that physicians infected nonsyphilitic patients with malaria in order to have a reservoir of pathogens for the treatment of syphilitic patients.

Physicians at Trenton State Hospital pursue surgery and fever therapy with patients: Andrew Skull details Cotton's use of surgical procedures in *Madhouse: A Tragic Tale of Megalomania and Modern Medicine* (New Haven, CT: Yale University Press, 2005). Robert G. Stone and J. B. Spradley discuss results of fever therapy with Trenton State patients not diagnosed with syphilitic disease in "Treatment of the Functional Psychoses with Fever Therapy: A Report of the Results of 1598 Cases," *Journal of the Medical Society of New Jersey* 32, no. 1 (November 1935): 650–53.

Stokes reports that risks associated with hepatitis are low ("the risk of serious"; "very small"): One-page typescript stamped March 23, 1944, NARA AEB Boards, Box 650, Folder: Commission on Measles and Mumps—Hepatitis Studies Including Religious Objectors.

Trenton hospital director welcomes hepatitis experiments ("it was to our advantage"): "Jaundice might be more effective than our present method by inoculations with malaria and injections of foreign proteins." Robert G. Stone, Report to the Board of Managers for March 1944, 1, NJSA Trenton Reports.

Trenton State patients classified as criminally insane are eligible for initial hepatitis studies: NJSA Board Minutes, Box 2, Binder: 1941–44, Minutes for March 28, 1944, 16.

Some researchers reject using impaired persons as subjects ("the insane"; "the feeble-minded"; "persons incapable of providing"): J. E. Moore to A. N. Richards (chair of the OSRD's Committee on Medical Research) February 1, 1943, NARA OSRD CMR General Records, Box 43, Folder: Human Experiments—V.D. Researchers selected a federal prison in Terre Haute, Indiana, as the site for the gonorrhea infection study. They aborted the experiment when attempts to infect inmates without using human carriers failed. For more extensive accounts of events and discussions surrounding the study, see Harkness, "Research behind Bars," 87–101; and Harry Marks, *The Progress of Experiment* (New York: Cambridge University Press, 1997), 100–105.

Moore later approves disease-inducing experiments with mental patients: Moore was chair of an NIH Syphilis Study Section that signed off on human infection studies with STDs in Guatemala begun in 1946 that enrolled prisoners, children, and mental patients. Susan M. Reverby, "'Normal Exposure' and Inoculation Syphilis: A PHS 'Tuskegee' Doctor in Guatemala, 1946–48," *Journal of Policy History* 23, no. 1 (January 2011): 6–28; Kayte Spector-Bagdady and Paul A. Lombardo, "'Something of an Adventure': Postwar NIH Research Ethos and the Guatemala STD Experiments," *Journal of Law, Medicine & Ethics* 41, no. 3 (Fall 2013): 697–710.

Penn investigators distinguish between volunteers and "volunteers": Two examples are found in John Neefe, Memo for Dr. Stokes, April 14, 1944,

NARA AEB Boards, Box 650, Folder: Commission on Measles and Mumps—Hepatitis Studies in Human Subjects; and a memo for the Commission on Viral and Rickettsial Diseases titled "Report on Hepatitis Studies in Philadelphia to 31st December, 1946," APS Stokes (unprocessed), Folder: Hepatitis #1 1946. Jon Harkness points to an earlier instance: Joseph Goldberger used *"volunteers,"* in quotes, when referring to prisoners enrolled in his 1915 study showing that the cause of pellagra is inadequate diet; see "Research behind Bars," 20.

Trenton Hospital physicians suppress information about hepatitis studies ("At the request of"): Robert G. Stone, Report to the Board of Managers for March 1944, 1, NJSA Trenton Reports. On the Board of Control keeping details confidential: NJSA Board Minutes, Box 2, Binder: 1941–44, Minutes for March 28, 1944, 15.

Stokes's group acknowledges assistance of CPS men but not of mental patients ("It is a pleasure to express"): John R. Neefe et al., "Hepatitis Due to the Infection of Homologous Blood Products in Human Volunteers," *Journal of Clinical Investigation* 23, no. 5 (September 1944): 854. The group mentions use of Trenton State's laboratory facilities in John R. Neefe, Sydney S. Gellis, and Joseph Stokes Jr., "Homologous Serum Hepatitis and Infectious (Epidemic) Hepatitis," *American Journal of Medicine* 1 (July 1946): 21.

Bayne-Jones insists on reviewing journal submissions ("You are required"): Bayne-Jones to Havens, November 8, 1944, WRAIR AEB, Folder: Commission on Neurotropic Virus Diseases, Jaundice, January 1944–December 1944.

Bayne-Jones requires changes in scientific paper ("as this appears"): Bayne-Jones to Neefe, March 6, 1945. An earlier communication on the matter was Bayne-Jones to Neefe, February 23, 1945. Both documents at WRAIR AEB, Folder: Commission on Measles and Mumps, Jaundice Studies, January–June 1945.

Interwar journal editor monitored descriptions of human experiments: Susan E. Lederer, "Political Animals: The Shaping of Biomedical Research Literature in Twentieth-Century America," *Isis* 83, no. 1 (March 1992): 61–79.

The OTSG reacts to an unauthorized press report ("volunteered to be a guinea pig"; "all blood banks are in continuous danger"): "War Objector Aids in Study of Jaundice," *Washington Evening Star*, June 29, 1943; "already caused trouble" is from Bayne-Jones to Francis Blake (AEB president), July 2, 1943. The clipping and letter are at NARA AEB Boards, Box 650, Folder: Commission on Measles and Mumps—Hepatitis Studies (Publicity). Another version of the newspaper entry in question appeared a day earlier in the *Baltimore Sun*, June 28, 1943. SCPC AFSC CPS, Neefe, 1943–1944.

Stokes explains the source of a leak to the press ("in direct defiance of"): Stokes to Bayne-Jones, July 3, 1943, NARA AEB Boards, Box 650, Folder: Commission on Measles and Mumps—Hepatitis Studies (Publicity).

AFSC distributes warning about leaks in telegram ("CURRENT NEWSPAPER PUBLICITY"): AFSC office to twelve CPS camps, July 1, 1943, SCPC AFSC CPS, Neefe, 1943–1944.

Bayne-Jones and Simmons converse through notes ("In the future Dr. Stokes"; "Col Bayne-Jones"): The notes were appended to Stokes's letter to Bayne-Jones dated July 3, 1943, NARA AEB Boards, Box 650, Folder: Commission on Measles and Mumps—Hepatitis Studies (Publicity).

The press covers OSRD experiments: Stories about the Norfolk prison fatality include "He Died for His Fellowmen," *Hartford Courant*, December 2, 1942; and Waldemar Kaempffert, "Science News in Review: Prison Guinea Pigs; Pardons Asked for Convicts Risking Lives for Science," *New York Times*, April 4, 1943. The *Cosmopolitan* piece is H. R. Baukhage, "They Fight without Weapons," April 24, 1943. Reports of malaria infection experiments in prisons include, among many others, "Convicts Volunteer to Find Malaria Cure," *Hartford Courant*, February 27, 1944; and "Malaria Remedy Tested in Prison," *New York Times*, July 23, 1944. The *Life* magazine article on the Minnesota starvation study is "Men Starve in Minnesota: Conscientious Objectors Volunteer for Strict Hunger Tests to Study Europe's Food Problem," *Life*, July 30, 1945, 43–46. Leah M. Kalm and Richard D. Semba discuss the experiment and accompanying press coverage in "They Starved So That Others Be Better Fed: Remembering Ancel Keys and the Minnesota Experiment," *Journal of Nutrition* 135, no. 6 (June 2005): 1347–52.

Bayne-Jones wants scientific papers to precede press accounts: Bayne-Jones to Gordon Dupee, December 31, 1943, NARA AEB Boards, Box 642, Folder: Commission on Influenza, Influenza Project—CO Camps and Army Posts.

Newspaper reports CPS men will participate in Connecticut hepatitis study: "18 Volunteers in Research on Jaundice: Conscientious Objectors at State Hospital to Aid Study and Cure of Disease," *Hartford Courant*, May 14, 1944.

Bayne-Jones releases information about hepatitis studies: Memo titled "Press Release on Army Work on Infectious Hepatitis," January 16, 1945, NARA AEB Boards, Box 676, Folder: Commission on Viral and Rickettsial Diseases—Jaundice Publications. Media coverage following the release included Waldemar Kaempffert, "Science in Review: Cause of Army Jaundice Is Now Discovered and the Means of Control Is Indicated," *New York Times*, January 21, 1945; "Jaundice in the Army," *Newsweek*, January 20, 1945; "Globulin vs. Jaundice," *Time*, February 5, 1945.

Bayne-Jones seeks to shape press reports: Bayne-Jones wrote to G. D. Fairbairn at the *Philadelphia Evening Bulletin* on February 16, 1945, with instructions about the tone and language to be used when describing hepatitis subjects. Bayne-Jones wrote to B. J. Waldemar Kaempffert, science editor at the *New York Times*, on January 17, 1945, to correct misinformation from an unapproved report originating in Italy. Both documents at NARA AEB Boards, Box 676, Folder: Commission on Viral and Rickettsial Disease—Jaundice Publications. Efforts to influence public depictions of human experiments were not new.

Depictions of heroes and martyrs of medical science: Discussions of medical experiments in popular culture include Susan E. Lederer, "Hollywood and Human Experimentation: Representing Medical Research in Popular Film," in *Medicine's Moving Pictures: Medicine, Health and Bodies in American Film and Television*, ed. Leslie J. Reagan et al. (Rochester, NY: University of Rochester Press, 2007), 282–306.

Newspaper article quotes interviews with draft objector subjects ("I feel that war is wrong"): Don Fairbairn, "Fighting the War on Disease," *Philadelphia Evening Bulletin*, February 27, 1945, SCPC AFSC CPS, Neefe, 1943–1944.

Chapter Three. Guinea Pig Camp

Timothy Haworth arrives in New Haven: George Mohlenhoff to Walter Havens, February 3, 1945, SCPC AFSC CPS, Part 1, Box 38a, Folder: Service Detached—Medical Research, New Haven Jaundice, January–July 1945 (referred to hereafter as SCPS AFSC CPS, NH Jaundice, January–July 1945).

Selective Service has a penchant for forms ("a bureaucratic passion for paper"): Mulford Q. Sibley and Philip E. Jacobs, *Conscription of Conscience: The American State and the Conscientious Objector, 1940–1947* (Ithaca, NY: Cornell University Press, 1952), 205.

Haworth submits a nonstandard biography ("Myself in Briefs"): May 5, 1943, SCPC AFSC CPS, Part 2, Box 75, Folder: Haworth, Timothy.

Haworth arranges for coverage of travel expenses ("palmed off"; "could produce no evidence"): Timothy Haworth to Mary Newman, February 12, 1945, SCPC AFSC CPS, NH Jaundice, January–July 1945.

Early recruitment flyer describes hepatitis risks ("Chances of Survival"; "There is a definite"): "Memo to All Camp Directors," SCPC AFSC CPS, Neefe, 1943–1944.

AFSC distributes New Haven recruitment circular ("FLASH: NEW OPPORTUNITY!"): CPS Personnel News, P-42, December 1, 1944, SCPC AFSC CPS, Part 1, Box 39d, Folder: Service Detached—Medical Research, New Haven Jaundice, 1944 (referred to hereafter as SCPC AFSC CPS, NH Jaundice, 1944).

Researchers report hepatitis death rate of one in one thousand cases: During the 1942 hepatitis B epidemic, officials found the death rate among hospitalized patients to be between two and three persons per one thousand hospitalized cases. The majority of infected personnel were not hospitalized and the mortality rate for all of those infected was lower.

Flyer describes likely course of illnesses ("The period of illness"): CPS Personnel News, P-42, December 1, 1944, SCPC AFSC CPS, NH Jaundice, 1944.

William Rhodes desires to serve in war conditions ("serve in areas of acute"): William E. Rhodes to Thomas P. Cope, July 11, 1942, SCPC AFSC CPS, Part 2, Box 169, Folder: Rhodes, William E.

Haworth is willing to die but not kill: Haworth's statement in "Special Form for Conscientious Objectors" (circa 1942). SCPC AFSC CPS, Part 2, Folder: Haworth, Timothy.

Peers influence Zimmerman's choice to participate in experiments ("One of my friends"): Interview with Howard "Paul" Zimmerman, August 25, 2003, in "Camp 56: An Oral History Project: World War II Conscientious Objectors and the Waldport, Oregon CPS Camp," 253, Lewis and Clark College Archives, Portland, OR.

Rhodes thinks experiments will alleviate suffering ("Thousands of cases"): William E. Rhodes to Lisle Crawford, June 4, 1945, SCPC AFSC CPS, Part 1, Box 40a, Folder: University of Pennsylvania Yellow Jaundice, Dr. Neefe, 1945–1946 (referred to hereafter as SCPC AFSC CPS, Neefe, 1945–1946).

New Haven men are highly educated: "Report of Projects and Incentives, June 23, 1945," SCPC AFSC CPS, Part 1, Box 60c (original processing), Folder: AFSC: Gory and Edwards. Sibley and Jacobs report that 55 percent of men in camps sponsored by the American Friends Service Committee had professional or technical training before their induction. *Conscription of Conscience*, 231–32, 171–72.

John Paul gets approval for men to take tutorials with Yale professors: Haworth to Sydney Lovett, Yale University chaplain, April 13, 1945, SCPC AFSC CPS, Part 1, Box 60d (original processing), Folder: Education: Statistics.

Haworth is pleased with camp assignees ("There is a truly terrific bunch"): Haworth to Ken Morgan, February 17, 1945, SCPC AFSC CPS, NH Jaundice, January–July 1945.

AFSC office staff circulates Haworth letter ("Your most recent"): Mohlenhoff to Haworth, March 8, 1945, SCPC AFSC CPS, NH Jaundice, January–July 1945.

Researchers and subjects meet ("Both Major Havens"): Haworth to Mohlenhoff, March 6, 1945, SCPC AFSC CPS, NH Jaundice, January–July 1945.

Haworth quips about female guests in the house ("Ah me, the college life!"): Haworth to Ken Morgan, February 17, 1945, SCPC AFSC CPS, NH Jaundice, January–July 1945.

Conscientious objectors hold "Pre-Inoculation Dance" ("The large room was cleverly"): Haworth to Mohlenhoff, March 6, 1945, SCPC AFSC CPS, NH Jaundice, January–July 1945.

Classic study finds gallows humor among research subjects: Renee C. Fox, *Experiment Perilous: Physicians and Patients Facing the Unknown* (Philadelphia: University of Pennsylvania Press, 1959), 175.

Goal of initial hepatitis inoculations at Yale: Havens reports on two four-month experiments at New Haven conducted between February 14 and October 31, 1945, with a total of thirty-four subjects. In the first, eighteen subjects were fed stool or inoculated with serum from an infectious hepatitis patient and specimens were taken at different points in the course of the patient's illness. Five participants contracted hepatitis. Walter P. Havens Jr., "Period of Infectivity with Experimentally Inducted Infectious Hepatitis," *Journal of Experimental Medicine* 83, no. 3 (March 1946): 251–58.

Researchers impose quarantine rules: Haworth to Mohlenhoff, February 17, 1945, SCPC AFSC CPS, NH Jaundice, January–July 1945.

New Haven men have varied work assignments: "Report of Projects and Incentives, June 22, 1945," SCPC AFSC CPS, Part 1, Box 60c (original processing), Folder: AFSC: Gory and Edwards.

Camp life includes arrangements for spare time study: Louis Schneider at the Friends Committee office commented on library privileges to Elton Atwater, CPS Camp 132, December 28, 1944, SCPC AFSC CPS, NH Jaundice, 1944. Haworth wrote Ken Morgan (February 17, 1945) and Mohlenhoff (March 6, 1945) that sixteen men wanted to take courses, and that auditing was prohibited but tutorials allowed. SCPC AFSC CPS, NH Jaundice, January–July 1945. Additional discussions of camp members' educational activities are at "Men in CPS #140 Taking Tutorial Work in Yale University," April 5, 1945; and "Memo to Mr. Lovett Re: Summer Courses for Jaundice Unit" (n.d.). Both documents at SCPC AFSC CPS, Part 1, Box 60d (original processing), Folder: Ed Sec, Yale University. "China Today Lecture Series" (circa August 1945); and "Proposed One Month Lecture Series (n.d.) are at SCPC AFSC CPS, Part 1, Box 60d (original processing), Folder: Co-ops and China Lecture Series.

Education secretary has a name for the camp's study program ("Jaundice College"): George Loveland, New Haven camp education secretary, to Richard C. Carroll, assistant dean, Yale University, June 20, 1945, SCPC AFSC CPS, Box 60c (original processing), Folder: Ed Sec, Yale University.

New Haven men produce the *Guinea Gazette:* SCPC AFSC CPS, Part 3, Box 18, Folder: Camp 140.

Haworth delivers a reprimand ("*YOU DID NOT SHOW UP*"): Document beginning "KNOW ALL MEN BY THESE PRESENTS," from Haworth to Al Votaw and Len Kenworthy, n.d., SCPC AFSC CPS, Part 1, Box 60d, Folder: Personnel.

Paul requests subjects for second round of experiments: John Paul to Aims McGuinness, Office of the Surgeon General–Army, April 3, 1945, SCPC AFSC CPS, NH Jaundice, January–July 1945.

New Haven men undertake letter-writing campaign for recruiting new men ("We now have"): Haworth to Mohlenhoff, May 10, 1945, SCPC AFSC CPS, NH Jaundice, January–June 1945.

Haworth and other assignees draft recruitment script ("Quotes from Veteran Pigs"; "Dr. Paul's direction"; "spirit of cooperation"): Four-page typescript beginning *"The Experiments"* (n.d.). Haworth attests to his authorship in the letter to George Mohlenhoff dated May 10, 1945. Mohlenhoff responds on May 12 saying that Haworth's statement has been dispatched to CPS camps. All documents at SCPC AFSC CPS, NH Jaundice, January–June 1945.

Yale researcher describes aim of the second round of inoculations: Havens wrote that in the second set of procedures at the Yale camp, researchers inoculated sixteen subjects with specimens (stool, nasal washings, urine, and serum) taken at different stages of the illness from the five subjects sickened earlier. Among second-round subjects, those who received stool and serum from the acute stage of the disease contracted hepatitis. Havens, "Period of Infectivity."

Researchers take subjects into their confidence ("A better job"): Haworth to Mohlenhoff, August 15, 1945, SCPC AFSC CPS, Part 1, Box 39d, Folder: Service Detached—Medical Research, New Haven Jaundice, August 1945–1946 (referred to hereafter as SCPC AFSC CPS, NH Jaundice, August 1945–1946). In a similar vein, Fox noted that, in the research unit she studied, investigators developed close relationships with their subjects and treated them as colleagues, collaborators, and "members of the family." Fox, *Experiment Perilous*, 87–92.

New illnesses raise camp morale ("The Chosen are dropping off like flies"): Haworth to Mohlenhoff, August 15, 1945, SCPC AFSC CPS, NH Jaundice, August 1945–1946.

Philadelphia flyer emphasizes possibilities for study ("Men interested"): Recruitment circular dated October 17, 1944, SCPC AFSC CPS, Neefe, 1943–1944.

Gallows humor is alive in the Philadelphia unit ("Hold everything"): Rhodes to Adrian Gory, April 10, 1945, SCPC AFSC CPS, Neefe, 1945–1946.

Stokes sends CPS work crew to Trenton State Hospital: McGuinness at the Office of the Surgeon General–Army to Imirie at Camp Operations of Selective Service, January 11, 1945, NARA AEB Boards, Box 650, Folder: Commission on Measles and Mumps—Hepatitis Studies Including Religious Objectors.

Draft objectors sought to humanize care of mental patients: Sources include Steven J. Taylor, *Acts of Conscience: World War II, Mental Institutions, and Religious Objectors* (Syracuse, NY: Syracuse University Press, 2009); Alex Sareyan, *The Turning Point: How Persons of Conscience Brought about Major Change in the Care of America's Mentally Ill* (Washington, DC: American Psychiatric Press, 1953); and Robert A. Clark and Alex M. Burgess, "The Work of Conscientious Objectors in State Mental Hospitals during the Second World War," *Psychiatric Quarterly Supplement* 22, part 1 (1948): 125–40.

Sawyer describes conditions at Byberry ("A few attendants"; "If you can convey"): Sareyan, *Turning Point*, 44.

Story in *Life* describes conditions in mental institutions: Albert Q. Maisel, "Bedlam 1946: Most U.S. Mental Hospitals Are a Shame and a Disgrace," *Life*, May 6, 1946.

Draft resisters object to lack of consent at Trenton State Hospital ("They were not getting"): Interview with Harold "Paul" Zimmerman, August 25, 2003, in "Camp 56," 253.

CPS men debate ethics of experiments with mental patients ("The constantly recurring question"): Philadelphia Unit announcement dated July 7, 1945. The typescript announcement noted, "Most likely the meeting of Dr. Stokes with those concerned will be set up." Handwritten: "Rhodes will keep us informed." SCPC AFSC CPS, Neefe, 1945–1946.

Protesting men meet with project researcher Gellis ("revolve around the actual"): Rhodes to Walton James, Trenton CPS Group, July 18, 1945, SCPC AFSC CPS, Neefe, 1945–1946.

Trenton hospital director is furious about meddling ("interesting themselves"): J. B. Spradley, letter to Board of Managers, July 1945, NJSA Trenton Reports.

Conscientious objectors refuse further work at the Trenton hospital ("Experimentation on mental patients"): Rhodes to Sydney Gellis, September 10, 1945. Rhodes also reported that "no more men would consent to work at Trenton." Several weeks later (October 22, 1945), Rhodes wrote in a typed message to Neefe: "Mr. Charles Ming informed me by telephone this morning that within a few days the number of men at Trenton will be reduced to one." He added in longhand: "The end of a long struggle" and signed with his initials. Charles Ming oversaw the laboratory facilities that Stokes maintained at Trenton State Hospital. All documents at SCPC AFSC CPS, Neefe, 1945–1946.

Haworth cancels requests for additional men: Haworth to Mohlenhoff, September 25, 1945, SCPC AFSC CPS, NH Jaundice, August 1945–1946. Haworth reported that five of the thirteen men remaining at the New Haven camp during its final months would participate in an immunity study and be infected with hepatitis viruses a second time.

Inoculations at Philadelphia continue after the war ends ("It appears"): Neefe to Bayne-Jones, October 29, 1945, WRAIR AEB, Folder: Commission on Measles and Mumps, Jaundice Studies, July 1945–.

Haworth comments on Warren Dugan's death ("laid down his life"): Haworth to Paterson and Rockford, August 28, 1945, SCPC AFSC CPS, Part 1, Box 60d (original processing), Folder: General Correspondences #140.

Haworth describes Paul's handling of Dugan's death ("truly wonderful"; "hit Dr. Paul"): Haworth to Paterson and Rockford, August 28, 1945, SCPC AFSC CPS, Part 1, Box 60d (original processing), Folder: General Correspondences #140.

Haworth reports curtailment of experiments at Yale ("The time is no longer ripe"; "I believe it is probable"): Haworth to Mohlenhoff, September 25, 1945, SCPC AFSC CPS, NH Jaundice, August 1945–1946.

Stokes requests permission to biopsy men with continuing symptoms ("in the further medical management"; "we can see"): Stokes to Bayne-Jones, September 17, 1945. Aims McGuiness conveyed Bayne-Jones's approval in a letter of September 21, 1945. Both documents at WRAIR AEB, Folder: Commission on Measles and Mumps, Jaundice Studies, July 1945–. The Philadelphia group conducted biopsies on two hepatitis subjects in October 1945.

Bayne-Jones approves biopsies on subjects in immunity studies: Bayne-Jones to Neefe, November 19, 1945, NARA AEB Boards, Box 650, Folder: Commission on Measles and Mumps—Hepatitis Studies on Human Subjects. Both Stokes and Neefe provided rationales for the surgical biopsies. In Stokes's words, "It was felt that the microscopic findings would be of particular importance in relation to the question of permanent injury to the liver from hepatitis." Report of the Commission on Mumps and Measles, July 1945–March 1946, NARA AEB Boards, Box 649, Folder: Commission on Measles and Mumps, Annual Reports.

Neefe wrote Bayne-Jones on November 12, 1945: "Biopsies on these cases may provide information concerning the debated question of the predisposing effect of hepatitis to cirrhosis." NARA AEB Boards, Box 650, Folder: Commission on Measles and Mumps—Hepatitis Studies on Human Subjects.

Biopsy from chronic patient is not normal ("subsiding inflammatory process"): Balduin Lucke, Army Institute of Pathology, to Neefe, October 23, 1945. Surgeon Jonathan Rhoads, who was present at the biopsy, thought the appearance of the liver suggested fibrous tissue. Neefe to Lucke, October 4, 1945. Both documents at NARA AEB Boards, Box 650, Folder: Commission on Measles and Mumps—Hepatitis Studies on Human Subjects.

Biopsies from cross-immunity subjects are indeterminate ("increased cellularity"; "obscure"): John R. Neefe, "Chronic Hepatitis in Volunteers," *Transactions of the Conference on Liver Injury* 5 (September 26-27, 1946): 104, 106. Several of the asymptomatic men had abnormal liver function tests.

Stokes requests discharges for two unrecovered subjects ("the need for consideration"): Stokes to Bayne-Jones, January 8, 1946, NARA AEB Boards, Box 650, Folder: Commission on Measles and Mumps—Hepatitis Studies on Human Subjects.

Bayne-Jones is displeased with request for medical discharges ("I will call your attention"): Bayne-Jones to Stokes, January 15, 1946, NARA AEB Boards, Box 650, Folder: Commission on Measles and Mumps—Hepatitis Studies Including Religious Objectors.

Stokes arranges care for unrecovered subjects through June: Stokes sought assistance from Alex Burgess, AFSC medical director, in making arrangements for continued medical care for the unrecovered. Burgess planned to speak with Colonel Prescott L. Brown of the Selective Service Medical Division about financial support for this purpose. Burgess to Stokes, February 22, 1946, APS Stokes, Folder: AFSC, Burgess, Alex, Re Experiments with Human Volunteers. At least some of the private funding Stokes secured was from the Donnor Foundation. Bayne-Jones, Memo for the file "Donnor Foundation Grant for Dr. Stokes's Work on Hepatitis," February 27, 1946, WRAIR AEB, Folder: Commission on Measles and Mumps, Jaundice Studies, July 1945–. In a letter of March 4, 1946, Neefe reported to Lewis Kosch at Camp Operations of Selective Service that the Philadelphia project was prepared to continue medical care for hepatitis subjects through June 30. NARA AEB Boards, Box 650, Folder: Commission on Measles and Mumps—Hepatitis Studies Including Religious Objectors.

Bayne-Jones orders transfer of unrecovered men ("As we agreed this morning"): Bayne-Jones to Neefe, March 13, 1946, WRAIR AEB, Folder: Commission on Measles and Mumps, Jaundice Studies, July 1945–.

Peace church elders regret inability to secure medical discharges ("Directors of camps reported"; "instruments for carrying out"): Clarence E. Pickett, *For More Than Bread Alone* (Boston: Little, Brown, 1953), 323. Sibley and Jacobs make similar observations in *Conscription of Conscience*, 291.

Neefe reports on three subjects with chronic hepatitis: Neefe, "Chronic Hepatitis in Volunteers," 90–106; and John R. Neefe, "Results of Hepatic Tests on Chronic Hepatitis without Jaundice," *Gastroenterology* 7, no. 1 (July 1946): 1–19.

Army researchers report the existence of chronic hepatitis: M. H. Barker, R. B. Capps, and F. W. Allen, "Chronic Hepatitis in the Mediterranean Theater: A New Clinical Syndrome," *JAMA* 129, no. 10 (November 3, 1945): 653–59.

Chapter Four. Nuremberg Notwithstanding

American tribunal conducts the Nuremberg Medical Trial: Literature on the Nuremburg Medical Trial is voluminous. My account draws heavily from Paul J. Weindling, *Nazi Medicine and the Nuremberg Trials* (New York: Palgrave Macmillan, 2004); and Paul J. Weindling, "The Origins of Informed Consent: The International Scientific Commission on Medical War Crimes and the Nuremberg Code," *Bulletin of the History of Medicine* 75, no. 1 (2001): 37–71.

Nuremberg Medical Trial addresses Nazi hepatitis infection experiments: A number of Medical Trial defendants were charged with responsibility for criminal conduct involving transmission of hepatitis to concentration camp prisoners. Only Karl Brandt was convicted on this charge. Prosecutors cited evidence that Eugen Haagen and Arnold Dohmen (neither defendants at the trial) performed hepatitis infection experiments at Sachsenhausen and Natzweiler concentration camps. Haagen, a trial witness, denied involvement. Harvard Nuremberg Digital: Trial Transcript for June 18, 1947. Brigitte Leyendecker and Gurghard F. Klapp write that Kurt Gutzeit was in charge of hepatitis research for the German army and approved hepatitis transmission studies that Hans Voegt conducted in 1941 with patients at a Breslau mental hospital and that Arnold Dohmen performed in 1944 on Jewish children at Sachsenhausen concentration camp. From Leyendecker and Klapp, "Human Hepatitis Experiments in the Second World War," *Zeitschrift fur gesamte Hygiene* 35 (December 1989): 756–60. Astrid Ley includes an eyewitness description of Dohmen's procedures at Sachsenhausen in "Children as Victims of Medical Experiments in Concentration Camps," in *From Clinic to Concentration Camp: Reassessing Nazi Medical and Racial Research, 1933–1945*, ed. Paul J. Weindling (London: Routledge, 2017), 209–20.

The trial defense submits reports of Stokes's hepatitis studies into evidence: Defense entries included abstracts of two papers from Stokes's group: John R. Neefe, Joseph Stokes Jr., and Sydney S. Gellis, "Homologous Serum Hepatitis and Infectious Hepatitis: Experimental Study of Immunity and Cross Immunity in Volunteers," *American Journal of Medical Sciences* 210, no. 5 (November 1945): 561–75; and John R. Neefe et al., "Disinfection of Water Containing Causative Agent of Infectious (Epidemic) Hepatitis," *JAMA* 128, no. 15 (August 11, 1945): 1076–80. Harvard Nuremberg Digital: Defense Documents, Brandt No. 105 and 108, Items No. 2758 and 2761.

Defense attorney invokes press coverage of U.S. malaria experiments: Servatius's example of malaria experiments in U.S. prisons drew from "Prison Malaria: Convicts Expose Themselves to Disease So That Doctors Can Study It," *Life,* June 4, 1945. Other reports of studies by American investigators cited by the trial defense included "The Conscientious Guinea Pigs," *Time,* December 10, 1945, 62.

Brandt's lawyer equates Nazi and U.S. malaria experiments: Weindling, *Nazi Medicine*; and Jon M. Harkness, "Nuremberg and the Issue of Wartime Experiments on U.S. Prisoners," *JAMA* 276, no. 20 (November 27, 1996): 1572–75.

Core provisions of the Nuremberg Code ("Where there is"; "The voluntary consent"): Posted at the website of the United States Holocaust Memorial Museum (www.ushmm.org) under online exhibitions.

The AMA hurriedly issues a statement on research ethics: The statement appears at "Supplementary Report of the Judicial Council, House of Delegates Meeting, December 9–11, 1946," *JAMA* 132, no. 17 (December 28, 1946): 1090.

Ivy testifies about AMA principles and U.S. malaria experiment: Discussion of Ivy's behind-the-scenes maneuvering and trial testimony is found in Advisory Committee on Human Radiation Experiments (ACHRE), *Final Report* (Washington, DC: Government Printing Office, 1995), 131–37, 147–50; Jon M. Harkness, "Research behind Bars: A History of Nontherapeutic Research on American Prisoners" (PhD diss., University of Wisconsin, Madison, 1996), 137–52; and Harkness, "Nuremberg and the Issue of Wartime Experiments."

Green Committee endorses Stateville malaria experiments ("as an example"; "can amount to undue"; "an act of good conduct"): Committee Appointed by Governor Dwight H. Green of Illinois, "Ethics Governing the Service of Prisoners as Subjects in Medical Experiments," *JAMA* 137, no. 7 (February 14, 1948): 457–58.

Ivy argues that consent from a guardian makes experiments with children and the impaired acceptable ("The ethical principles involved"): A. C. Ivy, "The History and Ethics of the Use of Human Subjects in Medical Experiments," *Science* 108, no. 2792 (July 2, 1948): 5.

American researchers have mixed reactions to the Nuremberg Code ("code for barbarians"): The full quote is "It was a good code for barbarians but an unnecessary code for ordinary physician-scientists." Jay Katz, "The Consent Principle of the Nuremberg Code: Its Significance Then and Now," in *The Nazi Doctors and the Nuremberg Code,* ed. George J. Annas and Michael A. Grodin (New York: Oxford University Press, 1992), 228. The symposium papers appeared as "The Problems of Experimentation on Human Beings," *Science* 117, no. 3035 (February 27, 1953): 205–15. Further discussion of the American research community's response to the Nuremberg Code is found in David J. Rothman, *Strangers at the Bedside* (New York: Basic Books, 1994), 62–63; and ACHRE, *Final Report,* 150–52.

The Reich issued written medical research guidelines in 1931: Ulf Schmidt and Andreas Frewer reprint the 1931 German regulations in Schmidt and Frewer, eds., *History and Theory of Human Experimentation: The Declaration of Helsinki and Modern Medical Ethics* (Stuttgart: Franz Steiner Verlag, 2007), 333–35. Michael A. Grodin also provides the text of the 1931 "Regulations on New Therapy and Human Experimentation" in "Historical Origins of the Nuremberg Code," in Annas and Grodin, *Nazi Doctors and the Nuremberg Code,* 130–31. Volker Roelcke discusses the origins and limited impact of the German guidelines in "The Use and Abuse of Medical Research Ethics," in Weindling, *From Clinic to Concentration Camp,* 33–50. The deaths of seventy-eight children from a contaminated tuberculosis vaccine triggered the Reich's 1931 circular. Christian Bonah and Philippe Menut discuss these events in "BCG-Vaccination around 1930: Dangerous Experiment or Established Prevention? Debates in France and Germany," in *Twentieth Century Ethics of Human Subjects Research,* ed. Volker Roelcke and Giovanni Maoi (Stuttgart: Franz Steiner Verlag, 2004), 111–27.

The WMA coalesces in response to the Medical Trial: Ulf Schmidt and Andreas Frewer, "History and Ethics of Human Experimentation: The Twisted Road to Helsinki," in *History and Theory,* 11–12.

European medical associations formulate guidelines on research ethics: In 1952, the French National Academy of Medicine distinguished interventions intended to benefit the individual patient and those conducted for the benefit of others. In 1955, the Public Health Council of the Netherlands drafted guidelines that disapproved of experiments with prisoners, children, and the mentally ill that would expose them to hazards or pain. Susan E. Lederer, "Research without Borders: The Origins of the Declaration of Helsinki," in Roelcke and Maoi, *Twentieth Century Ethics of Human Subjects Research,* 202–4; David A. Frenkel, "Human Experimentation: Codes of Ethics," in *Medical Experimentation,* ed. Amnon Carmi (Ramat Gan, Israel: Turtledove, 1978), 131–33.

Medical tradition distinguished therapeutic from nontherapeutic experiments: Sydney Halpern, *Lesser Harms: The Morality of Risk in Medical Research* (Chicago: University of Chicago Press, 2004), 4. Susan E. Lederer underscores different standards for securing consent for interventions with health subjects and therapeutic experiments with patients. Lederer, *Subjected to Science: Human Experimentation in America Before the Second World War* (Baltimore, MD: Johns Hopkins University Press, 1995), 9.

WMA committee formulates a draft research ethics code ("Persons retained in prisons"): Ethics Committee, World Medical Association, "Draft Code of Ethics on Human Experimentation," *British Medical Journal* 2, no. 5312 (October 27, 1962): 1119. Susan E. Lederer analyzes discussions surrounding early drafts in "Children as Guinea Pigs: Historical Perspectives," *Accountability in Research* 10, no. 1 (January–March 2003): 10–11.

WMA adopts research standards at its 1964 Helsinki meeting: The *British Medical Journal* printed the original Helsinki Code in 2, no. 5402 (July 18, 1964): 177. For nontherapeutic research, the code required free and fully informed consent of the subject or, if the person was not legally competent, the subject's legal guardian. It made no mention of "captive" subjects. Still, many scientists outside the United States and Canada disapproved of enrolling institutionalized persons in nontherapeutic medical research. A legal scholar at the Law-Medicine Research Institute at Boston University surveyed European medical scientists during the early 1960s about their use of prisoners in medical experiments. He reported that Europeans were averse to using prisoners as research subjects "because of the feeling that they are never free of duress and also because they represent a uniquely vulnerable group who should be protected, not used or possibly abused." Harkness cites this statement in "Research behind Bars," 176n5. The original source is Irving Ladimer, "Comparative Survey of Social Responsibility in Clinical Research, Summary Report from Trip to Europe, August 1961," Law-Medicine Research Institute papers, Center for Law and Health Sciences, Boston University.

Institutions become militarized in postwar America: Michael S. Sherry, *In the Shadow of War* (New Haven, CT: Yale University Press, 1995).

Notorious U.S. human experiments conducted during the early Cold War: Sources include ACHRE, *Final Report*; Jonathan D. Moreno, *Undue Risk: Secret State Experiments on Humans* (New York: Routledge, 2001); Gerald Kutcher, *Contested Medicine: Cancer Research and the Military* (Chicago: University of Chicago Press, 2009); Susan E. Lederer, "The Cold War and Beyond: Covert and Deceptive American Medical Experimentation," in *Military Medical Ethics*, ed. Thomas E. Beam (Falls Church, VA: Office of the Surgeon General–Army, 2003), 2:507–31; Jonathan D. Moreno, "Stumbling toward Bioethics: Human Experiments Policy and the Early Cold War," in *Dark Medicine: Rationalizing Unethical Medical Research*, ed. William R. Lafleur, Gernot Böhme, and Susumu Shimazono (Bloomington: University of Indiana Press, 2007), 140–45.

The OTSG designates hepatitis a research priority ("The Army placed liver disease"): William Stone, chair of the Army Medical Research and Development Command, made the statement at the first meeting of the NRC Subcommittee on Liver Disease. NAS Liver, Meeting Minutes, January 30, 1947.

World War II studies differentiated hepatitis A and B: Relevant publications include Joseph Stokes Jr., John R. Neefe, and Sydney Gellis, "Hepatitis: Immunological Studies," *Transactions of the Association of American Physicians* 59 (1945): 142–46; and, from John Paul's group, Walter P. Havens Jr., "Experiments in Cross Immunity between Infectious Hepatitis and Homologous Serum Jaundice," *Proceedings of the Society of Experimental Biology and Medicine* 59 (June 1945): 148–50.

Stokes heads the Committee on Allocation of Volunteers: A description of the committee—sometimes called a subcommittee—states that it worked closely with the NRC Committee on Sterilization of Blood. Report of the [AFEB] Commission on Liver Disease, April 1951–April 1952, NARA AFEB, Box 59, Folder Commission on Liver Disease, 1951–52.

Stokes resumes hepatitis infection studies with mental patients: "Report on Hepatitis Studies in Philadelphia to 31st December, 1946," APS Stokes (unprocessed), Folder: Hepatitis #1 1946. Also "Report on the Use of Infectious

Hepatitis and Serum Hepatitis in 297 Mental Patients," APS Stokes, Series VI, Folder: Hepatitis Study #1, 1944–48.

Stokes had long been testing vaccines in facilities for children: As early as 1936–37, Stokes conducted tests of cultivated influenza viruses with children at five facilities in New Jersey, including state colonies in New Lisbon, Skillman, and Vineland. Halpern, *Lesser Harms*, 74–76, 184n31. His wartime research included experiments with partially attenuated measles virus; for these, his teams enrolled children at seven facilities, among them state colonies at Skillman, New Lisbon, and Woodbine in New Jersey and Pennhurst State School in Pennsylvania. Joseph Stokes et al., "Studies in Measles IV. Results Following Inoculation of Children with Egg-Passage Measles Virus," *Journal of Pediatrics* 22, no. 1 (January 1943): 16. In 1942, Stokes wrote researcher John Enders saying that groups of children in state colonies had not had mumps and he was "anxious to see" whether a new preparation Enders had developed would immunize against that disease. Stokes to Enders, July 27, 1942, Yale Enders, Series I, Box 55, Folder: 1308 (Commission on Measles and Mumps, 1941–43). Joseph Stokes Jr. et al. discuss subsequent experiments in "Immunity in Mumps: VI. Experiments on the Vaccination of Human Beings with Formolized Mumps Vaccine," *Journal of Experimental Medicine* 84, no. 5 (November 1947): 407–28. Correspondence shows that subjects in the mumps vaccine trials included children at facilities in Skillman, New Lisbon, and Pennhurst. Correspondence at Yale Enders, Series I, Box 55, Folder: 1309 (Commission on Measles and Mumps). Allen M. Hornblum, Judith L. Newman, and Gregory J. Dober discuss Stokes's experiments with institutionalized children in *Against Their Will* (New York: Palgrave Macmillan, 2013). The broader literature on experimentation with children includes Lederer, "Children as Guinea Pigs," 1–16.

Stokes advises against publicly identifying Pennhurst as a study site ("should be used"; "If you use openly"): Stokes to James S. Dean, January 14, 1946; ("For the benefit"; "the advantages of"): Dean to Stokes, January 18, 1946. Both documents at APS Stokes, Series III, Folder: Pennhurst State School, 1945–55. Stokes's group reports measles challenge procedures at Pennhurst in Elizabeth P. Maris et al., "Studies in Measles. V. The Results of Chance and Planned Exposure to Unmodified Measles Virus in Children Previously Inoculated with Egg-Passage Measles Virus," *Journal of Pediatrics* 22, no. 1 (January 1943): 17–29.

During World War II, researchers used gamma globulin to stem hepatitis in children's institutions: Joseph Stokes Jr. and John R. Neefe describe their interventions in "The Prevention and Attenuation of Infectious Hepatitis by Gamma Globulin," *JAMA* 127, no. 3 (January 20, 1945): 144–45. Paul reported use of gamma globulin during outbreaks at two institutions in Annual Report of the Commission on Neurotropic Virus Disease, April 1944–March 1945, submitted March 27, 1945, NARA AEB Boards, Box 655, Folder AEB: Commission on Neurotropic Virus Disease, Annual Reports. A publication from one of the institutions is W. P. Havens and John R. Paul, "Prevention of Infectious Hepatitis with

Gamma Globulin," *JAMA* 12, no. 4 (September 22, 1945): 270–72. Melvin Berger discusses the origins and trajectory of fractionated blood products in "A History of Immune Globulin Therapy, from Harvard Crash Program to Monoclonal Antibodies," *Current Allergy and Asthma Reports* 2, no. 5 (September 2002): 368–78.

After the war, trials of gamma globulin against hepatitis continue in institutions for children: Joseph Stokes Jr. et al. discuss trials at New Lisbon, St. Vincent's, and Rosewood in "Infectious Hepatitis: Length of Protection by Immune Serum Globulin (Gamma Globulin) during Epidemics," *JAMA* 147, no. 8 (October 20, 1951): 714–19. In 1952, Stokes reported that, at the invitation of the U.S. Communicable Disease Center, AFEB scientists were working with state health departments in studying seven additional hepatitis outbreaks, some of these in community settings. In both community and institutional research, investigators conducted trials with gamma globulin, structuring its use to shed light on optimal timing and dosages. Stokes's Annual Report to the Commission on Liver Disease, February 28, 1952, NARA AFEB, Box 59, Folder: Commission on Liver Disease Reports, 1951–52. Miles E. Drake and Charles Ming report use of gamma globulin against hepatitis at a facility in Vineland in "Gamma Globulin in Epidemic Hepatitis: Comparative Value of Two Dosage Levels," *JAMA* 155, no. 15 (August 7, 1954): 1302–5.

Stokes's team transmits hepatitis to children at Pennhurst School: Multiple documents dated March through August 1947. APS Stokes, Series III, Folder: Pennhurst State School, 1945–55.

Stokes's team performs hepatitis virus challenges at New Lisbon: Stokes to C. T. Jones, March 8, 1949, APS Stokes, Series III, Folder: New Jersey State Colony, 1946–51.

Researchers administer hepatitis skin tests at multiple facilities for children: Use of hepatitis skin tests began in 1950 and involved multiple investigators, a broad range of institutions, and hundreds of subjects. The study sites included facilities in New Lisbon and Skillman Village in New Jersey, Rosewood in Maryland, and St. Vincent's orphanage in Chicago. Resulting publications include Miles Drake et al., "Studies on the Agent of Infectious Hepatitis, III. The Effect of Skin Tests for Infectious Hepatitis on the Incidence of the Disease in a Closed Institution," *Journal of Experimental Medicine* 95, no. 3 (February 29, 1952): 231–39.

Stokes says hepatitis skin test might contain live virus and function as a vaccine: Stokes discusses the possibility that skin test material contained live virus in his Annual Report for April 1952–March 1953, NARA AFEB, Box 60, Folder: Commission on Liver Disease, Progress Reports. His team suggested that the skin test material might produce at least partial immunity in Drake et al., "The Effect of Skin Tests," 238. In November 1952, Robert Graber, director of Skillman Village and one of Stokes's collaborators, sought approval from the New Jersey Board of Control for use of hepatitis skin test material at his facility under Stokes's supervision. Graber described the procedure as a "vaccine for hepatitis" involving "a scratch mark like the present day vaccination for small-pox." Minutes for November 25, 1952, 1–2, NJSA Board Minutes, Box 2, Binder: 1951–53.

Stokes requests access for challenge procedures after completing preventive measures ("Since these patients"): Stokes to C. T. Jones, March 8, 1949, APS Stokes, Series III, Folder: New Jersey State Colony—1946–51.

Stokes defends hepatitis transmission experiments with children ("point of ethics"; "except under the provision"; "well recognized pediatric practice"; "Epidemic hepatitis may be"): Stokes to Colin MacLeod, February 11, 1948, NARA AFEB, Box 54, Folder: Human Volunteers for Hepatitis Studies. Stokes does not state nor does other correspondence indicate who raised questions of ethics in 1948. Saul Krugman would later argue that his child subjects benefited from hepatitis infection studies, but his reasoning differed from Stokes's. Krugman maintained that his subjects gained immunity to a disease that, given its prevalence at Willowbrook, they would contract anyway; he did not suggest it was important that they acquire immunity before puberty.

Paul responds to Stokes's justification ("During the war"): Paul to Stokes, February 18, 1948, NARA AFEB, Box 54, Folder: Human Volunteers for Hepatitis Studies. In another passage of his letter, Paul wrote, "I understand that Dr. Ivy at the University of Illinois has been on some type of vigilance committee which has laid down certain principles about volunteers in order to protect this country from the criticisms brought up in Germany during the Nurnberg [*sic*] trials." Paul was mistaken about the purpose of Ivy's committee.

AFEB sends Stokes's justification for experiments with children up the ladder ("the advisability of"): C. J. Watson to Frank L. Bauer at the OTSG, March 11, 1948. The determination (a "resume for the record") came in a letter dated March 17, 1948, from Alfred P. Thom, chief of the Medical Research and Development Board, to Arthur Long, chief of Preventive Medicine at the OTSG. The relevant documents are at NARA AEB Boards, Box 648, Folder: Commission on Liver Diseases: Board Meetings, 1948.

In 1950, Koprowski tested live poliovirus using institutionalized children: Halpern, *Lesser Harms*, 76–79.

In response to Koprowski's depiction of child subjects as volunteers, *Lancet* editor invokes volunteer mice ("can only guess"; "Such a word"): "Poliomyelitis: A New Approach," *Lancet* 259, no. 6707 (March 15, 1952): 552. The controversial vaccine trials are reported in Hilary Koprowski, George Jervis, and Thomas Norton, "Immune Response in Human Volunteers upon Oral Administration of a Rodent-Adapted Strain of Poliomyelitis Virus," *American Journal of Hygiene* 55, no. 1 (1952): 108–26.

Rivers objects to Koprowski's experiments with children ("I personally did not"; "you might even say"; "The law winks"): Saul Benison, ed., *Tom Rivers: Reflections on a Life in Medicine and Science* (Cambridge, MA: MIT Press, 1967), 465–66, 187.

Chapter Five. Tales of Redemption

A regime of prison experimentation grows: The figure of twenty thousand inmate-subjects is from Alvin Bronstein, director of the National Prison Project of the American Civil Liberties Union Foundation. Victor Cohn quotes Bronstein in "Medical Research on Prisoners, Poor Defended, Hit," *Washington Post*, February 20, 1975, 3. Sources on twentieth-century medical research in prisons include Jon M. Harkness, "Research behind Bars: A History of Nontherapeutic Research in American Prisons" (PhD diss., University of Wisconsin, Madison, 1996); and Allen M. Hornblum, *Acres of Skin* (New York: Routledge, 1998). Anthony R. Hatch discusses more recent developments in prison experimentation in *Silent Cells: The Secret Drugging of Captive America* (Minneapolis: University of Minnesota Press, 2019).

The AMA rejects medical experiments with violent criminals ("heinous crimes"; "commendatory citations"): "Resolution on Disapproval of Participation in Scientific Experiments by Inmates of Penal Institutions," *JAMA* 150, no. 17 (December 27, 1952): 699. Harkness links the AMA resolution to Leopold's commutation in "Research behind Bars," 159–62.

The outcome of Stokes's first hepatitis experiment with prisoners: Neefe reported that of fifteen inmate-subjects, five ingested pooled feces, five ingested liver tissue from biopsies, and five ingested pooled serum. Some of them became ill, but none developed jaundice and available laboratory tests failed to confirm that they had hepatitis. John R. Neefe, "Chronic Hepatitis in Volunteers," *Transactions of the Conference on Liver Injury* 5 (September 26–27, 1946): 90–91.

Report suggests Gellis was responsible for prisoner's escape ("made promises to prisoners"): "Office Memorandum" submitted to Commissioner Bates by R. Spencer Smith, May 14, 1946, NJSA Commissioner, Box 1, Folder: Trenton State Prison 1946. Gellis responded in a letter to Stokes dated May 21, 1946. APS Stokes, Series I, Folder: Gellis, Sydney #1, 1944–52.

The AFEB arranges access letters for Mirick and Gordon: On September 26, 1951, AFEB president Colin MacLeod wrote to Frederick Knoblauch at the OTSG asking about the status of letters from the surgeons general to the governors. The AFEB had originally asked that the secretary of defense write letters to governors, but this request was refused. Hilton W. Rose to MacLeod, July 25, 1951. Documents at NARA AFEB, Box 56, Folder: Liver Disease.

Schley feels that with the war's end, hepatitis experiments in New Jersey facilities should cease ("now that the war"): Stokes to William Stone, chair of the Army Medical Research and Development Board, October 2, 1946, APS Stokes (unprocessed), Folder: Hepatitis #7.

The OTSG requests access to Rahway reformatory for hepatitis studies ("We have every reason to believe"): Stone to Sanford Bates, October 7, 1946, APS Stokes (unprocessed), Folder: Hepatitis #7. Stone also dispatched an appeal to Reeve Schley on October 7, 1946, APS Stokes (unprocessed), Folder:

Hepatitis #3. In December 1946, Bates wrote Stokes to say that the Board of Control would allow hepatitis experiments at Rahway.

Deputy Commissioner Bixby signs letters to Stokes as "Bix": Dr. F. Lovell Bixby to Stokes, January 15, 1953, APS Stokes (unprocessed), Folder: New Jersey Department of Institutions and Agencies #1.

Stokes secures letters of support for access to inmates at Clinton Farms: Stone to Bixby, February 16, 1949. Emlen Stokes's letter to Schley read in part, "I was very disturbed to hear you say that you disapprove of all such investigations in our institutions. I am afraid you cannot fully appreciate the tremendous contribution which our department has made in many such fields of investigation. If it were stopped, we would be taking a very backward step." S. Emlen Stokes to Reeve Schley, January 27, 1949. Documents at APS Stokes (unprocessed), Folder: Department of Institutions and Agencies #2.

Stokes cultivates Clinton Farms' manager and board: Stokes to Edna Mahan, October 27, 1948, APS Stokes (unprocessed), Folder: Clinton Farms Project #5. Stokes's social connections again facilitated access. The Stokes family had a summer house in the Poconos near the vacation home of Anita Mary Quarles, a longtime member of Clinton Farms' board of managers. Mary Q. Hawkes mentions ties between the Stokes and Quarles families in *Excellent Effect: The Edna Mahan Story* (Laurel, MD: American Correctional Association, 1994), 109–10.

Stokes forwards a patriotic appeal for Clinton Farms managers and adds an ironic aside ("great service to"; "I trust it makes the eagle scream"): Stokes to Mahan, December 14, 1948, APS Stokes (unprocessed), Folder: Clinton Farms Project #5.

Hepatitis subjects at Annandale receive credit in reformatory canteen: Winslow Bashe (on Stokes's research team) to Mr. Dempsey, New Jersey Reformatory for Men (Annandale), September 26, 1952, APS Stokes (unprocessed), Folder: New Jersey Reformatory, Bordentown.

Clinton Farms requires parental consent for subjects under twenty-one: A parental consent document accompanied a letter from Mahan to Stokes's secretary Dorothy Melville, January 27, 1955, APS Stokes (unprocessed), Folder: Clinton Farm Project #3.

Stokes urges the OTSG to allow insurance for injuries ("assurances that if"; "apparently not virulent"; "always, however"): Stokes to Stone, October 15, 1947, APS Stokes (unprocessed), Folder: Rahway Reformatory. Stokes would continue to pursue the matter of disability insurance for subjects with the AFEB and the Army Surgeon General's Office, but without success. Relevant discussion at NARA AFEB, Box 56, Folder: Liver Disease.

Research sponsors other than the OTSG addressed insurance for human subjects: For OSRD scientists' deliberations about insurance for inmate-subjects in the 1942 bovine-albumin study, see Harkness, "Research behind Bars," 79–80. While government agencies declined to approve insurance for subjects, some private research sponsors required that researchers provide it. See

Sydney A. Halpern, *Lesser Harms: Morality of Risk on Medical Research* (Chicago: University of Chicago Press, 2004), 102–4.

New Jersey Board of Control accepts statement that injuries are unlikely ("medical authorities representing"): Bates to Stokes, December 9, 1946, APS Stokes, Series III, Folder: New Jersey Department of Institutions and Agencies, 1946–57.

Prison professionals embrace "penal welfarism": David Garland, *Culture of Control* (Chicago: University of Chicago Press, 2001). Discussions of the rehabilitation ethos more broadly include Francis A. Allen, "Criminal Justice, Legal Values, and the Rehabilitative Ideal," *Journal of Criminal Law and Criminology* 50, no. 3 (Fall 1959): 226–32; and Francis A. Allen, *Decline of the Rehabilitative Ideal: Penal Policy and Social Purpose* (New Haven, CT: Yale University Press, 1981).

Sanford Bates insists that medical experiments are rehabilitative ("What must take place"): Sanford Bates to Harold Murray, March 17, 1953, APS Stokes (unprocessed), Folder: New Jersey Department of Institutions and Agencies #1.

Army surgeon general commends Clinton Farms' cooperation with hepatitis studies: R. W. Bliss, Major General, to Mahan, June 16, 1949, APS Stokes (unprocessed), Folder: Clinton Farms Project #3. Bliss sent copies of his letter to Sanford Bates, Reeve Schley, and Joseph Stokes.

Clinton Farms managers respond to army surgeon general ("gracious and enthusiastic"; "It is a source of"): L. B. Wescott to Bliss, July 7, 1949, NARA AFEB, Box 56, Folder: Folder: Human Volunteers for Hepatitis Studies.

Bordentown superintendent writes inmate's mother about son's participation in experiments ("utmost medical attention"; "a very real problem"; "inmost knowledge"; "Danny is doing"): Albert C. Wagner to Mrs. G., July 20, 1951, APS Stokes (unprocessed), Folder: New Jersey Reformatory, Bordentown.

Mirick's waiver form promises a future certificate of merit: The form was titled "Agreement with Volunteer" and read in part, "I understand that at the conclusion of my satisfactory participation in the study, I am to be furnished an appropriate Certificate of Merit and a statement of my voluntary cooperation in the study. The fact that I have thus rendered voluntary service to humanity will be placed in my official record." The document accompanies a letter of January 2, 1952, from Mirick to Adam Rapalski, AFEB administrator. NARA AFEB, Box 56, Folder: Human Volunteers for Hepatitis Studies.

Origins and uses of certificates of merit ("would be an aid to morale"): Bayne-Jones to Francis Blake, July 4, 1945, NARA AEB Boards, Box 642, Folder: Commission on Influenza—Jaundice, Dr. Thomas Francis. A copy of Francis's statement is in the same location. Sabin's certificates of service and related correspondence are at Winkler Sabin, Series V (Military Service), Subseries VC (Dengue), Box 15, Folder 3: Correspondence, Waiver and Release Forms and Certifications of Service, 1944–45. The origins and uses of commendations receive virtually no attention in the historical literature. I did find mention of an adaptation: in 1958, PHS investigator issued certificates of appreciation to

Tuskegee Study subjects. James H. Jones, *Bad Blood: The Tuskegee Syphilis Experiments* (New York: Free Press, 1981), 187. Susan M. Reverby includes a photo of the certificate in Reverby, ed., *Tuskegee's Truths: Rethinking the Tuskegee Syphilis Study* (Chapel Hill: University of North Carolina Press, 2000), 187.

Commendations are on official letterhead or are embossed: Gordon corresponded with AFEB administrator Adam Rapalski about certificates for prisoners in Maryland state facilities on February 5, March 26, and April 21, 1952. Mention of two commendations is in Gordon's letter of April 21. Mirick requested AFEB letterhead like Gordon's in a communication dated March 26, 1952. These documents are at NARA AFEB, Box 56, Folder: Human Volunteers for Hepatitis Studies. In a letter dated June 1, 1950, Stokes wrote the University of Pennsylvania vice president in charge of medical affairs about affixing the university seal on awards of appreciation for subjects at Clinton Farms. APS Stokes (unprocessed), Folder: Clinton Farms Project #6.

Stokes participates in celebration at Bordentown recognizing inmate-subjects: Wagner to Stokes, August 20, 1951, and Stokes to Wagner, August 22, 1951, APS Stokes (unprocessed), Folder: New Jersey Reformatory, Bordentown.

Stokes is to provide certificates of merit and attend Clinton Farms' award ceremony: Mahan to Stokes, May 24, 1949, APS Stokes (unprocessed), Folder: Clinton Farm Project #3. Hawkes notes Henle's role at the 1951 ceremony in *Excellent Effect* 135–36.

The *Spectator* extols inmates who participated in hepatitis experiments ("Volunteers Praised"): "Inmates Told Yellow Jaundice Test Is as Important as Any War Work, Volunteers Praised for Cooperative Spirit," *Spectator*, March 24, 1945, 1; ("heroes—as brave"; "With no promises"): "Experimental Tests with Inmates Here Aided War Effort and Science, Heroic Prisoners Lauded in Report" *Spectator*, December 15, 1945, 1. The *Spectator* (Jackson, MI) is available at the New York City Public Library.

Clinton Farms newsletter lauds hepatitis subjects ("splendid results"; "not only in the United States"; "had the fullest"; "the girls who are"): "Clinton Farms Volunteers Help to Combat Infectious Hepatitis," *US Personified*, July 1949, APS Stokes (unprocessed), Folder: Clinton Farms Project #4.

Clinton Farms playbill reveals Stokes's patronage ("Jaundice Follies"; "PLEASE ACCEPT"): Playbill titled "Hungry Hill Play House Presents." ("Jaundice Unit Members"): Thank-you notes for Stokes's patronage accompany his RSVP to Wittpen Dorm dated August 8, 1949. All documents at APS Stokes (unprocessed), Folder: Clinton Farm Project #6.

Few records are available on the race of inmate-subjects: Hatch comments on the paucity of archival materials—even from the 1960s and early 1970s—on the race of inmate-subjects. Hatch, *Silent Cells*, 73–74. Harkness suggests that African American prisoners were underrepresented among inmates serving as research subjects; he argues that discrimination led to relatively low percentages of inmates of color having access to a route for parole or institutional privileges. Harkness, "Research behind Bars," 2–3. Harriet A. Washington, however, suggests that the number of African Americans enrolled in prison research may be underestimated. Washington, "Caged Subjects: Research on Black Prisoners," in *Medical Apartheid* (New York: Broadway Books, 2006), 244–70.

Mahan desegregated Clinton Farms dormitories in 1947: Hawkes, *Excellent Effect*, 110–13. Another source on Mahan's leadership is Mary Q. Hawkes, "Edna Mahan: Sustaining the Reformatory Tradition," *Women and Criminal Justice* 9, no. 3 (1998): 1–21. I found no information on racial dynamics surrounding the hepatitis experiments at Clinton Farms or in the facility more broadly.

Reformatory census and research participation at Clinton Farms: Census from NJSA Clinton, Folder: 1948–51 Triannual Report. Number of hepatitis subjects from NJSA Clinton, Folder: 1951–53 Biennial Report. A lone document reports the ages of twenty of Clinton Farms' hepatitis subjects: Charles and Mary Ming to Miles Drake, May 18, 1951, APS Stokes (unprocessed), Folder: Clinton Farms Project #5.

Clinton Farms reformatory had a nursery: Census of babies from NJSA Clinton, Folder: 1948–51 Triannual Report. Desegregation of Clinton Farms extended to the facility's nursery.

Stokes recognizes that blood-borne hepatitis could be transmitted from mother to infant ("on rare occasions"; "on one occasion"): Stokes to Bixby, February 16, 1952, APS Stokes (unprocessed), Folder: NJ Department of Institutions and Agencies #2. In this letter Stokes states, "We have been careful to use only epidemic hepatitis virus in the girls at Clinton Farms and not the serum hepatitis virus." The earlier document showing that Stokes's team was planning procedures with blood-borne hepatitis at Clinton Farms—using serum from a donor thought to be a hepatitis carrier—is C. J. Watson, Minutes of the Annual Meeting, Commission on Liver Disease, October 15, 1949, 3–4, NARA AFEB, Box 53, Folder: Commission on Liver Disease Meetings, March 23, 1950.

Stokes's team transmitted blood-borne hepatitis to female psychiatric patients: In interventions conducted in 1949 or 1951, eleven female patients of childbearing age at Trenton State Hospital received inoculations with serum hepatitis virus. "Report of the Use of Infectious Hepatitis and Serum Hepatitis in 297 Mental Patients," circa 1953, APS Stokes, Series VI, Folder: Hepatitis Study #1, 1944–48.

Bordentown superintendent asks Stokes about allowing press coverage: Wagner to Stokes, January 5, 1951. A handwritten version of Stokes's response accompanies it. APS Stokes (unprocessed), Folder: New Jersey Reformatory, Bordentown.

Writer for *Welfare Reporter* accedes to Stokes's requirements ("This is in keeping"): Donald Benson to Stokes, October 23, 1946, APS Stokes (unprocessed), Folder: Department of Institutions and Agencies #3. Commissioner Bates was also to review the draft.

New Jersey officials veto story for the *Philadelphia Inquirer* ("The Board feels"): Bixby to Hugh Scott at the *Inquirer,* January 15, 1953, APS, Stokes (unprocessed), Folder: New Jersey Department of Institutions and Agencies #1.

Stokes wrote his letter suggesting *Inquirer* coverage on May 20, 1952; Bixby's response to Stokes is dated June 27. The latter two documents at APS Stokes (unprocessed), Folder: New Jersey Department of Institutions and Agencies #2.

Newspapers cover hepatitis infection experiments in prisons: "Women Inmates Take Jaundice Cure Tests," *Philadelphia Bulletin*, July 19, 1949 (Clinton Farms); "Serum Tests by Inmates," *Trenton Evening Times*, July 19, 1951 (Bordentown); "46 in Reformatory Volunteer to Test Jaundice Shots," *Philadelphia Bulletin*, November 1, 1951 (Annandale); "Prisoners Volunteer in Jaundice Research," *Washington Post*, February 13, 1952 (Breathedsville Reformatory, Maryland).

***New York Times* reports experiments at Clinton Farms** ("been offering"; "one of the Army's"): "Women Prisoners Aid Jaundice Test: 200 at Clinton Farms, N.J., Infected with the Disease, May Help Conquer It," *New York Times*, September 4, 1950.

***Reader's Digest* story portrays rehabilitated inmate** ("he knew it was"; "close to miraculous"; "If I were in charge"): John L. O'Hara, "The Most Unforgettable Character I've Met," *Reader's Digest*, May 1948. Other magazine articles lauding the altruism of research subjects include Thomas Koritz, "I Was a Human Guinea Pig," *Saturday Evening Post*, July 25, 1953; Don Wharton, "Prisoners Who Volunteer Blood, Flesh—and Their Lives," *American Mercury*, December 1954, 51–55; Don Wharton, "'A Treasure in the Heart of Every Man,'" *Reader's Digest*, December 1954; Alvin Shuster, "Why Human 'Guinea Pigs' Volunteer," *New York Times Magazine*, April 13, 1958.

Stokes wrote a letter supporting Duncan's parole: Stokes to Court of Pardons, Trenton, NJ, May 15, 1946, APS Stokes (unprocessed), Folder: New Jersey State Prison #2.

Duncan experienced a relapse of hepatitis after serving as a research subject ("Two weeks after"; "some method must be"): James E. Duncan to Surgeon General's Office, Washington, DC, October 14, 1952. Duncan received a response from Adam Rapalski on October 22, 1952. Documents at APS Stokes (unprocessed), Folder: New Jersey, Department of Institutions and Agencies #1.

Shortened sentences for inmate-subjects were a reality: Robert Howard reports special considerations for Stateville subjects in "445 Guinea Pig Convicts May Win Clemency," *Chicago Daily Tribune*, February 1, 1947, 10. That subjects in malaria experiments received two-year reductions in sentences is from George Wright, "Leopold Seeks Shorter Term in Parole Plea," *Chicago Daily Tribune*, April 23, 1949, 13. Bernard E. Harcourt discusses the reduced sentences in "Making Willing Bodies: The University of Chicago Human Experiments at Stateville Penitentiary," *Social Research* 78, no. 2 (Summer 2011): 450.

Nathan Leopold reports his reasons for enrolling in malaria studies: Nathan F. Leopold, *Life Plus 99 Years* (New York: Doubleday, 1958), 330–32.

Leopold describes motivations of other inmate-subjects ("Many took part"): Leopold, *Life Plus 99 Years*, 329. Harkness discusses Leopold's remarks in "Research behind Bars," 106–7.

Mainstream press portrays human experiments in prisons as all-American ("as American as apple pie"): Depiction of postwar press coverage from Advisory Committee on Human Radiation Experiments, *Final Report* (Washington, DC: U.S. Government Printing Office, 1995), 152. Also see Sydney Halpern, "Constructing Moral Boundaries: Public Discourse about Human Experimentation in Twentieth-Century America," in *Bioethics in Social Context*, ed. Barry Hoffmaster (Philadelphia: Temple University Press, 2001), 69–89.

Chapter Six. Cold War Calculations

Oliphant had reported that irradiation disables hepatitis in blood: John W. Oliphant and Alexander Hollaender, "Homologous Serum Jaundice: Experimental Inactivation of Etiological Agent in Serum by Ultraviolet Irradiation," *Public Health Reports* 61, no. 17 (April 26, 1946): 598–602.

The NIH biologics lab requires that government-licensed plasma be irradiated: "Historical Background," a one-page typescript on the hepatitis contamination problem. NARA AFEB, Box 81, Folder: Commission on Viral Infections, Project: Roderick Murray (referred to hereafter as NARA AFEB, Murray). The NIH unit overseeing biologics underwent multiple name changes: from Division of Biologics Control (1937–44) to Laboratory of Biologics Control (1944–55) to Division of Biologics Standards (1955–72).

JAMA announces irradiated blood products were triggering hepatitis: *JAMA* 144, no. 3 (September 16, 1950): 224–29, 241–43.

Reports reveal hepatitis is prevalent among plasma recipients: Officials reported that 20 to 25 percent of plasma recipients returning from Korea were developing hepatitis. "Commission on Liver Disease, Annual Report to the AFEB, April 1951–April 1952," NARA AFEB, Box 59, Folder: Commission on Liver Disease, Reports 1951–52.

The Truman administration centralizes blood collection and distribution: President Harry Truman announces the Office of Defense Mobilization will coordinate the national blood program in a memo to the Heads of Executive Departments and Agencies, December 10, 1951, NARA SOD, Entry 351 (AFMPC, DOD Blood Program Historical File, 1948–52), Box 50, Binder Vol. VI, May–June 1952; and "Summary Report of the Health Advisory Committee, Office of Defense Mobilization, August 1950–August 1952," NARA SOD, Entry 348 (AFMPC, General Decimal File 1949–52), Box 21, Binder 334.

The NRC sets up advisory committees on blood: The NRC created the Committee on Blood and Blood Derivatives in the late 1940s—renamed, in 1952, the Committee on Blood Related Programs. This body convened conferences and a panel on blood sterilization. In 1951, the panel became the Subcommittee on Sterilization of Blood and Plasma. Meeting minutes of these bodies span from July 1949 through June 1953.

The defense secretary alerts the president to the problem of hepatitis in plasma ("To eliminate the causative agent"): Robert A. Lovett to President

Truman, June 11, 1952. In the memo, Lovett objected to plans for allocating plasma developed by the Health Resources Advisory Committee of the Office of Defense Mobilization. NARA SOD, Entry 351 (AFMPC, DOD Blood Program, Historical File), Box 50, Binder Vol. VI, May–June 1952.

Hepatitis contamination threatens the entire blood program: A statement to this effect from Milton C. Winternitz, head of the NAS Division of Medical Science, is recorded in Meeting Minutes, NAS Sterilization, September 28, 1951, 2.

Federal agencies collaborate in a project to sterilize blood: Roderick Murray, "Annual Report: Public Health Services Hepatitis Studies," February 27, 1952, NARA AFEB, Box 59, Folder: Commission on Liver Disease, Reports 1951–52; "Defense Activities of the NIH, 1950–1952," May 13, 1952, NARA NIH Planning, Box 2, Folder: Defense, 1951–53.

NIH's agenda includes advancing nuclear preparedness: Documents in which NIH officials elaborate the agency's Cold War national security agenda include Kenneth Endicott, NIH Division of Research Grants, to David Price, NIH associate director, July 10, 1951, NLM NIH Director, Box 7, Folder 7; "Defense Activities of the National Institutes of Health, 1950–1952," May 13, 1952, NARA NIH Planning, Box 2, Folder: Defense 1951–53; and "National Defense Aspects of Public Health Research," August 7, 1950, NARA NIH Planning, Box 6, Folder: Research Planning Council, Defense Projects, 1950.

Oliphant's career trajectory after work at Lynchburg: Documents from Department of Health and Human Services FOIA #15-0347.

Stokes plays a role in the blood sterilization project: Murray notes Stokes's leadership of an NIH ad hoc committee that endorsed and helped shape the study. "Annual Report," February 27, 1952, at NARA AFEB, Box 59, Folder: Commission on Liver Disease Reports 1951–52.

Scientists formulate expansive goals for the project: A meeting at the NIH set out ambitious aims for the study: "Recommendations of the Committee on Sterilization of Blood and Blood Derivative," circa December 1950, NARA SOD, AFMPC General Subject Files, 1949–53, Entry 349, Box 46, Folder: Research Grants and Fellowships (NIH).

Prison paper reports recruitment pitch given to McNeil Island inmates ("admitted frankly"; "permanent disability"; "consideration"; "There are definitely not"; "advance the science"; "contribute in a magnificent"; "unsung heroes"): C. C. Barker, "SUBJECT: Hepatitis," *Island Lantern*, August 1951, 6–7. This and other cited issues of the *Island Lantern* are in Special Collections, University of Washington Library, Seattle.

Inmates enroll as subjects in large numbers: Figures are from Murray, "The Hepatitis Research Program," December 5, 1952, 6, NARA AFEB, Murray.

The wording of the project's waiver and release statement ("the risks to"; "the potential benefits"; "I understand"; "I am convinced of"): From the waiver document used at Lewisburg with the heading, "Federal Security Agency, Public Health Service, National Institutes of Health," NARA AFEB, Murray.

Oliphant reports disappointing study outcomes: Meeting Minutes, December 5, 1951, NAS Sterilization. The NRC now recommended that units of fresh plasma used to make pools for storage be reduced to a minimum. Milton Winternitz to W. R. Lovelace, chair of the Armed Forces Medical Advisory Council, December 13, 1951, NARA SOD, Entry 349 (AFMPC General Subject Files, 1949–53), Box 42, Binder: 742, 1951.

Newspapers announce Oliphant's untimely death: The *Washington Times-Herald*'s story appeared January 11, 1952, under the headline "Dr. Oliphant Was Director at Bethesda." Other press accounts include "Dr. John W. Oliphant, Authority on Viruses, Found Dead in Garage," *Evening Star*, January 11, 1952; and "PHS Expert on Blood Plasma Is Found Dead in His Garage," *Washington Post*, January 11, 1952.

NIH officials scurry in response to Oliphant's death: Officials at the scene of death from memos of January 11, 1952, in Department of Health and Human Services FOIA #15-0347. The newsletter report is "NIH Saddened by Death of John Oliphant," *NIH Record* 4, no. 2 (1952): 3.

Kirschstein describes Roderick Murray, Oliphant's successor ("He was a consummate"; "they told him"): Oral history interview with Ruth L. Kirschstein conducted by Victoria Harden, October 29, 1998, 3–4, available at the website of the Office of History, National Institutes of Health: www.history.nih.gov.

Hepatitis inmate-subjects Higgins and Wood die at McNeil Island: "M'Neil Convict Dies as Result of Germ Test," *Seattle Post-Intelligencer*, May 6, 1952 (Higgins); "McNeil Inmate Forfeits Life in Medical Test," *Tacoma News Tribune*, October 6, 1952 (Wood); and "Second Human Guinea Pig Dies in Drug Tests," *Chicago Tribune*, October 7, 1952 (both Higgins and Wood). Murray noted that the two men had recovered from experimentally induced hepatitis and then relapsed in "Summary of Results Obtained to Date," 6, NARA AFEB, Murray.

Advisory committees examine McNeil Island deaths ("a picture of complete atrophy"): "Report of Dr. Murray on Hepatitis Study among Volunteers," transcript of October 13, 1952. The description of Wood's autopsied liver is on p. 61. Meeting of October 13–14 1952, NARA AFEB, Box 53, Folder: Commission on Liver Disease.

Warden lauds deceased inmates ("a real nice fellow"): "M'Neil Convict Dies"; ("died in the service"): "McNeil Inmate Forfeits Life."

Veteran researchers visit Lewisburg to examine comatose subjects: "Report of Visit to the Federal Penitentiary at Lewisburg, Pa, December 13, 1952," NARA AFEB, Murray.

Lewisburg inmate-subject John Gavin dies: John McKelway, "Convict, 23, Dies in Research Project on Yellow Jaundice," *Washington Evening Star*, December 17, 1952; "Convict Told of Dangers in Fatal Tests," *Washington Post*, December 18, 1952, 20; and "U.S. Pen Magazine Eulogizes Inmate," *Union County Standard* (Lewisburg, PA), January 15, 1953.

Prison papers publish eulogies for deceased hepatitis subjects ("Officials of the Bureau"): "Dedicated to the Memory of John F. Gavin, American Patriot," *Periscope*, Christmas 1952, 1–2; ("John Gavin died"): "The Experiment," *Periscope*, Spring–Summer 1953, 14. Eulogies for the men at McNeil Island are "In Memoriam" (Walter Harvey Wood), *Island Lantern*, November 1952, 1; and "Obituary" (Richard Henry Higgins), *Island Lantern*, June 1952, 1.

Commendations of inmate-subjects appear in the prison press: "Honor Roll," *Island Lantern*, January 1953, 1; ("in grateful appreciation"): *Periscope*, Spring–Summer 1953, 15.

Murray compares estimated and actual death rates in the blood sterilization project ("The danger of possible fatalities"): Meeting Minutes, February 4, 1953, 2, NAS Sterilization. Murray based his computation on the number of subjects who contracted hepatitis rather than the number inoculated with the virus. He had noted a month earlier that ninety-six inmates had developed hepatitis. Meeting Minutes, Subcommittee on Allocation of Volunteers, January 4, 1953, NARA AFEB, Box 54, Folder: Commission on Liver Disease.

Researchers had been sustaining viral strains by passages through subjects: Cecil Watson would later express concern that, with a halt on human experiments, it might be difficult to obtain specimens for work with tissue cultures. Meeting Minutes, April 16, 1953, 11, NARA AFEB, Box 50, Folder: Committee on Allocation of Volunteers. Henle reported in 1954 that stores of known specimens were nearly depleted: Werner Henle, Annual Progress Report, March 1, 1953–February 28, 1954, 3. APS Stokes (unprocessed), Folder: Commission on Liver Disease. David D. Rutstein, professor of preventive medicine at Harvard, later voiced the opinion that, even in the absence of an animal host, "it is not ethical to use human subjects for the growth of a virus for any purpose." Rutstein, "The Ethical Design of Human Experiments," *Daedalus* 98, no. 2 (Spring 1969): 529.

Deceased subjects received specimens from suspected carriers: John Neefe, Annual Progress Report, February 28, 1952, NARA AFEB, Box 59, Folder: Commission on Liver Disease, Reports 1951–52. Additional discussion of the implicated specimens is at "Carrier Problem," Meeting Minutes, February 4, 1953, NAS Sterilization.

Researchers discuss "silent carriers": Stokes and others on his team were using the term *silent carrier* in advisory committee meetings during 1951 and 1952. One such discussion concerned possible sexual transmission by silent carriers. Meeting Transcript, Report of the Subcommittee on Allocation of Volunteers, 128–31, NARA AFEB, Box 53, Folder: Commission on Liver Disease Meeting, October 13–14, 1952. Three papers on hepatitis carriers appeared in *JAMA* 154, no. 13 (March 27, 1954): 1059–74. Stokes was lead author on the first paper, Neefe on the second, and Murray on the third.

Scientists are concerned about "street viruses": Annual Report of the Commission on Liver Disease, Section IV, May 1, 1953, NARA AFEB Accession NN3 334 09 001, Box 4, Folder: Commission on Liver Disease, Progress Reports, 1952–53.

Committee on Human Volunteers makes recommendations ("Even though no one"; "In order to proceed"): Meeting Minutes, Subcommittee on

Allocation of Volunteers, January 4, 1953, 7, NARA AFEB, Box 54, Folder: Commission on Liver Disease.

Officials consider the problem of hepatitis in blood too urgent to abandon research ("well-considered studies"): Adam Rapalski's words as reported in Meeting Minutes, February 4, 1953, 5, NAS Sterilization. He was relaying the outcome of the Epidemiology Board meeting held on January 30, 1953.

The Epidemiology Board scales back the project: Murray, Annual Progress Report, April 1, 1952–March 15, 1953, 18, under "Reorientation of the Program." NARA AFEB, Box 60, Folder: Commission on Liver Disease, Reports, 1952–53.

Additional meetings address the fate of the hepatitis program: On March 24, 1953, Murray sent background material to Colonel John Wood at the OTSG for the meeting set for March 28. NARA AFEB, Murray. On April 16, Murray noted that a decision was "pending from a committee determining the future of human volunteers studies by the NIH USPHS group." NARA AFEB, Box 50, Folder: Committee on Allocation of Volunteers, Meeting Minutes, April 16, 1953, 9.

The Epidemiology Board halts its entire hepatitis program: As Murray stated, "Transmission studies involving the use of serum hepatitis were terminated on June 30, 1954." "Analysis of NIH Program Activities," for Murray's "Studies on Serum and Infectious Hepatitis," NARA NIH Planning, Box 10, Intramural Research Projects, 1955, Folder 30–39: Lab of Biologics Control.

No official statement is available on the termination of all hepatitis infection studies: If the Epidemiology Board issued an official rationale for halting human infection studies, the statement did not become part of the available archival record. Minutes of a board meeting in the winter of 1953 are conspicuously missing from repository folders.

The Defense Department adopts the Nuremberg Code: A reprint of the Wilson Memo appears in Advisory Committee on Human Radiation Experiments (ACHRE), *Final Report* (Washington, DC: Government Printing Office, 1995), 105–7. Melvin Casberg, AFMPC chair, reported the October 13 decision to recommend the code's adoption and added, "As soon as the policy has been coordinated with interested agencies, it will be submitted to the Secretary of Defense for approval." Casberg to the defense secretary, November 10, 1952, NARA SOD, Entry 348, General Decimal Files, 1949–52, Box 21, Binder: AFMPC. AFMPC members included university medical leaders and high-level medical officers in the army, navy, and air force. On the body's original composition, see "Armed Forces Medical Advisory Committee," *JAMA* 139, no. 3 (January 15, 1949): 157.

Historians explain DOD's decision to adopt Nuremberg principles: ACHRE, *Final Report*, 101–12; Jonathan D. Moreno and Susan E. Lederer, "Revising the History of Cold War Research Ethics," *Kennedy Institute of Ethics Journal* 6, no. 3 (1996): 230–33; Jonathan D. Moreno, *Undue Risk* (New York:

Routledge, 2001), 157–88; and Jonathan D. Moreno, "Stumbling toward Bioethics: Human Experiments Policy and the Early Cold War," in *Dark Medicine: Rationalizing Unethical Medical Research*, ed. William R. Lafleur, Gernot Böhme, and Susumu Shimazono (Bloomington: University of Indiana Press, 2007), 140–45.

U.S. supports international human rights in words if not deeds ("intended to be a beacon"): Barbara J. Keys, *Reclaiming American Virtue: The Human Rights Revolution of the 1970s* (Cambridge, MA: Harvard University Press, 2014), 22.

Soviet scientist criticized U.S. prison experiments: "Experiments on Prisoners," *Science News Letter*, February 21, 1948, 117.

The pope issues a statement on human experimentation: The pope delivered the address "Moral Limits of Medical Research and Treatment" at the First International Congress of Histopathology of the Nervous System on September 14, 1952. ACHRE, *Final Report*, 154–55.

Rivers states the pope's research ethics address had wide impact ("That speech had"): Saul Benison, ed., *Tom Rivers: Reflections on a Life in Medicine and Science* (Cambridge, MA: MIT Press, 1967), 498. Cited in ACHRE, *Final Report*, 155. In 1952, Rivers was director of the hospital at Rockefeller Institute for Medical Research. A year later he became director of the entire Rockefeller Institute, a position he held until 1955.

The Wilson Memo adopting Nuremberg principles was top secret: But some heard of its existence. In 1952, Henry K. Beecher—not a member of the hepatitis research community—wrote Melvin Casberg, chair of the Armed Forces Medical Policy Council, requesting a copy of the new document. Susan E. Lederer, "'Ethics and Clinical Research' in Biographical Perspective," *Perspectives in Biology and Medicine* 59, no. 1 (Winter 2016): 26–27.

Researchers are particularly concerned about a provision in the code ("No experiment should be conducted"): Provision 5 of the original Nuremberg Code.

Attorney clarifies death or disabling injury provision ("the question of whether"): Rapalski, AFEB administrator, recounting Stephen Jackson's interpretation in response to MacLeod's request for clarification. Rapalski discussed the matter in a letter of March 2, 1953, to Howard Karsner, a senior medical officer in the navy. NARA AFEB, Box 54, Folder: Commission on Liver Disease, Committee on Allocation of Volunteers.

Arrangements protect the defense secretary from responsibility for decisions about medical experiments ("gave instructions that"; "firmly delegated to"; "that the Secretary"): Rapalski to MacLeod, March 2, 1953, NARA AFEB, Box 54, Folder: Commission on Liver Disease, Committee on Allocation of Volunteers. Rapalski was recounting directives he received from the Office of the Secretary of Defense.

Stokes had sought approval for insuring hepatitis subjects: Stokes's initial request was in a letter to William Stone, Office of the Surgeon General, October 15, 1947, APS Stokes (unprocessed), Folder: Rahway Reformatory. He continued to advocate for reimbursing research injuries in Stokes to Colin Mac-Leod, February 11, 1948, in NARA AFEB, Box 56, Folder: Commission on Liver Disease. Discussion of the matter was on the agenda for a March 20, 1948, meeting of the Liver Disease Commission; NARA AEB Boards, Box 648 Folder: [AFEB] Commission on Liver Disease Meetings, 1948.

The OTSG allowed payment for deceased subject's burial costs: Adam Rapalski to comptroller regarding obligation of funds, February 2, 1953, NARA AFEB, Murray. This practice was apparently long-standing. Jon Harkness notes that the OSRD covered burial costs for Arthur St. Germaine, who died in the 1942 bovine-albumin study; that payment also was drawn from the investigator's research account. See Harkness, "Research behind Bars: A History of Nontherapeutic Research on American Prisoners" (PhD diss., University of Wisconsin, Madison, 1996), 87.

Researchers get unwelcome news about their liability for research injuries: Watson to MacLeod, April 5, 1948. In a letter to Watson, April 14, 1948, John Paul concurred that the individual researcher was the legally responsible party. Both documents at NARA AFEB, Box 56, Folder: Commission on Liver Disease, Human Volunteers for Hepatitis Studies. This folder also includes a memo of April 14, 1948, from MacLeod to OTSG legal counsel asking that office to obtain information about legal outcomes in Massachusetts where Arthur St. Germaine had died while a subject in the bovine-albumin study. In 1952, Congress passed a bill allowing the Defense Department to indemnify contractors. This would permit the agency to reimburse researchers for legal costs, but would not prevent a legal suit from occurring. ACHRE, *Final Report*, 101. Rapalski discussed the implications of the bill for medical researchers in "Applicability of Section 5, Public Law 557—82nd Congress," in ACHRE, *Final Report Supplement*, vol. 1, 260–61 (ACHRE Document No. NARA-012395-A).

Family retains legal counsel after Lewisburg death ("Legal representatives"): Irving Ladimer, "Ethical and Legal Aspects of Medical Research on Human Beings," *Journal of Public Law* 3, no. 1 (Spring 1954): 472.

Defense lawyer views the voluntariness of prisoners' participation as not in question: Jackson proposed the amendment in a memo to Casberg dated December 4, 1952. ACHRE, *Final Report Supplement*, vol. 1, 302 (ACHRE Document No. NARA 101294-A-3). The Wilson Memo included a proscription against experiments with prisoners of war and no statement about experiments with prisoners more generally.

MacLeod wants reassessment of experiments with wards of the state ("only those practices"; "I think it would be"): MacLeod to Stokes, November 24, 1952. It was in a letter to Stokes dated December 1, 1952, that MacLeod urged Stokes to have the Committee on Allocation of Volunteers do more than coordinate scientific work and subject access. Both documents at NARA AFEB, Box 54, Folder: Commission on Liver Disease.

Rivers was known for delivering stinging criticism: Richard Shope, "Thomas Milton Rivers," *Journal of Bacteriology* 84, no. 3 (September 1962): 387.

Rivers criticizes Stokes's experiments with children ("At a recent meeting"): Stokes to Cecil Watson, February 4, 1953, APS Stokes, Series II, Folder: Army Epidemiology Board #30, 1953 January–March. Rivers's comments about children not being free agents are at Benison, *Tom Rivers*, 467.

Stokes distributes exposition on research ethics: "A Clarification of the Question of 'Ethical Responsibility' in the Exposure of Human Beings to Certain Infectious Agents" accompanies Stokes letter to Cecil Watson of February 4, 1953. APS Stokes, Series II, Folder: Army Epidemiology Board #30, 1953 January–March. Stokes had distributed an earlier "point-of-ethics" statement addressing virus transmission procedures with children. Stokes to Colin MacLeod, February 11, 1948, NARA AFEB, Box 56, Folder: Commission on Liver Disease. A statement from a major pediatric society at least partially corroborates Stokes's claim that child specialists saw it as beneficial to expose youngsters to some infectious diseases before puberty. According to a panel of experts, "Girls should have rubella [German measles], wherever possible, before their childbearing period." "Report of the Committee on Immunization and Therapeutic Procedures for Acute Infectious Diseases," American Academy of Pediatrics, Evanston IL, 1952, 55.

Henle describes Rivers as a bully ("As so often happens"): NLM Henle, 99–100.

Document reports outcome of experiments with mental patients: "Report on the Use of Infectious Hepatitis and Serum Hepatitis in 297 Mental Patients," circa 1953, APS Stokes, Series VI, Folder: Hepatitis Study #1, 1944–48. A letter among Stokes's papers indicates that the report's authors were doctors Robert E. Bennett and Robert S. Garber, both affiliated with the New Jersey State Hospital at Trenton. The relevant correspondence reads in part: "I am in receipt of a letter from Dr. Bashe asking when Dr. Garber and I were going to start our psychiatric follow-up, and advising me to contact you in regard to this matter." The letter goes on to say that the report would be based on review of patient files. Robert E. Bennett, New Jersey State Hospital's assistant medical director, to Stokes, January 23, 1953, APS Stokes, Series III, Folder: New Jersey State Prison, 1946–53.

A general criticizes the program's record and asks whether other researchers should be studying hepatitis ("Great amount of time"): Memo for the record dated January 3, 1952. The author, A. H. Schwichtenberg, wrote that he had discussed the matter with Dorlan Davis, an infectious disease specialist at the NIH who was not involved with the blood sterilization study. NARA SOD, Entry 351, AFMPC DOD Blood Program Historical File, Box 50, Binder vol. 4, December 1951–March 1952.

John Paul laments the lack of scientific progress: Report of the director, Hepatitis Group of the Viral Infection Commission, 3, NARA OTSG R & D, Accession 67-D-4813, Box 57, Folder: Dr. John R. Paul. Commission director W. McD. Hammon noted that Paul was author of the Hepatitis Group's report. Commission on Viral Infections Director's Report, 1957, NARA AFEB Meetings, Box 57 (Meeting Files, May–December 1958), Folder: Spring Docket, May 1958.

Epidemiology Board shuts down its Liver Commission: Documented in a letter from MacLeod to Stokes dated March 19, 1954, and a memorandum, "Activities of Commission on Liver Diseases," dated December 30, 1954. Both documents at APS Stokes (unprocessed), Folder: Armed Forces Epidemiology Board, #5. Earlier MacLeod had announced the redirection of hepatitis research from human experiments to propagation of the virus in animals and tissue cultures. Meeting Minutes, Commission on Liver Disease, April 17, 1953, NARA AFEB, Box 50, Folder: Commission on Liver Disease, General Correspondence, 1953.

Future studies would need a higher bar for results to justify risks ("any future study"): Statement by Murray, Meeting Minutes, May 31, 1957, NAS Blood Related.

Stokes leaves hepatitis transmission research: In a February 1953 communication to Stokes, Winslow Bashe, a physician on Stokes's project, noted that arrangements were being made to discontinue work at Trenton State Hospital. "Hepatitis Volunteer Studies, January 16, 1953 to February 24, 1953," APS Stokes (unprocessed), Box: Hepatitis no. 3, Folder: Hepatitis Studies: Misc. Notes, Reports. Stokes reported the termination of his broader program in a letter of May 28, 1953, to Harold S. McGee, then superintendent of Trenton State Hospital. APS Stokes (unprocessed), Folder: New Jersey State Prison #1.

Stokes moves on to testing live polio vaccine: The subjects in these studies included women and babies at Clinton Farms. Relevant documents include Stokes and Hilary Koprowski, "Progress Report on Immunization with Living Attenuated Poliomyelitis Virus of Infants and Inmates at Clinton Farms," May 21, 1957, APS Stokes (unprocessed), New Jersey Reformatory for Women. Publications from this research include Stanley A. Plotkin, Hilary Koprowski, and Joseph Stokes Jr., "Clinical Trials in Infants of Orally Administered Attenuated Poliomyelitis Viruses," *Pediatrics* 23, no. 6 (June 1959): 1041–62.

Henle takes over Stokes's hepatitis contract: Henle, now principal researcher, reported that Stokes had resigned as the responsible investigator, that human interventions were discontinued, and that work on cultivating hepatitis virus in chick embryos was largely discontinued in favor of growth in tissue cultures. Annual Progress Report, Werner Henle, March 1, 1953–February 28, 1954, APS Stokes (unprocessed), Folder: Commission on Liver Disease. Also reported in NLM Henle.

Neefe loses AFEB funding: "While it was generally agreed that Dr. Neefe's study of carriers had contributed ... important knowledge, some doubt was expressed as to how the study could continue unless volunteers were used and that they probably should not be used for this type of transmission of what amounts to unknown or 'street viruses.'" Annual Report of the Commission on Liver Disease, May 1, 1953, 7, NARA AFEB Accession NN3 334 09 001, Box 4, Folder: Commission on Liver Disease Progress Reports, 1952–53.

Kirschstein comments on Murray's involvement with deaths ("an unfortunate experience"): Kirschstein's oral history interview of October 29, 1998,

4. Nicholas Wade commented on the weakness of Murray's leadership in "Division of Biologic Standards: The Boat That Never Rocks," *Science* 175, no. 4027 (March 17, 1972): 1225–29.

Press announcements of research deaths become more common: Susan E. Lederer, "Dying for Science: Historical Perspectives on Research Participants' Deaths," *AMA Journal of Ethics* 17, no. 12 (December 2015): 116–71.

Post **quotes officials saying America's adversaries might depict the experiments as atrocities for propaganda purposes** ("in admittedly hazardous"; "be twisted"; "Every effort was made"): Nate Haseltine, "Convicts Give Lives in War on Dread Disease," *Washington Post*, September 6, 1953, B1.

Post **declares subjects had full knowledge of risks** ("Convict Told of Dangers in Fatal Tests"—headline without byline; "I'm very proud"): *Washington Post*, December 18, 1952, 20.

Editorial adds to praise of deceased subject Gavin ("of his own free will"): "He Also Served," *Washington Post*, December 18, 1952, 12 (no byline).

Journalist reports inmates insist they were not coerced ("All insisted unequivocally"): N. S. Haseltine, "Scientists Make Progress in Fight on Jaundice Virus," *Washington Post*, September 8, 1953.

Other coverage depicts prisoners as motivated by patriotism ("for his courage"): "U.S. Pen Magazine Eulogizes Inmate"; ("These men, ineligible"): Walter Ruch, "Prisoners in Heroic Fight against Dread Disease," *Harrisburg Patriot-News*, November 27, 1952, reprinted in Lewisburg prison's *Periscope*, Spring–Summer 1952, 18–19; Don Wharton, "Prisoners Who Volunteer Blood, Flesh—and Their Lives," *American Mercury*, December 1954, 51–55.

Journalist quotes PHS officials saying public sentiment will determine whether prison experiments continue ("whether or not"): Haseltine, "Scientists Make Progress," 13.

Chapter Seven. Science on the Cusp

The AFEB resumes hepatitis infection research ("a fresh start"; "one of the largest"): R. W. Babione to the chief, Navy Bureau of Medicine and Surgery, November 19, 1956, NARA AFEB, Box 87, Folder: Committee on Viral Infections, Project: Saul Krugman. Babione was a captain in the Navy Medical Corps.

Eight hundred children pass through the NYU hepatitis research unit: Saul Krugman repeated this estimate in several places, including AFEB Minutes, December 15, 1972, Committee on Viral Infections, Dr. Scherer, NARA AFEB Accession NN3 334 09 003, Box 15, Folder 7, Minutes of AFEB Meetings 1972, 71.

NYU researchers were invited to Willowbrook to help with infectious diseases: "Dr. Robert Ward and I were invited to join the staff of Willowbrook as consultants in infectious disease." Saul Krugman, "The Willowbrook Hepatitis Studies Revisited: Ethical Aspects," *Review of Infectious Diseases* 8, no. 1 (January–February 1986): 158.

Physicians advised parents to institutionalize impaired children: Allison C. Carey, *On the Margins of Citizenship* (Philadelphia: Temple University Press, 2009), 90–91. Sources on the postwar expansion in institutions for the developmentally impaired and accompanying social movements include Carey's book as well as James W. Trent Jr., *Inventing the Feeble Mind: A History of Mental Retardation in the United States* (Berkeley: University of California Press, 1994).

The severity of impairments among Willowbrook's residents: Krugman, "Willowbrook Hepatitis Studies Revisited," 158. David J. Rothman and Sheila M. Rothman describe characteristics of the facility's residents in *The Willowbrook Wars* (New York: Harper & Row, 1984), 23–25.

The NYU team's initial studies at Willowbrook focused on rubella: Robert Ward discussed experiments with rubella in "Progress Report to the Commission on Virus and Rickettsial Disease, July 1–December 31, 1953," NARA AFEB Accession NN3 334 09 004 Box 9, Folder: Commission on Viral Infections, April 1952–March 1953. The team's published work on rubella included Krugman et al., "Studies on Rubella Immunization. 1. Demonstration of Rubella without Rash," *JAMA* 151, no. 4 (January 24, 1953): 285–88.

Saul Krugman describes the flow of children into the hepatitis unit: Statement by Krugman in Dr. Scherer's AFEB Minutes, December 15, 1972, Committee on Viral Infections, NARA AFEB Accession NN3 334 09 003, Box 15, Folder 7, Minutes of AFEB Meetings 1972, 71.

Willowbrook had multiple buildings and multiple units for children: David Goode et al. describe the institution's physical layout in *A History and Sociology of the Willowbrook State School* (Washington, DC: American Association on Intellectual and Developmental Disabilities, 2013), 131–37.

Race and ethnicity of a group of ten Willowbrook hepatitis subjects: Saul Krugman to Walter Paul Havens, September 6, 1960, NARA AFEB, Box 87, Folder: Commission on Viral Infections, Projects: Saul Krugman. Rothman and Rothman note that in the facility overall, one-third of residents were from minority groups and two-thirds were white. *Willowbrook Wars*, 25.

NYU researchers describe their early goal of extending immunity to hepatitis A: In the group's initial research proposal, the aim was to generate "passive-active immunity"—a notion proposed earlier by Stokes—in which gamma globulin suppresses symptoms while exposure to the virus generates protective antibodies. "Hepatitis in a State Institution for Mental Defectives: A Plan to Attempt to Immunize the Population at Willowbrook State School," 3–4. This document accompanies a letter of February 8, 1956, from Ward to Babione. NARA AFEB, Box 87, Folder: Commission on Viral Infections, Project: Saul Krugman.

The AFEB Virus Commission initially rejects experiments with hepatitis B: John Paul stated, "General Wood asked the Commission to consider the possibility of resuming volunteer studies to get an early firm answer to the plasma sterilization problems. Members have held two conferences, one here and one in Philadelphia on this question. The majority of Commission members are strongly against use of human volunteers, at least with SH virus." AFEB Minutes of December 2, 1955, NARA AFEB Accession NN3 334 09 003, Box 15, Folder: Minutes of AFEB Meetings, January 1951, May 1955, and December 1955, 1.

Virus Commission approves experiments at Willowbrook with hepatitis A: John Paul reported the Virus Commission's unanimous approval of early interventions at Willowbrook in a report to the AFEB submitted March 5, 1956. NARA AFEB Accession NN3 334 09 004, Box 9: Folder: Annual Report of the Commission on Viral Infections, March 1954–February 1956.

The commission allows other interventions deemed to be low risk ("back-log of high priority projects"): William McD. Hammon, Director's Report—1958, Commission on Viral Infections, NARA AFEB Meetings, Box 8 (December 1958–May 1959), Folder: Docket Spring Meeting 1959, Commission on Viral Infections.

The AFEB approves testing of Enders's tissue culture at Willowbrook ("within the scope"; "a benign strain"): AFEB Meeting Minutes, May 2–4, 1957, NARA AFEB Accession NN3 334 09 003, Box 15, Folder 2: Minutes of Meetings 1957, 1959. A decade earlier, Enders led a team that introduced a non-neurological tissue culture for poliovirus that laid the groundwork for development of polio vaccines. Enders's group won a Nobel Prize in 1954 for that work.

Detroit-6 culture touted by some researchers likely contained metastasized cancer cells: Investigators who introduced the Detroit-6 culture described it in Lawrence Berman, Cyril S. Stulberg, and Frank H. Ruddle, "Long-Term Tissue Culture of Human Bone Marrow," *Blood* 10 (1955): 896–911; and Cyril S. Stulberg, Lawrence Berman, and Frank H. Ruddle, "Detroit-6 Strain of Human Epithelial-like Cells: Virus Susceptibilities," *Proceedings of the Society of Experimental Biology and Medicine* 89 (July 1955): 438–41. The scientists were from the Wayne State College of Medicine in Detroit. On burgeoning use of cell lines, including human cell lines, during the late 1940s and 1950s, see Hannah Landecker, *Culturing Life: How Cells Became Technologies* (Cambridge, MA: Harvard University Press, 2007).

Yale lab was unable to grow hepatitis in Detroit-6 culture: "R. W. Mc-Collum's Discussion of Dr. McLean's paper," NARA AFEB Accession 71A 3159 (AFEB Office of the Executive Secretary) Box 5, Folder: Commission on Viral Infections, General 1961. Also, Annual Report of John Paul's Project to the Commission on Viral Infections, February 1956, 8, NARA OTSG R & D, Accession 67A 4813, Box 57, Folder: Dr. John R. Paul, Yale University.

Virus Commission rejects tests of Detroit-6 culture at Willowbrook ("The use of Detroit-6"; "The probable risk"): Report of the Commission on Viral Infections, AFEB Meeting Minutes, May 8–10, 1958, NARA AFEB Accession NN3 334 09 003, Box 15, Folder 2: Minutes of Meetings 1957, 1959.

***New England Journal* publishes letter critical of Willowbrook studies** ("the feeding of live virus"; "lack of feeling"; "work with live virus"): John B. De-Hoff, "Correspondence: Human Experimentation," *New England Journal of Med-*

icine 257, no. 9 (August 29, 1957): 431. The report in *Scope Weekly* appeared in vol. 2, no. 27 (July 3, 1957).

AFEB scientists arrange for a supportive editorial in *New England Journal* ("The suggestion was made"): John Paul's full statement about actions taken in response to the De Hoff letter is as follows. "Dr. Ward and his colleagues produced a manuscript in short order and this was submitted to the New England Journal at once. At the same time Drs. Dingle and Enders were kind enough to consult with Dr. Garland, Editor of the New England Journal and the suggestion was made, with which their Board of Editors agreed, that an Editorial be written to appear in the same issue of the journal in which the paper by Dr. Ward and his colleagues appeared." "Report of the Director of the Hepatitis Group of the Viral Infections Commission" (1957–58). Paul comments further on the arrangements in "Report of the Director of the Hepatitis Group of the Viral Infections Commission," under Report of the Commission on Viral Infections, AFEB Minutes, December 9, 1957. Both documents at NARA OTSG R & D, Accession 67A 4813, Box 57, Folder: Dr. John R. Paul, Yale University.

Editorial on scientific paper from Willowbrook studies appears in *New England Journal*: "Regarding Infectious Hepatitis," *New England Journal of Medicine* 258, no. 9 (1958): 451. The scientific paper was Robert Ward et al., "Infectious Hepatitis: Studies of Its Natural History and Prevention," *New England Journal of Medicine* 258, no. 9 (February 27, 1958): 407–16.

Virus Commission advises Krugman to include justifications in publications: Hammon wrote Krugman, July 30, 1959, "I note that it has been recommended by Dr. R. J. McKay Jr., Recorder of the American Pediatric Society, to include this [justification] with the published paper." NARA AFEB, Box 87, Folder: Commission on Viral Infections, Project: Saul Krugman, 1953–62.

Augusta McCoord criticizes Willowbrook studies: In a letter to Krugman dated July 30, 1959, Hammon refers to both criticism from McCoord and to Krugman's written response. Neither the McCoord nor the Krugman letter accompanies Hammon's. NARA AFEB, Box 87, Folder: Commission on Viral Infections, Project: Saul Krugman, 1953–62.

Internist complains about experiments to Willowbrook director ("the incidence"): J. H. Hutchinson to Harold Berman, January 20, 1960, Bentley Francis, Box 31, Folder: AFEB President's Files 1958–60, Commission on Viral Infections.

Krugman responds to Huchinson's complaint ("We too"): Krugman to Berman, January 27, 1960, Bentley Francis, Box 31, Folder: AFEB President's Files, 1958–60, Commission on Viral Infections.

Virus Commission sends letters of protest and Krugman's responses up the ladder: On March 21, 1960, Hammon wrote Krugman saying that, at the recommendation of the Virus Commission, copies of the correspondence were being forwarded to Thomas Francis (AFEB president), Colonel John Rizzolo (AFEB executive secretary), and Major Thomas Dunne (chief, Preventive Medicine Division, Army Medical R & D Command). Hammon went on to say no further action would be taken unless Hutchinson communicated with the army surgeon general either directly or through the governor of New York. Bentley Francis, Box 31, Folder: AFEB President's Files, 1958–60, Commission on Viral Infections. Krugman elaborated his justification for the Willowbrook studies to Dunne in a letter of August 30, 1960; this was in response to an August 16 request from the OTSG. NARA AFEB, Box 87, Folder: Commission on Viral Infection, Project: Saul Krugman. When controversy surrounding the Willowbrook studies intensified in the late 1960s, Krugman included an ethical rationale for the research in his funding proposals. Krugman's Application for Research, January 12, 1968, NARA AFEB Accession 71A 3159 (Army OTSG AFEB Ex Sec), Box 1, Folder: Docket Spring Meeting, AFEB Commission on Viral Infections, 1969.

The AFEB has no qualms about hepatitis experiments at Willowbrook ("This matter of carrying on"): Hammon to Krugman, March 21, 1960, Bentley Francis, Box 31, Folder: AFEB President's Files, 1958–60, Commission on Viral Infections.

The Virus Commission writes the New York State commissioner in support of experiments at Willowbrook ("This is to counteract any"): Hammon's report on the activities of the Commission on Viral Infections, May 20–22, 1963, AFEB Meeting Minutes, NARA AFEB Accession NN3 334 09 003, Box 15, Folder 4: Minutes of AFEB Meeting, 1963–65.

Experiments at Joliet are done largely in secret ("a hush-hush atmosphere"): "Doctors Hail Vaccine Test for Hepatitis," *Chicago Daily Tribune*, May 5, 1961.

Parke-Davis researchers report success in growing hepatitis in Detroit-6 culture: W. A. Rightsel et al., "Tissue-Culture Cultivation of Cytopathogenic Agents from Patients with Clinical Hepatitis," *Science* 124, no. 3214 (August 3, 1956): 226–28.

Joseph Boggs describes recruitment at Joliet and subjects' race: Description of recruitment from "Infectious Hepatitis: Importance of the Route of Administration," n.d., 2. Two documents provide information on the race of some participants in studies conducted at Joliet Penitentiary in the late 1960s: "Application for Renewal of Research Contract," November 1970, 4–11 (describing eight subjects); and "Joliet Prison Study," September 17, 1969 (describing sixteen subjects). The percentage of inmates of color in these listings is 25 and 44 percent, respectively. All documents at TMC Melnick, Series III, Box 4, Folder: Boggs, 1969–71. In 1970, 43 percent of inmates admitted to state correctional facilities were black. In 1960, that figure had been substantially lower, at 34 percent. Patrick A. Landan, "Race of Prisoners Admitted to State and Federal Institutions, 1926–86," from the Bureau of Justice Statistics, U.S. Department of Justice, 1991, available at the Bureau of Justice Statistics website, www.bjs.gov.

Parke-Davis announces human transmission of hepatitis grown in tissue culture: "Status Report on Tissue-Culture Cultivated Hepatitis Virus," *JAMA* 177, no. 10 (September 9, 1961): 671–82. Rightsel was first author on part

1 of this report; Boggs was first author on part 2. The Joliet prison newspaper reported that in July 1961 the state medical society bestowed commendations for the hepatitis studies upon two hundred Joliet inmates, the study's investigators, Joliet's wardens, and the current and past Illinois governors. "Illinois State Medical Society Lauds Joliet Inmates," _Joliet-Stateville Time_, August 1961, 8–9. The _Time_ is available at the Richard J. Daley Library, University of Illinois, Chicago.

Life magazine covers hepatitis experiments at Joliet: Keith Wheeler, "Lurking Risks of Transfusion," _Life_, February 15, 1963, 70–80.

Robert McCollum reacts to claims of Parke-Davis researchers: About Parke-Davis withholding its cell line McCollum remarked, "The reason for this is quite manifest. The bitter taste left by the experience of five and six years ago is still on the tips of several fingers." McCollum to Hammon, November 17, 1961. On October 11, 1961, John Paul (in a communication to members of the Hepatitis Group) commented on the Virus Commission's reaction to Parke-Davis's reports: "In recent weeks there has been some agitation regarding new findings presented by the Parke Davis (Detroit and Chicago) group." Both documents at NARA AFEB, Accession 71A 3159 (Army OTSG AFEB Executive Secretary), Box 5, Folder: Commission on Virus Infections, General, 1961. Paul described efforts at Yale to grow hepatitis in Detroit-6 culture in Annual Project Report of the Commission on Virus Infections, March 1955–February 1956, 8, NARA OTSG R & D, Accession 67A 4813, Box 57, Folder: Dr. John R. Paul, Yale University.

The military moves ahead with developing a hepatitis vaccine grown in new cell lines: Minutes of the Subcommittee on Plasma, November 21–22, 1961, 4, NAS Blood Related. The source was Henry T. Gannon from the NRC Division of Medical Sciences.

The R & D Command reorganizes its hepatitis research efforts: Military medical officers discussed the reorganization of the R & D Command's support of hepatitis research at the December 4, 1962, AFEB meeting. NARA AFEB Accession NN3 334 09 003, Box 15, Folder 3: Minutes of AFEB Meetings, 1960–62.

The OTSG creates a new Advisory Committee on Liver Disease: Multiple documents of the AFEB and R & D Command refer to a meeting of the committee on November 1, 1961, at which plans to move forward with hepatitis vaccines were to be discussed. Further records of the Advisory Committee on Liver Disease (also referred to as the Subcommittee on Liver) are at NARA OTSG R & D, Accessions 69A 2608 and 71A 3158.

The army increases medical research funding five-fold: _USAMRMC: 50 Years of Dedication to the Warfighter, 1958–2008_ (Fort Detrick, MD: U.S. Army Medical Research and Materiel Command, 2008), 30.

Targeted increases for research include funding for hepatitis prevention: The Advisory Committee on Liver Disease had a growing budget; early in 1966, the committee was allocating $518,000 toward research projects ($4 million in today dollars). The AFEB was allocating another $195,000 to research on liver disease. Memo for the Record, March 1996, Subject: Hepatitis Research Program, NARA OTSG R & D, Accession 69A 2608 (Project Control Files, 1961–65), Box 40, Folder: Correspondence Files, Hepatitis Program, 1966.

U.S. soldiers in Vietnam were contracting hepatitis: Marcel Conrad reported in 1969 that seven thousand military personnel in Vietnam had contracted hepatitis. Transcript of the Eighteenth Meeting, June 23, 1969, 101, NAS Plasma.

R & D Command awards a contract to Parke-Davis scientists: Donald Howie, assistant chief of medical research, wrote on June 29, 1962, in a memo for the record that the R & D Command would be funding researchers at Parke-Davis so long as an arrangement could be reached about patenting. NARA OTSG R & D, Accession 71A 3158 (R & D Project Control Files), Box 7, Folder: Truffelli, G. T., Hepatitis Research, Parke Davis.

Boggs is to administer hepatitis specimens from Korea to Joliet subjects: Minutes of the Subcommittee on Liver, November 4, 1964 (distributed March 22, 1965) report that Boggs had administered sera from Korea to Joliet inmates. NARA OTSG R & D, Accession 71A 3158, Box 8, Folder: Hepatitis Committee Meeting 1966. Records of Boggs's contract show that support was ongoing in May 1965. NARA OTSG R & D (Science and Tech Info Division), Accession 67A 4813, Box 41, 1303–17 (Technical Report Record Files, 1964–66), Folder: Boggs Dr. Joseph D. MD 2645. Liver Committee members hoped that in the process of testing "candidate viruses," researchers would also isolate diagnostic antigens that would allow the identification of blood donors who carried hepatitis B.

Liver Disease Committee reluctantly renews Parke-Davis contract ("failed thus far"): Bulletin #2, Communication 80, the Surgeon General's Subcommittee on Liver, June 15, 1966, NARA OTSG R & D, Accession 71A 3158, Box 7, Folder: Truffelli, Hepatitis Research, Parke Davis.

Liver Disease Committee member voices more dissatisfaction about Parke-Davis research ("no way out"): Comments of review A, Subcommittee on Liver Disease, Bulletin 2, Communication 44, Surgeon General's Subcommittee on Liver, July 16, 1965, NARA OTSG R & D, Accession 71A 3158, Box 7, Folder: Truffelli, Hepatitis Research, Parke Davis.

Liver Disease Committee takes over the project at Joliet: Reaction to Boggs's research methods and the army's corrective action are discussed in the Minutes of the Subcommittee on Liver Disease of May 27–28, and in minutes of the Liver Disease Steering Committee, November 11, 1966. NARA OTSG R & D, Accession 71A 3158, Box 8, Folder: Hepatitis Committee Meeting 1966. After the Liver Committee took over, Boggs was no longer in charge of cultivating viruses for research interventions.

Viruses being propagated in Detroit-6 culture were not hepatitis: A memo of April 13, 1971, reports that one pathogen being grown was a parvovirus. "Working Conference on the Use of Detroit-6 Cells for Isolation of Agents from Patients with Infectious Hepatitis," TMC Melnick, Series III, Box 2,

Folder: NIH Hepatitis Committee Reports, Bureau of Biologics Meetings, 1971–73. Conrad remarked on this and other problems with research at Joliet in Transcript of the Eighteenth Meeting, June 23, 1969, 101, NAS Plasma.

Exact end date of experiments at Joliet is unclear: Hepatitis studies were still ongoing at the prison in the fall of 1970. "Joliet MS-1 Study" and "Joliet FK 30 Study," TMC Melnick, Series III, Box 4, Folder: Joliet, 1970. In September 1970, Boggs applied for an additional year of support to carry the project through the fall of 1971. TMC Melnick, Series III, Box 4, Folder: Boggs—Hepatitis, 1969–71. The trail of archival documents on experiments at Joliet ends there.

Information on numbers of biopsied inmate-subjects at Joliet: On the biopsies of Joliet inmates, see Hans Popper to Robert M. Glickman at the OTSG, March 25, 1969, TMC Melnick, Series III, Box 4, Folder: Joliet I.

What is known about number of inmates who participated in experiments at Joliet: The total number of Joliet prisoners who were hepatitis infection subjects is unclear. Boggs compiled a nineteen-page typescript summarizing hepatitis interventions at the prison between 1959 and 1969 that lists well over 300 subjects. "Previous Projects," TMC Melnick, Series III, Box 4, Folder: Joliet III Hepatitis. In 1961, the prison warden stated that 350 inmates participated in hepatitis research. Frank J. Pate, "Illinois State Penitentiary," in *1961 Annual Report, Department of Public Safety* (Springfield: State of Illinois, 1961), 25. Neither figure includes inmates enrolled in studies conducted at Joliet after October 1969.

The OTSG reports its position on approving studies transmitting hepatitis B: "The Department of the Army will continue to exercise its best judgment on an individual basis as studies are proposed." Under "Attitude of the Military Medical Service concerning the Use of Human Subjects in Studies on Post Transfusion Hepatitis," Meeting Minutes of November 25, 1964, 7, NAS Plasma. A record of deliberations preceding experiments at Willowbrook with the blood-borne pathogen was unavailable. Krugman's AFEB project files for the years 1963–66 were not among the documents available at the National Archives.

Studies at Willowbrook confirm the existence of two hepatitis strains ("whose parents gave"): Saul Krugman, Joan P. Giles, and Jack Hammond, "Infectious Hepatitis: Evidence for Two Distinct Clinical, Epidemiological and Immunological Types of Infection," *JAMA* 200, no. 5 (1967): 365–73; ("that would have been impossible"): The accompanying editorial is "Is Serum Hepatitis Only a Special Type of Infectious Hepatitis?" *JAMA* 200, no. 5 (May 1, 1967): 406–7.

The availability of MS-1 and MS-2 is a boon for hepatitis researchers: This and "pedigreed" specimens are from personal communication with Robert Purcell, April 2013.

Willowbrook investigators test heat-inactivated hepatitis B serum: Resulting publications included Saul Krugman, Joan P. Giles, and Jack Hammond, "Hepatitis Virus: Effect of Heat on the Infectivity and Antigenicity of the MS-1 and MS-2 Strains," *Journal of Infectious Diseases* 122, no. 5 (November 1970): 432–36; Saul Krugman, Joan P. Giles, and Jack Hammond, "Viral Hepatitis Type

B (MS-2 Strain): Studies in Active Immunization," *JAMA* 217, no. 1 (July 5, 1971): 41–45.

Blumberg's group reports discovering Australia antigen: Baruch Blumberg, Harvey J. Alter, and Sam Visnich, "A 'New' Antigen in Leukemia Sera," *JAMA* 191, no. 7 (February 15, 1965): 101–6; Baruch Blumberg et al., "A Serum Antigen (Australia antigen) in Down's Syndrome, Leukemia and Hepatitis," *Annals of Internal Medicine* 66 (May 1967): 924–31.

Researchers identify Australia antigen as the antigen of hepatitis B: Publications on this matter included Alfred M. Prince, "An Antigen Detected in the Blood during the Incubation Period of Serum Hepatitis," *Proceedings of the National Academy of Sciences* 60, no. 3 (July 15, 1968): 814–21; and Alfred M. Prince, "Relation of Australia and SH Antigens," *Lancet* 292, no. 7565 (August 24, 1968): 462–63. The confirming study with Willowbrook specimens was Joan Giles et al., "Viral Hepatitis: Relation of Australia/SH Antigen to Willowbrook MS-2 Strain," *New England Journal of Medicine* 281, no. 3 (July 17, 1969): 119–22; McCollum and Krugman were among the authors of this paper.

Group introduces marmoset model for hepatitis A: F. Deinhardt et al., "Studies on the Transmission of Human Viral Hepatitis to Marmoset Monkeys. I. Transmission of Disease, Serial Passages and Description of Liver Lesions," *Journal of Experimental Medicine* 125, no. 4 (April 1967): 673–88. This group received funding from the R & D Command.

Scientists formulate serum-based vaccine for hepatitis B: Eugene B. Buynak et al., "Vaccine against Hepatitis B," *JAMA* 235, no. 26 (June 28, 1976): 2832–34; R. Palmer Beasley, "Development of Hepatitis B Vaccine: Summary of the Original Article," *JAMA* 302, no. 3 (July 15, 2009): 322–24. Paul A. Offit points to contention over credit for the design of the first hepatitis B vaccine. Baruch Blumberg claimed the idea was his in *Hepatitis B: The Hunt for a Killer Virus* (Princeton, NJ: Princeton University Press, 2002). In Offit's account, Maurice Hilleman accomplished all the work on the vaccine's development that followed identification of the hepatitis B surface antigen. Offit, *Vaccinated: One Man's Quest to Defeat the World's Deadliest Disease* (New York: Smithsonian/Collins, 2007), 135–36.

Willowbrook heated serum was a prototype hepatitis B vaccine ("the first prototype"): Krugman, "Willowbrook Hepatitis Studies Revisited," 161. "Proof of principle" is from Robert Purcell, personal communication, April 2013.

Discovery of the hepatitis B antigen is a watershed ("After a long and arid period"): Saul Krugman (quoting Enders), in "Viral Hepatitis: Overview and Historical Perspectives," *Yale Journal of Biology and Medicine* 49, no. 3 (July 1967): 202.

Interest in research with hepatitis surges ("In summer of 1969"): Robert McCollum's remarks, NRC Committee on Viral Hepatitis, Meeting Minutes of September 8, 1971, 1, TMC Melnick, Series III, Box 2, Folder: NRC 1971–72, Committee on Viral Hepatitis.

Chapter Eight. Backlash

Protesters disrupt Krugman's ACP award ceremony: Harold M. Schmeck, "Researcher, Target of Protest, Is Lauded at Physician's Parley," *New York Times*, April 18, 1972, 33; and "Doc Honored, Hit on Tests at Willowbrook," *New York Daily News*, April 18, 1972. The *Daily News* quoted demonstrators saying, "Poor and working class people should be guaranteed adequate treatment and not be forced to turn their children into guinea pigs to obtain treatment." Several weeks earlier, the MCHR's New York chapter had sent the ACP president a telegram dated April 4, 1972, demanding time to present their position on the Willowbrook studies at the award ceremony for Saul Krugman. Telegram dated April 4, 1972, NYU Krugman, Folder: Willowbrook I.

Scuffle takes place outside the Krugmans' hotel room: Saul and Sylvia Krugman interview with Jonathan Soffer, May 23, 1995, 31–33, Division of Library and Archival Services, American Academy of Pediatrics, Itasca, IL.

Protesters mount additional multiple actions against Krugman: Daniel S. Gillmor reported demonstrators outside the entrance to Bellevue Hospital in "How Much for the Patient, How Much for Medical Science?" *Modern Medicine*, 42, no. 1 (1974): 30. Sources related to action on October 14, 1972, at the pediatric meetings in New York City include "Join the MCHR at the American Academy of Pediatrics," Penn MCHR, Box 54, Folder: Krugman Protests 1972. Krugman discusses demonstrators at the San Francisco meeting in the Krugmans' Soffer interview, 30. Promotional material on protest actions during March and April 1972 includes "Human Experiments at Willowbrook," leaflet from Mount Sinai MCHR (another version of this leaflet names supporters from Bellevue Hospital); "The Willowbrook Experiments: Medical Fascism," leaflet from Progressive Labor Party; "Stop the Racist Beast of Willowbrook, Atlantic City, April 17," leaflet from Students for a Democratic Society. These documents are located at CSI McCourt, Box 1, Folder 4: Hepatitis Program, 1958, 1969–79. Additional materials from the months of March and April 1972 are located at NYU Krugman, Folder: Willowbrook I. This includes "Against Inhuman Experimentation," leaflet from the Bellevue Hospital MCHR; "Meet Saul Krugman, 'Doctor of the Year,'" leaflet from the Einstein Peace Committee; "Censure Dr. Krugman," leaflet from the New York chapter of MCHR; and "Confront the Racist Beast at Willowbrook," leaflet from Boston Regional Students for a Democratic Society.

Krugman reacts to the onslaught from dissidents ("It was a very traumatic"): Krugmans' Soffer interview, 31.

1960s activism fosters "generalization of rights": Paul Starr coined and elaborated this term in *The Social Transformation of American Medicine* (New York: Basic Books, 1982), 388–93. Starr notes that ongoing efforts included claims for rights *in* health care: the right to informed consent, to refuse treatment, to see one's records, and to participate in medical decisions.

Young health-care professionals embrace radical causes: Naomi Rogers, "'Caution: The AMA May Be Dangerous to Your Health': The Student Health Organizations (SHO) and American Medicine, 1965–1970," *Radical History Review* 80 (Spring 2001): 5–34.

U.S. court rulings define informed consent: Ruth Faden and Tom Beauchamp, *A History and Theory of Informed Consent* (New York: Oxford University Press, 1986). Martin Pernick discusses notions of consent prior to the late 1950s in "The Patient's Role in Medical Decisionmaking: A Social History of Informed Consent in Medical Therapy," in *Making Health Care Decisions*, ed. President's Commission for the Study of Ethical Problems in Biomedical and Behavioral Research (Washington, DC: U.S. Government Printing Office, 1982), 3:1–35. Wendy Mariner provides commentary in "Informed Consent in the Post-modern Era," *Law and Social Inquiry* 13, no. 2 (Spring 1988): 385–406.

Early bioethicist sees continuity with rights movements ("I moved easily"): Statement by Robert Veatch, quoted in Albert R. Jonsen, *Birth of Bioethics* (New York: Oxford University Press, 1998), 387. Veatch was involved in antiwar and civil rights activism.

Pappworth decries experiments with patients and rejects parental consent ("Parents may have"): Maurice H. Pappworth, "Human Guinea Pigs: A Warning," *Twentieth Century* 171, no. 1015 (Autumn 1962): 71. An editorial in a British medical publication noted that Pappworth's article "provoked widespread comment." See "Experimental Medicine," *British Medical Journal* 2, no. 5312 (October 27, 1962): 1108. Pappworth expanded his arguments in *Human Guinea Pigs: Experimentation in Man* (London: Routledge & Kegan Paul, 1967). He did not identify researchers in his magazine article but did so in this book. Jenny Hazelgrove examines debates in postwar Britain over medical experiments with hospital patients in "British Research Ethics after the Second World War: The Controversy at the British Postgraduate Medical School, Hammersmith Hospital," in *Twentieth Century Ethics of Human Subjects Research*, ed. Volker Roelch and Giovanni Maio (Stuttgart: Franz Steiner Verlag, 2004), 181–97; and Jenny Hazelgrove, "The Old Faith and the New Science: The Nuremberg Code and Human Experimentation Ethics in Britain, 1946–73," *Social History of Medicine* 15, no. 1 (2002): 109–35.

British Medical Research Council questions the legality of parental consent: Medical Research Council, "Responsibility in Investigations on Human Subjects," *British Medical Journal* 2, no. 5402 (July 18, 1964): 178–80.

Groups used as human subjects are perceived as vulnerable: Nancy D. Campbell and Laura Stark comment on this development and its implications in "Making Up 'Vulnerable' People: Human Subjects and the Subjective Experience of Medical Experiments," *Social History of Medicine* 28, no. 4 (November 2015): 825–48.

Medical news magazines spread information: The publications included *Scope Weekly* from Upjohn Co., which was first to report hepatitis experiments at Willowbrook. Two other newly created outlets for practicing physicians were the

Medical Tribune, established by Arthur Sackler, and *Medical World News*, whose founding editor was Morris Fishbein.

JCDH dissidents invoke Nazi medical experiments ("acts which belong more properly in Dachau"): Affidavit from attending physician Hyman Strauss, November 23, 1963, reprinted in Jay Katz, *Experimentation in Human Beings* (New York: Russell Sage, 1972), 16. Lawyer William A. Hyman recounted statements about Nazi experiments and the Nuremberg Trial made at the September 30 meeting of the JCDH hospital board in Petition to the Supreme Court of New York Kings County, dated December 12, 1963 reprinted in Katz, *Experimentation*, 12.

New York state board censures Southam and Mandel ("fraud and deceit"): Elinor Langer, "Human Experimentation: New York Verdict Affirms Patient's Rights," *Science*, February 11, 1966, 663. Barron H. Lerner discusses the decision in "Sin of Omission—Cancer Research without Informed Consent," *New England Journal of Medicine* 351, no. 7 (August 12, 2004): 628–30.

Mainstream press follows JCDH controversy: James P. McCaffrey, "Hospital Accused on Cancer Study: Live Cancer Cells to Patients without Their Consent, Director Tells Court," *New York Times*, January 21, 1964, 31; Alexander Burnham, "Tests on Cancer to Need Consent," *New York Times*, January 23, 1964, 28; John A. Osmundsen, "Many Scientific Experts Condemn Ethics of Cancer Cell Injection," *New York Times*, January 26, 1964, 70; "Suit Seeks Data in Cancer Tests," *New York Times*, February 8, 1964, 50; James P. McCaffrey, "Cancer Test Data Granted by Court," *New York Times*, February 28, 1964, 34; "Ruling Is Upset on Cancer Test," *New York Times*, July 8, 1964, 32.

Beecher repudiates unethical medical experiments: Henry K. Beecher, "Ethics and Clinical Research," *New England Journal of Medicine* 274, no. 24 (June 16, 1966): 1354–60. Beecher received assistance with the article from the *Journal*'s editor at that time, Joseph Garland. *JAMA* had declined to publish the article. David J. Rothman discusses the significance of Beecher's paper in "Ethics and Human Experimentation: Henry Beecher Revisited," *New England Journal of Medicine* 317, no. 19 (November 5, 1987): 1195–99; and in Rothman, *Strangers at the Bedside* (New York: Basic Books, 1991), 15–18.

Beecher conducted hazardous human experiments for defense agencies: Susan E. Lederer, "'Ethics and Clinical Research' in Biographical Perspective," *Perspectives in Biology and Medicine* 59, no. 1 (Winter 2016): 25–26; and George Mashour, "From LSD to the IRB: Henry Beecher's Psychedelic Research and the Foundation of Clinical Ethics," *International Anesthesiology Clinics* 45, no. 4 (Fall 2007): 105–11.

Beecher communicated with Pappworth before releasing his exposé: Allan Gaw, "Exposing Unethical Human Research: The Transatlantic Correspondence of Beecher and Pappworth," *Annals of Internal Medicine* 156, no. 2 (January 17, 2012): 150–55.

Fellow scientists sharply criticize Beecher's paper: Lara Freidenfelds, "Recruiting Allies for Reform: Henry K. Beecher's 'Ethics and Clinical Research,'" *International Anesthesiology Clinics* 4, no. 4 (Fall 2007): 92–96.

The mainstream press reports on Beecher's exposé: Lara Freidenfelds describes Beecher's releases to the press in "Recruiting Allies for Reform," 85, 89. Media coverage of Beecher's 1965 conference presentation included John Osmundsen, "Physician Scores Test on Humans," *New York Times*, March 24, 1965, 35; Herbert Black, "Are Humans Used as Guinea Pigs Not Told?" *Boston Globe*, March 24, 1965, 1, 3; Harry Nelson, "Human Guinea Pigs? Doctor Challenges Ethics in Experiments," *Los Angeles Times*, March 24, 1965; and William M. Carley, "Fight Flares over Role of Human Volunteers in Some Medical Studies," *Wall Street Journal*, June 10, 1965, 1, 14. Carley addressed both the JCDH controversy and Beecher's conference presentation. Press reports on Beecher's *New England Journal* article include "Medical Testing without Consent Involved 100 Humans, Doctor Says," *Washington Post*, June 17, 1966; Jane E. Brody, "Some Drug Tests on People Scored: Professor at Harvard Hits Ethics of Experiments," *New York Times*, June 17, 1966, 17; and Jane E. Brody, "Experiments and Risk," *New York Times*, June 19, 1966, 17E.

Thaler repudiates experiments at public hospitals including Willowbrook ("thousands of patients"; "being used daily"): Ronald Matorana, "Thaler Says Poor in City Hospitals Are 'Guinea Pigs,'" *New York Times*, January 11, 1967, 94.

Citing Beecher, Thaler escalates charges concerning Willowbrook ("unethical, immoral and illegal"): Terence Smith, "'Smear and Scare' Charged to Thaler by City Doctors," *New York Times*, January 13, 1967, 1. In an editorial titled "Senator Thaler's Charges," the *New York Times* questioned the accuracy of Thaler's allegations (January 14, 1967), 30. Thaler later rescinded his objections: "Project on Hepatitis Now Praised by State Critic," *New York Times*, March 24, 1971, 20.

Critic insists consent of Willowbrook parents was coerced ("high-pressure method"; "desperate to institutionalize"): Gootzeit's assertions are reported in "Studies with Children Backed on Medical, Ethical Grounds," *Medical Tribune*, 8, no. 19 (February 20, 1967): 23. A week earlier, Thaler had charged that children were admitted to Willowbrook only if their parents agreed to their participation in the research program. Reported in "Willowbrook Defended by Parents' Unit," *Staten Island Advance*, February 15, 1967, CSI Clippings, Box 1, Folder 5.

Willowbrook director objects to depiction of the impact of dual letters on parents ("a complete misinterpretation"): Hammond's statement from "Studies with Children Backed on Medical, Ethical Grounds," 23.

Krugman defends his team's procedures for securing parental consent: Krugman included descriptions of parental consent in many of his publications. He noted that the team's approach to handling the consent process changed over time. At first, parents received information about the studies by letter; later, a social worker would interview parents, after which a group of parents would attend a meeting with research staff where questions could be asked and answered. Saul Krugman, "The Willowbrook Hepatitis Studies Revisited: Ethical Aspects," *Review of Infectious Disease* 8, no. 1 (January–February 1986): 159–60. Very little documentation on the group's consent procedures remains. A lone surviving document is a 1958 letter from the Willowbrook director asking parents whether they were interested in having their child admitted to the hepatitis research unit. It states that by participating in the research, their youngster would experience either "no attack or only a minor attack of hepatitis," which "may give the child immunity against the disease for life." The letter instructs parents to fill out and return an enclosed permission form. I found no copy of this form. Letter from H. H. Berman to parents, November 14, 1958, CSI McCourt, Box 1, Folder 4: Hepatitis Program 1958, 1969–79.

Krugman reports that he enrolled no wards of the state ("We decided at the start"): "Studies with Children Backed on Medical, Ethical Grounds," 23.

Krugman contacted Beecher to discuss studies as Willowbrook ("Krugman invited Beecher"): AFEB meeting minutes, May 14, 1970, referring to events taking place seven years earlier. NARA AFEB Accession NN3 334 09 003, Box 15, Folder (6): Minutes of Meetings (AFEB) 1970–71, under Commission on Viral Infections.

Leader of parents' group denies consent was coerced: Statements by Mrs. Israel Epstein reported in "Willowbrook Defended by Parents' Unit."

Leaders of advocacy groups defend Krugman ("In recognition of"): Presented to Saul Krugman on May 13, 1967. NYU Krugman, Folder: Willowbrook I; ("the individual love"): Letter from William A. Fraenkel, Association for the Help of Retarded Children, to Dr. Jack Hammond, February 24, 1967, NYU Krugman, Folder: Correspondence—Willowbrook.

Ingelfinger takes aim at Willowbrook critics ("medical knowledge"): David E. Rogers et al., eds. *Yearbook of Medicine, 1967–1968* (Chicago: Year Book Medical Publishers, 1968), 430. Louis Goldman attributed the quoted remarks to Franz J. Ingelfinger, one of the *Yearbook*'s editors, in *When Doctors Disagree* (London: Hamish Hamilton, 1973), 69. In his *Yearbook* comments, Ingelfinger went on to say that the "zealots" pursuing "one-track efforts to protect the rights of the individual" at Willowbrook "are in fact depriving that individual of his right to good medical care." Ingelfinger was editor of the *New England Journal of Medicine* from 1967 to 1977.

***Daedalus* authors defend experiments at Willowbrook** ("no greater risk"): Geoffrey Edsall, "A Positive Approach to the Problem of Human Experimentation," *Daedalus* 98, no. 2 (Spring 1969): 471–72. The other author, Louis Lasagna from Johns Hopkins University, agreed: "Everyone admitted to the school appears to develop hepatitis anyway during the first six to twelve months." Lasagna, "Special Subjects in Human Experimentation," *Daedalus* 98, no. 2 (Spring 1969): 458. David J. Rothman rejected Edsall's argument in "Were Tuskegee and Willowbrook 'Studies in Nature'?" *Hastings Center Report* 12, no. 2 (April 1982): 5–7.

Mainstream media questions standards for human experiments: John Lear, "Do We Need New Rules for Experiments on People?" *Saturday Review*, February 6, 1966, 61–70; John Lear, "Experiments on People—The Growing

Debate," *Saturday Review*, July 2, 1966, 41–43; Walter Goodman, "Doctors Must Experiment on Humans but What Are the Patient's Rights?" *New York Times Magazine*, July 2, 1967, 12–13, 29–32.

Supporters argue that hepatitis is mild in children: It was a widely shared perception that hepatitis was a milder disease in children than in adults. Researchers were not yet aware that children exposed to hepatitis B—particularly young children—are much likelier than adults to become long-term carriers.

Beecher challenges the claim that children at Willowbrook would inevitably get hepatitis: Henry K. Beecher, *Research and the Individual* (Boston: Little, Brown, 1970), 122–27. When Beecher was preparing his book, he sent Krugman an advance copy of his critical commentary. Letter from Beecher to Krugman, October 1, 1968, Countway Beecher, Box 12, Folder 13. According to AFEB records, this time "Krugman did not respond to the written comments of Beecher." Minutes of May 14, 1970, under Commission on Viral Infections; NARA AFEB Accession NN3 334 09 003, Box 15, Folder (6): Minutes of Meetings (AFEB), 1970–71. Joel D. Howell and Rodney A. Hayward further examine the assertion that children at Willowbrook were bound to contract hepatitis in "Writing Willowbrook, Reading Willowbrook: The Recounting of a Medical Experiment," in *Useful Bodies: Humans in the Service of Medical Science in the Twentieth Century*, ed. Jordan Goodman, Anthony McElligott, and Lara Marks (Baltimore, MD: Johns Hopkins University Press, 2003), 190–213.

Ramsey argues scientists should have cleaned up conditions at Willowbrook: Paul Ramsey, *Patient as Person* (New Haven, CT: Yale University Press, 1970), 47–58. He calls institutionalized children a "captive population" on p. 41.

Lancet **publishes warring letters about the Willowbrook studies** ("could not justify"): The *Lancet* editor's criticism of the ethics of Willowbrook studies is in 294, no. 7702 (April 10, 1971): 749. Stephen Goldby's letter "Experiments at the Willowbrook State School" appears on the same page. The authors of other letters were Saul Krugman (May 8), Samuel Shapiro (May 8), Edward Willey (May 22), Benjamin Pasamanick (May 22), Joan Giles (May 29), Maurice Pappworth (June 5), Henry Beecher (June 5), and Geoffrey Edsall (July 10).

Lancet **and** *JAMA* **spar over Willowbrook studies** ("Mission accomplished!"; "pious tone"; "*Lancet*'s editor's"): *JAMA*'s rebuke is in "Prevention of Viral Hepatitis: Mission Impossible?" *JAMA*, 217, no. 1 (July 5, 1971): 71. The scientific paper that the *JAMA* editorial refers to is Saul Krugman, Joan P. Giles, and Jack Hammond, "Viral Hepatitis, Type B (MS-2 Strain): Studies on Active Immunization," *JAMA*, 217, no. 1 (July 5, 1971): 41–45.

Medical press outlets turn critical ("This is not true"): "Was Dr. Krugman Justified in Giving the Children Hepatitis?" *Medical World News* 12, no. 38 (1971): 25. Louis Goldman also provided critical commentary in "The Willowbrook Debate," *World Medicine*, September 22, 1971, 17–25. *World Medicine* was published in Britain.

Protests targeting conditions at Willowbrook intensify: David J. Rothman and Sheila Rothman, *Willowbrook Wars* (New York: Harper & Row, 1984).

Robert F. Kennedy condemns conditions at Willowbrook ("snake pit"): "Retarded Children in 'Snake Pits,' Kennedy Says," *New York World Telegram and Sun*, September 9, 1965, 3; ("living in filth"): "Excerpts from Statement by Kennedy, *New York Times*, September 10, 1965, 21. Additional coverage is John Sibley, "Kennedy Charges Neglect in State Care of Retarded," *New York Times*, September 10, 1965, 1, 21. Rothman and Rothman discuss Kennedy's excoriation of the Staten Island facility in *Willowbrook Wars*, 23–25. James W. Trent Jr. provides a more general description of the rise of advocacy groups seeking to improve institutional conditions in *Inventing the Feeble Mind: A History of Mental Retardation in the United States* (Berkeley: University of California Press, 1994), 239–61.

Staten Island Advance reports staff shortages at Willowbrook: "Willowbrook Staff Down 300," *Staten Island Advance*, August 30, 1971. Personnel shortages were not new. Several years earlier (May 24, 1968), the *Advance* ran an article with the headline: "Willowbrook Heads List of Most Understaffed Facilities." CSI Clippings holds these and other *Advance* articles about problems at Willowbrook.

Citizens' Board of Visitors writes the governor in protest ("shocked and appalled"): Gene Spagnol, "Child Neglect in Job Freeze Stirs Willowbrook Fund Rally," *New York Sunday News*, November 14, 1971, CSI Clippings, Box 2, Folder 1.

The Advance covers Willowbrook firings and parents' protests: Jane Kurtin, "Parents Protest Cutbacks at State School," *Staten Island Advance*, November 15, 1971, CSI Clippings, Box 2, Folder 1. Additional coverage includes Jane Kurtin, "Willowbrook Head Fires 2 Who Spoke Out," *Staten Island Advance*, January 7, 1972; and Jane Kurtin, "Willowbrook Protesters Turn Rally into Bedlam," *Staten Island Advance*, January 12, 1972. Both at CSI Clippings Box 2, Folder 2.

Michael Wilkins brings Geraldo Rivera to Willowbrook: Transcripts of interviews with Dr. Michael Wilkins (August 19, 2007) and William Bronston (August 18, 2007) are part of the Civil Service Employee Association's oral history project at the Department of Special Collections, University at Albany Library, State University of New York. Available under Digital Selections at www.archives.albany.edu.

Newspapers cover Rivera's TV reporting: John J. O'Connor, "Willowbrook State School: 'The Big Town's Leper Colony,'" *New York Times*, February 2, 1972. The *New York Daily News* printed an advertising notice on February 2 for WABC-TV with an image of naked Willowbrook residents and a caption reading, "Tonight, as a public service, we're going to make you sick," CSI Clippings, Box 2, Folder 2.

Scientist objects to notion that Krugman should clean up Willowbrook ("I do not doubt"): Stanley A. Plotkin to Robert Morrow (representing the Mount Sinai MCHR), March 15, 1972, NYU Krugman, Folder: Correspondence—Willowbrook. Plotkin identified himself as a MCHR member.

Willowbrook activists initiate class action lawsuit and win consent decree: Rothman and Rothman, *Willowbrook Wars*.

Krugman reports his research unit's impending closure: Krugman, Annual Report, June 1971–May 1972, NARA AFEB Accession NN3 334 009 004, Box 9, Folder: Commission on Virus Infections, 1954–72. In minutes of the AFEB meeting of December 15, 1972, Krugman reported that hepatitis transmission procedures at Willowbrook had ended; Krugman stated that he intended in the future to mine specimens in storage and follow patients forward. NARA AFEB Accession NN3 334 09 003, Box 15, Folder (7), Minutes of AFEB Meetings 1972, under Commission on Viral Infections. The end of hepatitis studies at Willowbrook coincided with the termination of all of the AFEB's research commissions. As of 1973, the AFEB ceased research and operational functions and become an advisory body only. Theodore E. Woodard, *The Armed Forces Epidemiology Board* (Falls Church, VA: Office of the Surgeon General–Army, 1990).

Krugman was stung by condemnations of his hepatitis studies: Personal communication with Robert Purcell, April 2013. Joseph Dancis describes Krugman's distress at the attacks in a 1996 interview with Norman J. Sissman, Oral History Project, Division of Library and Archival Services, American Academy of Pediatrics, Itasca, IL.

Krugman defended the program at an NYU symposium: *Proceedings of the Symposium on Ethical Issues in Human Experimentation: The Case of Willowbrook State Hospital Research*, sponsored by the Student Council of New York University Medical School (New York: Urban Health Affairs Program, New York University Medical Center, May 7, 1972), 4–12. Colleagues rallied around Krugman as the Willowbrook project was ending. A pediatrician who said she had known Krugman for years described him as "a warm, humane, concerned and conscientious physician." He pursued the experiments, she continued, with concern for the patients' welfare, and his methods for obtaining consent were well in advance of the practices of the day. Elaine L. Allen to Medical Committee on Human Rights, October 5, 1972, NYU Krugman, Folder: Correspondence—Willowbrook. This document is also at Penn MCHR, Box 54, Folder: Krugman Protests, 1972.

The Tuskegee Syphilis Study becomes headline news: Jean Heller, "Syphilis Victims in U.S. Study Went Untreated for 40 Years," *New York Times*, July 26, 1972, 1, 8.

Newspapers nationwide condemn the Tuskegee study (multiple newspaper headlines): James H. Jones, *Bad Blood: The Tuskegee Syphilis Experiment* (New York: Free Press, 1981), 10–14, 243n21.

What the public took away from coverage of experiments at Tuskegee ("was the need"): Jones, *Bad Blood*, 14. On racial dimensions of the Tuskegee Study, see Allan M. Brandt, "Racism and Research: The Case of the Tuskegee Syphilis Experiment," *Hastings Center Report* 8, no. 6 (December 1978): 21–29; and Susan M. Reverby, ed., *Tuskegee's Truths: Rethinking the Tuskegee Syphilis Study* (Chapel Hill: University of North Carolina Press, 2000).

Critics raise objections to experiments with prisoners: Jessica Mitford, "Experiments behind Bars," *Atlantic Monthly*, January 1973, 64–73. Mitford expanded her critique in *Kind and Usual Punishment* (New York: Knopf, 1973). Jon M. Harkness follows the growing resistance in "Research behind Bars: A History of Nontherapeutic Research on American Prisoners" (PhD diss., University of Wisconsin, Madison, 1996), 248–325.

The JCDH controversy triggered initial human subjects guidelines: When New York state agencies were investigating the allegations against Chester Southam and Emanuel Mandel, the state attorney general had asked the PHS whether the two had violated agency regulations; PHS responded that there were no regulations governing extramural research. Langer, "Human Experimentation," 666. Sources on the development of federal human subjects oversight include Eugene A. Confrey, "PHS Grant Supported Research with Human Subjects," *Public Health Reports* 83, no. 2 (February 1968): 127–33; Mark S. Frankel, "Public Health Service Guidelines Governing Research involving Human Subjects: An Analysis of the Policy Making Process," Monograph no. 10, Program in Policy Studies in Science and Technology, George Washington University, 1972; and Mark S. Frankel, "The Development of Policy Guidelines Governing Human Experimentation in the United States: A Case Study of Public Policy-Making for Science and Technology," *Ethics in Science and Medicine* 2, no. 1 (1975): 43–59. Laura Stark provides a more recent account of NIH's decision-making regarding research regulations in *Behind Closed Doors: IRBs and the Making of Ethical Research* (Chicago: University of Chicago Press, 2012). The PHS released an initial version of its guidelines in February 1966 and a revised version with expanded applicability on July 1, 1966. The latter is William H. Stewart, "Surgeon General's Directive on Human Experimentation" (PPO #129), available at www.history.nih.gov.

Edward Kennedy holds hearings on human experimentation: Proceedings of Hearings before the Subcommittee on Health, Committee on Labor and Public Welfare, U.S. Senate, 93rd Congress, *Quality of Health Care—Human Experimentation, 1973* (Washington, DC: U.S. Government Printing Office, 1973). Testimony on the Tuskegee study (March 8 and April 30) is found in part 3, 1033–43, and part 4, 1187–1253. Testimony on experiments with prisoners (March 7 and 8) is in part 3, 793–809, 822–86, 897–942, 977–1024, and part 4, 1025–33. The Kennedy hearings did not include testimony on experiments at Willowbrook.

Ingelfinger hopes for only limited restrictions on research with children ("neither observed nor"; "Perhaps as a result"): Franz J. Ingelfinger, "Ethics of Experiment on Children," *New England Journal of Medicine*, 288, no. 15 (April 12, 1973): 791–92.

DHEW releases human subjects policies as formal regulation: *Federal Register* 29, no. 105, part 2 (May 30, 1974): 18913–20. In this iteration, provisions for informed consent prohibited waiver clauses in consent documents.

National Commission makes recommendation on research with categories of vulnerable persons: The resulting publications included *Research Involving Prisoners* (October 1, 1976); *Research Involving Children* (September 7,

1977); and *Research Involving Those Institutionalized as Mentally Infirm* (February 2, 1978). All available online at www.repository.library.georgetown.edu.

Illinois halts human infection research in prisons ("immoral and unethical"): Allyn Sielaff, director of the Illinois Department of Corrections, quoted in "Prison Official in Illinois Halts Malaria Research on Inmates," *New York Times*, April 28, 1974, 50; ("Our stand is based"): Brenda Stone, quoting Sielaff, in "Malaria Tests Vital, 'but Just Not for Prisons,'" *Chicago Tribune*, June 9, 1974, 46. The *Chicago Tribune* also published a long piece written by one of the malaria researchers: Paul E. Carson, "Prison Project Being Closed: A Lethal Blow to Malaria Research," (August 24, 1974) section 1, p. 10.

Stateville prisoners object to ending malaria experiments ("a vital force"; "the only program"): Brenda Stone, "Malaria Tests Vital."

Policy actors outside DHEW move to restrict experimentation in prisons: Harkness, "Research behind Bars," 255–91.

DHEW releases codes restricting studies with children and prisoners: Robert J. Levine reprints parts C and D of the code in *Ethics and the Regulation of Clinical Research* (Baltimore, MD: Urban & Schwarzenberg, 1986), 408–12.

Authors argue that hepatitis studies at Willowbrook were ethical ("Willowbrook in such"): Walter M. Robinson and Brandon T. Unrah, "The Hepatitis Experiments at the Willowbrook State School," in *Oxford Textbook of Clinical Research Ethics*, ed. Ezekiel Emanuel et al. (New York: Oxford University Press, 2008), 84.

In the 1970s, individualism triumphs in public health and bioethics: Deborah Stone observes a shift from collectivist to individualist orientation in multiple arenas of public health policy. "The Resistible Rise of Preventive Medicine," *Journal of Health Politics, Policy and Law* 1, no. 4 (1986): 671–96. Paul Wolpe writes that individualism explains in large measure the dominance of autonomy as a principle in American bioethics. "The Triumph of Autonomy in American Bioethics: A Sociological View," in *Bioethics and Society: Constructing the Ethical Enterprise*, ed. Raymond DeVries and Janardan Subedi (Upper Saddle River, NJ: Prentice-Hall, 1998), 38–59.

Chapter Nine. An Ending
without Closure

Early warning signs of long-term hepatitis sequelae: An initial paper on chronic hepatitis was M. H. Barker, R. B. Capps, and F. W. Allen, "Chronic Hepatitis in the Mediterranean Theater," *JAMA* 129, no. 10 (November 3, 1945): 653–59. Neefe discussed abnormal liver function tests among patients with a history of hepatitis in J. R. Neefe and C. H. Kurtz, "Studies of Liver Function following Localized Outbreak of Virus Hepatitis," A Progress Report, Appendix B of Minutes of Fifth Meeting, November 3, 1948, 75, NAS Liver. Early reports linking hepatitis to cirrhosis include Henry G. Kunkel and Daniel Labby,

"Chronic Liver Disease following Infectious Hepatitis, II. Cirrhosis of the Liver," *Annals of Internal Medicine* 32, no. 3 (March 1950): 433–50. Oliphant's disclosure of a 1 to 2 percent disability rate from hepatitis is reported in C. C. Barker, "SUBJECT: Hepatitis," *Island Lantern*, August 1951, 6.

Parents of susceptible school children object to mainstreaming youngsters who became carriers at Willowbrook: David J. Rothman and Sheila Rothman, *Willowbrook Wars* (New York: Harper & Row 1984), 271–72.

Epidemiologists link liver cancer to hepatitis B: The many population studies included R. Palmer Beasley et al., "Hepatocellular Carcinoma and Hepatitis B Virus," *Lancet* 318, no. 8256 (November 21, 1981): 1129–33.

Authors report carrier rates for hepatitis B and C: Joanne C. Imperial, "Natural History of Chronic Hepatitis B and C," *Journal of Gastroenterology and Hepatology*, 14 Suppl. (1999): S1–S5; Leonard B. Seeff, "Natural History of Chronic Hepatitis C," *Hepatology*, November 2002, S35–S46; and Ankar Chugh et al., "Viral Hepatitis in Children: A through E," *Pediatric Annals* 45, no. 12 (December 2016): e420–e426.

Researchers find hepatitis C in specimens from NIH's blood sterilization study: Jay Hoofnagle et al., "Transmission of Non-A, Non-B Hepatitis," *Annals of Internal Medicine* 87, no. 1 (July 1977): 14–20.

CDC estimates that one-quarter of hepatitis B carriers die prematurely: U.S. Centers for Disease Control and Prevention, "Chapter 10: Hepatitis B" (Section on Complications: Chronic HBV Infection), in *Epidemiology and Prevention of Vaccine-Preventable Diseases* (Pink Book), 13th ed. (1915), 152, available at the CDC website: www.cdc.gov.

NIH group followed blood sterilization subjects after study ended: Hoofnagle et al., "Transmission of Non-A, Non-B Hepatitis," 17.

Oliphant said PHS would care for subjects with continuing symptoms ("The Public Health Service"): From Barker, "SUBJECT: Hepatitis," 7.

The AFEB allowed payment of burial costs for deceased subjects: Adam J. Rapalski to comptroller, February 2, 1953, NARA AFEB, Murray. The wartime Army Epidemiology Board permitted scientists to provide workmen's compensation insurance for conscientious objectors who performed duties on research projects or in university laboratories; this insurance did not cover medical research injuries.

Neefe planned follow-up studies of hepatitis infection subjects: Neefe proposed a study of persistent hepatic disturbance after an outbreak of hepatitis at a summer camp in 1944. For comparative purposes, he hoped to include both veterans in the Philadelphia area and conscientious objectors who had served as subjects in Stokes's hepatitis infection studies. Minutes of Fifth Meeting, November 3, 1948, NAS Liver.

Researchers study long-term health of veterans who had hepatitis B: Publications included Leonard B. Seeff et al., "A Serologic Follow-up of the 1942 Epidemics of Post-vaccination Hepatitis in the United States Army," *New England Journal of Medicine* 316, no. 16 (April 16, 1987): 965–70; and Gilbert W.

Beebe and A. Hiram Simon, "Cirrhosis of the Liver Following Viral Hepatitis, a Twenty-Year Mortality Follow-up," *American Journal of Epidemiology* 92, no. 5 (November 1970): 279–86.

The U.S. government has redressed some research injuries: Fred Gray discusses the Tuskegee settlement in "The Lawsuit," in *Tuskegee's Truths: Rethinking the Tuskegee Syphilis Study*, ed. Susan M. Reverby (Chapel Hill: University of North Carolina Press, 2000), 473–88. Numerous reports on atomic veterans include "Atomic Veterans, 1946–1962," Atomic Heritage Foundation, available at the organization's website (www.atomicheritage.org). On deliberations about compensation for injuries from chemical warfare experiments, see Constance M. Pechura and David P. Rall, eds. *Veterans at Risk: Health Effects of Mustard Gas and Lewisite* (Washington, DC: National Academies Press, 1993).

Ethicists and policy makers advocate a program for compensating injured subjects: James F. Childress, "Compensating Injured Research Subjects: I. The Moral Argument," *Hastings Center Report* 6, no. 6 (December 6, 1976): 21–27. Childress bases his advocacy on the notion of compensatory justice, in this case a moral obligation to restore injured parties harmed in research conducted for the public good, whether fault was involved or not. A more recent proposal based on this concept is found in Leslie M. Henry, Megan E. Larkin, and Elizabeth R. Pike, "Just Compensation: A No-Fault Proposal for Research-Related Injuries," *Journal of Law and the Biosciences* 2, no. 3 (November 2015): 645–68.

Presidential Commission recommends more study of compensation for research injuries: Presidential Commission for the Study of Bioethical Issues, *Moral Science: Protecting Participants in Human Subjects Research* (Washington, DC, 2011), 8. The 1982 policy statement is in President's Commission for the Study of Ethical Problems in Medicine and Biomedical and Behavioral Research, *Compensating for Research Injuries*, vol. 1 (Washington, DC: U.S. Government Printing Office, 1982).

Scholars note changes in the conduct of clinical research: Adriana Petryna, "Globalizing Human Subjects Research," in Adriana Petryna, Andrew Lakoff, and Arthur Kleinman, eds., *Global Pharmaceuticals: Ethics, Markets, Practices* (Durham, NC, Duke University Press, 2006), 33–60; Jill A. Fisher, *Medical Research for Hire: The Political Economy of Pharmaceutical Clinical Trials* (Piscataway, NJ: Rutgers University Press, 2009); and Jill A. Fisher, *Adverse Events: Race, Inequity, and the Testing of New Pharmaceuticals* (New York: New York University Press, 2020). In *Adverse Events*, Fisher notes the prevalence of minority group members in experiments conducted with healthy subjects.

NAS advisory committees favor relaxing restrictions on experiments with children and prisoners: Marilyn J. Field and Richard E. Behrman, *Ethical Conduct of Clinical Research Involving Children* (Washington, DC: National Academies Press, 2004); and Lawrence O. Gostin et al., *Ethical Consideration for Research Involving Prisoners* (Washington, DC: National Academies Press, 2007).

Epilogue

C. Everett Koop was highly influential as surgeon general ("widely regarded as"): Holcomb B. Noble, "C. Everett Koop, Forceful U.S. Surgeon General, Dies at 96," *New York Times*, February 25, 2013.

Koop published a memoir: C. Everett Koop, *Koop: The Memoirs of America's Family Doctor* (New York: Random House, 1991). Koop was a surgical resident at Pennsylvania Hospital between 1942 and 1945. It was in 1945 that he performed liver biopsies on conscientious objectors serving as research subjects.

Neil Hartman and Koop discuss the hepatitis program ("I wrote him a fan letter"; "I was introduced"): Script of *The Good War and Those Who Refused to Fight It: The Story of Conscientious Objectors in World War II*, directed and produced by Judith Ehrlich and Rick Tejada-Flores, 2000. Koop mentions serial biopsies; Joseph Stokes Jr. originally requested approval for serial biopsies on CPS men. According to the documents I located, the Office of the Surgeon General–Army withheld approval for more than one surgical procedure per subject.

In 2000, Koop doubts IRBs would approve hepatitis infection studies: Koop may be correct about hepatitis infection interventions, but in 2000, transmission experiments with other disease pathogens were taking place with approval from IRBs. See David L. Evers et al., "Deliberate Microbial Infection Research Reveals Limitations to Current Safety Protections of Health Human Subjects," *Science and Engineering Ethics* 21, no. 4 (2015): 1049–64.

Scientific publications report on interventions with Hartman: John R. Neefe et al., "Hepatitis Due to the Infection of Homologous Blood Products in Human Volunteers," *Journal of Clinical Investigation* 23, no. 5 (September 1944): 836–55; John R. Neefe, Joseph Stokes Jr., and Sydney S. Gellis, "Homologous Serum Hepatitis and Infectious (Epidemic) Hepatitis: Experimental Study of Immunity and Cross Immunity in Volunteers," *American Journal of the Medical Sciences* 210 (November 1945): 561–75.

Hartman puzzles over the shift in moral sensibilities ("We had much more ethical discussion"): "Panel on Ethics and the Guinea Pig Experiments," in *Friends in Civil Public Service: Quaker Conscientious Objectors in World War II Look Back and Look Ahead* (Wallingford, PA: Pendle Hill, 1996), 176.

Index

Page numbers in *italics* refer to illustrations.

State Prison), 110; *US Personified*
(Clinton Farms Reformatory),
110
prisons as locations for medical experiments: at Norfolk Prison, 49, 224n;
prison experimentation as a regime,
101, 102–3; at Stateville
Penitentiary, 86–87; at Terre
Haute Federal Prison, 222n. *See
also* hepatitis infection experiments
in prisons
psychotic disorder therapies, 51–52, 73,
133
Public Health Service (PHS): hepatitis
infection experiments and, 4, 31–34,
36, 119–21, 131–32, 137; human-
subject regulations and, 176–77,
270n; institutional access and, 120,
121; military biomedical elite and,
3, 36; yellow fever vaccination and,
27, 29, 33
public narratives of hepatitis experiments: eclipse of sympathetic accounts in the 1960s, 161–62,
164–66, 179–80; laudatory depictions in the 1940s and 1950s, 56–58,
112–16, 136–37; patriotism and
common good invoked in, 5–6, 41,
105, 115–16, 121–22, 125–26; sup-
pression of studies with children
and the disabled, 6, 53–54, 95–98,
151. *See also* moral frameworks, rise
and fall of; patriotism in research
narratives; press coverage
public relations as problem for military,
5, 26–27, 36, 54

Quakers, 43–45, 64, 78. *See also*
American Friends Service
Committee

race of hepatitis subjects, 1, 5, 111, 145,
152, 182, 205n, 207n, 219–20n,
241–42n, 254n, 257n

Rahway Reformatory, 104–6
Ramsey, Paul: *The Patient as Person*, 169
Rapalski, Adam, 128, 241n
recruitment of subjects: conscientious
objectors, 8–9, 47, 62–63, 70, 71;
from marginalized groups, 5–6,
46–47, 62; prisoners, 108, 152, 184;
regulations on, 176. *See also* institutional access
Reed, Walter, 30
rehabilitative ethos, 5; apparent adoption by prisoners, 115–16, 178; Ivy
on, 88; in press coverage of hepatitis
experiments, 112–14; promoted by
prison professionals, 106–8, 114;
researchers as stewards of inmate
transformation, 108–12; Stokes and,
103
research controversies, 5; experiments
with children, 96–100, 132–34,
148–50, 161, 163; intra-professional
vs. public, 164–66; Jewish Chronic
Disease Hospital, 164–65, 168,
175–76; Tuskegee Syphilis study,
174–77; Willowbrook experiments
and, 146–51, 159–61, 164, 166–70,
179–80
researchers as stewards of inmate
transformation, 108–12
research ethics activism, 6; by conscientious objectors, 72–74, 229n; by
Pius XII, 129; by protesters in the
1970s, 160–63
research ethics guidelines: AMA's 1946
statement, 87–88; early written
codes, 89; Reich Health Council
standards (1931), 89–90; therapeutic
vs. nontherapeutic studies in, 89–90,
98, 187–88, 233–34n. *See also*
Declaration of Helsinki; human
subject regulations; Nuremberg
Code
research injuries. *See* legal liability
Rhoads, Jonathan, 76, 230n